STAYING ALIVE

BY THE SAME AUTHOR

The Family Through Divorce: How You Can Limit the Damage

Love Life: Making Your Relationship Work

Sexual Arrangements: Marriage, Monogamy and Affairs

STAYING ALIVE

A FAMILY MEMOIR

Janet Reibstein

BLOOMSBURY

First published in Great Britain 2002
This paperback edition published 2003

Bloomsbury Publishing Plc, 38 Soho Square, London W1D 3HB

A CIP catalogue record is available from the British Library

ISBN 0 7475 6470 1

10 9 8 7 6 5 4 3 2 1

Typeset by Palimpsest Book Production Limited,
Polmont, Stirlingshire
Printed in Great Britain by Clays Ltd, St Ives plc

Acknowledgements

The kindness of friends, family, and colleagues helped make this private story public. The book really began with the legacy left to me of my mother's unfinished journal, its next step a gentle suggestion from my agent, Araminta Whitley, to try a journal of my own. Like Topsy, it growed and growed. Araminta and her colleagues at Lucas, Alexander, and Whitley have been my cheerleaders, their cheers a tonic throughout. My husband, Stephen Monsell, and then my friend, Michelle Spring, each read a fledgling version of *Staying Alive*. Their warm encouragement meant that this first version did not remain locked in a drawer, unfinished and messy. Early versions and sections were read, in turn, by many friends and family – including my brothers, my sisters-in-law, Cathy and Lauren Reibstein and Stephanie Brody, and my cousins. While too numerous to name them all here, I hope each friend and family member will recognise his or her contribution. Some of them also gave me important information or verified facts. Notably these include my brothers, Gene, Rick, and Mark Reibstein, my cousins, Joyce Pomerance, Barbara Klein, and Jerrilyn Marston, and my mother's and my dear friends, Phyllis and Irvin Stock, Evelyn Prieto, and Dr Leona Laskin. I also benefited from medical friends' input, including Drs Ashley Moffett, Jill Haslehurst and Vanessa Lloyd-Davies, and Professor Theresa Marteau, and from an enlightening consultation with the clinical geneticist, Dr James McKay. My thanks to all who helped and encouraged me feels a paltry exchange for their belief in both me and the book.

Various medical journals and books helped me try to make sense of the medical aspects of my story. Particularly helpful were the books *Breakthrough: The Race to Find the Breast Cancer Gene* by Kevin Davies and Michael White (NY: Wiley, 1995); *The Breast Cancer Wars: Hope, Fear, and the Pursuit of Care in Twentieth Century America*, by Barron H. Lerner (Oxford: Oxford University Press, 2001), and *Dr Susan Love's Breast Book: Second Edition*, by Susan M. Love with Karen Lindsey (Reading, Massachusetts: Addison-Wesley, 1995) as well as the editorial entitled, 'Prophylactic Mastectomy for Women with BRCA1 and BRAC2 Mutations: Facts and Controversy' (*New England Journal of Medicine: Vol. 345*, July 19, 2001, pp. 207–208).

At various stages certain people made key suggestions that substantially directed its course or shaped its progress. They include my friend, Angela Neustatter, and also Marsha Rowe and Gideon Weill. But most of all, my amazing editorial team at Bloomsbury – Alexandra Pringle, Marian McCarthy, and Chiki Sarkar, and my chief supporter in the US, Karen Rinaldi – pulled out of me a book immeasurably better as a result of their acute and sensitive work. I hope it has earned their pride as much as they have earned my thanks.

Finally, I hope this book repays my family's and relatives' support, and that I have succeeded in balancing their right to privacy with the demands of the story I have tried to tell.

Janet Reibstein, Exeter, UK, March 2002

A NOTE ON THE AUTHOR

Janet Reibstein is a university lecturer, clinician, writer and broadcaster on the psychology of relationships. Born in America, she lives in the UK with her husband and two sons, and is currently teaching at the University of Exeter.

CONTENTS

To the next generation:

Adam and Daniel Monsell; Zack and Luke Reibstein; Josiah and Rebecca Reibstein; Lena Reibstein; and Tim and Lynn Kaufman

Prologue

In November 1995 I stood alone in my bedroom in front of the mirror and scrutinised my naked body. It was slim, not in bad shape for its age, if marked by ragged tracks – scars from a Caesarian birth and infertility surgery. Sags were beginning to soften its edges. It was a body of middle age, its shape shifted both by the babies it had carried and by the gravity of years. Those years, and those babies sucking with their fierce, tiny mouths, had pulled and lowered my once firm breasts. I had loved my breasts, the source once of sexual ecstasy as well as maternal bliss. Now they were my enemies. Soon I would defeat them. This was to be their last day on earth. Out loud I bade them farewell. 'Well, guys, that's it,' I said, then I turned from the mirror, the ritual done. I dressed, collected my bags, and went downstairs for my last breakfast as the woman I was. I was due at the hospital.

I am a member of a breast cancer family, the most recent woman in it to face that fact. Like rising numbers of women today (but still too few), I have defeated breast cancer. I am no longer waiting to die of it, no longer living with the conviction that my killer is known to me, lurking inside, waiting to strike. The threat of that killer is now virtually erased. I learned what my options were. I took charge. It was possible because I live when, where and how I do. Tragically, this wasn't so for my two aunts or my mother. Today women, even those without a known cancer gene, can and do take charge. Increasingly, those who do so early enough survive.

In the time of my mother, Regina Reibstein, in the time of my aunts, Mary Kaufman and Fannie Pomerance, women with breast cancer died. Today breast cancer is not all-powerful. It does not have to be a killer.

PART I

INNOCENCE

I

Three Sisters

Paterson, New Jersey, January 1920

In the winter of 1920, Paterson, New Jersey, was a town of mainly greys and browns – brown trees, grey pavements, brown and grey painted on to the wood-frame and brick houses lining the new streets of its comfortable Jewish East Side. Neat, small squares of scraggly green grass stood, like sentries, fronting proud new homes. Weeds had not yet pushed through the few cracks in the pavements. Square, sturdy houses hid, like pigeons, behind the peacocks of thrusting white mansions with sculpted hedges and long lawns. Within twenty years Paterson, the old mill town – briefly famous when the newly arrived Jews led the Paterson silk strikes – had grown moderately prosperous. On this dingy spot along the Passaic river, just west of Ellis Island where they'd first landed, the now better-off Jews built these homes.

On January 20, 1920, outside Barnert Hospital, Mary and Fannie Smith, aged eight and five respectively, were being led home by their Aunt Bertha. Her older sister, Rose, their exhilarated mother, lay in her hospital bed with their new baby sister, Rebecca. The little girls wore smart, matching red dresses, dark brown tweed coats and little red berets, which brought out their high colour – rosy cheeks, black curls and large, inky eyes. Rose had made the drop-waisted dresses from velvet which the girls' father, Isidore, had brought home from his mill. The girls had handed pins and stood like mannequins while Rose pressed fabric against their thin bodies. Diligent Fannie had observed the dextrous movements, then precisely threaded pins into fabric, her mother nodding approvingly.

Beautiful Mary was fidgety and flighty, like a trapped bird, dropping pins and giggling, to her mother's exasperation.

Today both were angels. With his normally bustling wife out of action, Isidore remained at the hospital, taking charge. They left him handing out cigars in the waiting room, wryly enquiring whether there were any rich males among the newborns: he joked that for them he had a job lot of impoverished, pretty brides. Baby Rebecca would soon become Regina. Mary had once been Miriam. Smith had once been Schmidt. Rose had once been Yetta, and still was to Isidore, Bertha, and their Polish friends and relations. But not to the American world of which the family had become part.

On the walk home Mary and Fannie chattered about the baby. Rose, endlessly busy, would surely assign her to the girls' care. A truncated childhood, her parents dead in a disease-swept shtetl, had schooled Rose to delegate, her younger sister put in charge of a younger brother. By the time she was fifteen she had organised a passage to America, settled herself and siblings in Paterson, and a few years later found a mate – the socialist Isidore. She mothered her daughters with dutiful love, though frail Fannie elicited tenderness. Frothy Mary was Isidore's. The baby would belong to the sisters. Already they'd got out a cradle, installed dolls, and cleared her a space in their room.

Although Rose and Isidore had become American citizens, and although their daughters were born in Paterson, the spectre of Poland hovered over each birth: these girls would know neither hunger nor oppression. These girls were Americans.

Paterson, 1928: Regina

On a rainy, cold winter night Regina Smith lay alone, in bed, in the dark, in the room she shared with her sisters. Her day had been nastier than the wintry weather itself and she tossed about, trying, but failing, to be soothed by the domestic murmurings below.

In the pale-blue-walled kitchen the radio crackled, while sixteen-year-old Mary bellowed along with the singer: 'Five foot two!

Eyes of blue! Oh what those two eyes can do!' She pictured Mary dancing, black eyes merry, blue worsted skirt flapping, hips swinging, hands circling daintily, cheeks sucked in so that her eyes bulged, round and popping; Regina pictured her mother knitting, tuning Mary out. Their father was half listening, peering through wire-rimmed glasses, hunched over the kitchen table, and working at figures. She heard him chuckle. Then Mary's large 'Mmmmmmmwahh!' erupted, as she threw her arms round him and collapsed in giggles. Their silent mother knitted on.

In the silence after Mary's kiss she heard Fannie, almost fourteen, in the sewing room, using the gleaming black Singer treadle machine. Her knees pumped rhythmically up and down, feeding through the machine the pink silk their father had brought home, mating one side to another till the elegant top of a scoop-necked party dress began to emerge. Fannie would look beautiful in it, though she wouldn't know it. Not in the way Mary would. Fannie wore her chic dress as if she were merely a hanger, while Mary glided around as if she were the silk itself. The sewing room Fannie was working in was always strewn with pattern pieces, decapitated, limbless paper dolls.

Regina hated sewing. Her attempts ended in bad temper: her mother exasperated, the clowning Mary, trying to cheer Regina, banished, and Fannie summoned to salvage Regina's uneven hems and jagged cutting. If her father were home and overheard, he would creep into her room later when she was in bed, and wordlessly place a small Hopje – their favourite coffee-flavoured boiled sweet – in her fist, kiss her forehead, and leave.

Whenever she couldn't sleep, like tonight, she stared at the pink cabbage roses splodged in a repeating pattern on the brown wallpaper. The paper was an accompanying theme to her life, announcing she was home, in her cosy room, soon to snuggle near her sisters. Tonight it provoked her: she found herself trying to remember a time when it wasn't there – her first home, an apartment; they had moved when she was two. Her two sisters would share a memory: 'Remember when . . .' and Regina couldn't giggle with them. They teased her about it – 'Oh, you're so little.

Your life's only in single numbers' – and grabbed her and kissed her messily, as if gobbling up her cheeks.

'Isn't she adorable?' Mary used to demand of the myriad friends she dragged home after school. Mary and Fannie liked to dress her up in costumes their mother had sewed, or to arrange her hair in elaborate styles. Expertly they brushed back her thick black curls, their deft, comforting fingers sweeping across her scalp as they scooped the curls into ringlets. Then Mary would turn Regina round carefully, like a waxwork doll, preserving their work of art, inviting applause: ta da! Cute, pliable Regina.

When Regina was four Fannie taught her to read. Before bedtime Fannie would park her tiny sister on her lap. Holding her tight and kissing the top of her head, she'd point to a word. Word reproduced, both Fannie and Mary would delightedly sweep Regina into their soapy-smelling arms. Then one would read to her. Or Mary would stretch next to her, murmuring made-up adventures. Proud of their protégée, the older two moved on to family recitals, schooling her in orations they themselves had learned. At family gatherings she recited *Hiawatha*, or the Gettysburg Address. Sometimes Mary inserted gibberish; 'Four score and seven years ago,' Regina once warbled to assembled relatives, 'our mothers brought forth on this continent a new baby', while Mary and Fannie fell about. No matter what, Mary and Fannie clapped loudest and longest of all.

As well as Mary's numerous friends, and Fannie's fewer but constant ones, her parents' cronies from the Old Country were in and out of the house. The men played pinochle and canasta, ate pistachios, and drank schnapps from shot glasses. The grown-ups spoke Yiddish, which to Regina was background noise. Her parents did not teach the girls Yiddish, though Mary and Fannie could understand some because before Regina's birth her parents, unsteady in English, spoke Yiddish to them despite themselves. Now they spoke strictly English to their American girls. Regina was guiltily ashamed of her parents' accents. Why couldn't they hear that 'very' is not 'wery'? That 'this' is not 'dis'?

The bracing blast of her mother shouting 'Vot you saying you haf no verk, Mary? No homeverk? You nefer haf no verk?' bounced her out of her reverie. She flopped around angrily, pushing the bedclothes about, wishing for sleep, but instead was pursued by visions of the humiliation she'd suffered that day at school. She'd never been reprimanded before – only boys were told off, or the one bad girl, Adele Rosenberg. Last year's teacher had nominated her 'most diligent'. She yearned for lightning to strike this year's teacher. Little Miss Moskowitz was the dark opposite of her lumpy sister, Big Miss Moskowitz. Both taught at Regina's school. One was kindly but dull. The other delighted in making children quake as she strutted her tiny frame about her high-ceilinged, blank-walled classroom. Little Miss Moskowitz had today unleashed her venomous tongue upon Regina.

Regina's shame was so great that she wanted no one – not Fannie, not Mary, certainly not her parents – to know. With none of her usual reluctance she went to bed before her sisters, relieved to be alone at last. In the snatched privacy before Fannie and Mary came to bed, Regina at last released the tears she had stored up all day. Her sobs were so absorbing that she did not hear Fannie's soft footsteps coming down the corridor. Fannie reached out to the small, shaking body, and began rubbing gently in ever-increasing circles on Regina's back. 'Shah,' she soothed and soon Regina's resolve broke, first making Fannie swear not to tell their mother. To which Fannie promised, 'I'll handle Ma,' which was all Regina needed to hear. She knew Fannie could, indeed, manage Ma.

Slightly calmer, Regina sat up, her black curls a wiry halo round her small face, a face remarkably like Mary's and Fannie's, but with rounder, softer features, lighter, pinker skin – as if any sharpness the others might possess had been removed from her. She raced through her tale, hoping speed would blur its ugliness.

Miss Moskowitz had accused Regina of dipping Bernice Malkin's pigtail into her inkwell. Meekly but still indignantly Regina protested that the offending, swinging pigtail had dipped accidentally. The frightened class tittered. Like a fox Miss Moskowitz thrilled as she sniffed fear. An evil smile crossed her bony face and she delivered the sentence. Regina was to stay after school. But first she was to stand at the blackboard till her fingers ached, and scratch 'I will be a good girl' in white chalk one hundred times. Regina pleaded for justice. Miss Moskowitz smiled wordlessly. Under the glare of Miss Moskowitz's triumphant, unyielding gaze, Regina bravely fought back tears as if she would burst. And then she did burst. To the sound of her teacher's harsh 'Tut tut', Regina felt a shaming tell-tale warm trickle down her leg, and the class howled with laughter as it spread below her in a pale yellow pool.

Fannie had to catch her breath. How dare that tyrant! She gazed with determination at her sister's wet almond eyes. She was only eight! She carried on rubbing and assured Regina – she was lying – that she wouldn't tell anyone.

The next morning Regina pretended she had a stomach ache. Fannie, dressed, kissed her cheek and urged, 'Come on. Out of bed.' Mary tickled her ribs under the bedclothes and whispered, 'Up you get.' Finally Ma bustled in. She gently forced Regina's nightgown over her head, dressing her as if she were a baby. Regina went limp.

At her seat with the offending inkwell Regina morosely pushed her pen across columns of numbers, hoping for the usual buzz she got from solving puzzles, when suddenly the door to the silent classroom flew open. The class shot up in their seats, startled. Bursting in was – Oh my God – her short, broad-bosomed mother.

'Miss Moskovitz,' her mother boomed, staring at the teacher in her thick brown chair, 'shame on you.' She paused. There was no sound, apart from Mrs Smith's sterterous breath. 'Bullying a chi-ilt!' Regina's eyes widened. 'Nefer again.' Her mother shook her fist. The class was hushed. No titters today. Miss Moskowitz stretched her small frame as if to gain a height advantage. Her stammered protest was drowned by an indignant '*No excuses!*' Yesterday's enormity diminished to tininess, Miss Moskowitz stared stupidly at Mrs Smith, who turned on her heel, marched down the aisle and gently coaxed her daughter out of her seat.

'She leaves mit me.' Regina rose. At the door her mother hissed a final shot: 'Da principal next.' Today Regina was a heroine, reflected in her mother's glory.

* * *

'Haf votefer.' Her mother gestured magnanimously, positioning herself on the swivelling red leather stool at the drugstore counter. There were clear glass domes over plates filled with slices of seven-layer chocolate cakes, apple and cherry pies, ruggelach and other Jewish pastries. 'An egg cream? Yes?' Regina had hardly spoken. She nodded. Her mother ordered two.

'Ma,' Regina eventually said, between sips of exquisitely mixed sharp seltzer, milk and sweet chocolate, 'thank you.' She fought the hated tears. She was a crier. Her sisters were tougher. Her mother smiled, pleased by her pride. 'Mammele. No vun bullies a Smit.'

That afternoon and evening Regina was buoyant. After the drugstore she immediately wrote a story, which came out in a rush. When Fannie arrived they made a cover for the book. When Mary, a wonderful artist, came home she drew illustrations. Fannie presented it to their mother as she was putting a chicken in the oven. Ma wiped her hands, reached for her glasses, and sat down at the table. 'Vell! Wery nice,' she clucked. She thumbed through it, pausing every few pages. Regina rested her chin on her mother's shoulder, and read silently along, savouring the look of the words on the page. When they finished, her mother regarded the book as if it were a specimen, turning it over and back again. 'Wery nice. Fannie, you make dis?' she asked, pointing to the cover.

Fannie winced. 'Yeah, Ma, but it's Regina's story,' she prompted. 'Wery nice,' their mother repeated, to no one in particular. 'Mary! Dat face – dat, dat . . .' she gestured in circles round her head, to show curls, 'you tink dat's me?' she joked. Mary appeared discomfited. She put her arm round her mother, and pecked her on the cheek. 'It's a swell story, isn't it, Ma?'

Regina waited. 'Wery nice. Yah, wery nice.' Her mother was already turning her back, on her way to check the chicken; absent-mindedly she patted the top of Regina's head.

Years later, when it was my mother, Regina Reibstein, who cuddled her small children – my brothers and me – on her lap, stroking our hair, nuzzling our necks, telling bedtime stories, our favourites were the 'when you were little, Mommy' ones. Most requested was the story of Little Miss Moskowitz. She told it with gusto, the teacher evil incarnate, her mother bold and strong. The story had a moral like a fairy tale. It started with Miss Moskowitz's twisted accusation, skipped straight to the next thrilling day, omitting Fannie's intervention, and ended with the happy embrace at the soda fountain. Over time, facts from other relatives filled spaces I didn't know were there. Fragments from a different narrative, they didn't fit the official bedtime story.

Paterson, January 1934: Fannie

Another cold day; Fannie, recovering from what seemed to be her millionth cold of the season, lolled in the large, claw-footed bath. Bathing during the late afternoon was a sneaky, ridiculous luxury. She'd also stolen her father's razor, hers lost in a clutter of cosmetics, most left behind by Mary. The house was much quieter now, though considerably less alive, for Mary had recently married and moved to a terrible, dirty tenement in the Bronx, with views of ribbed metal garbage cans and fire escapes winding into dark alleys.

To add to the gloom, Mary had that weekend jubilantly announced her pregnancy. No one begrudged her the impending child – they shared her joy. The problem was her husband, Murray, an undependable earner and an intermittently faithful husband. The rest of the family had recognised 'bounder' at once, as if it were printed in neon on his forehead, but Mary had always failed to spot envy, meanness or ill motives in anyone.

Despite Fannie's warnings, not to mention their mother's, and even Regina's baffled question 'But why, Mary? You're too good for him', Mary had fallen in love with and married Murray, whom she'd met at a dance the year before her graduation. Murray himself never graduated. In her innocence Mary had even tried to fix Fannie up with Murray's good-looking, long-limbed younger brother. The conversation between them ran out after two sentences: the first about the weather and the next about their engaged siblings. Mysteriously to Mary, Fannie preferred quieter men. Mary's final year of high school, when she knew she would be getting married, had been marked by their mother's wailing pleas to finish, just finish, just get the diploma, while Mary insouciantly blanked her out. But Mary clearly possessed an uncommon intelligence, for, in spite of her selective attendance and her erratic reading, on graduation day there she was, on stage with the other new graduates. She'd triumphantly squeaked through.

Now Fannie had graduated from high school, her romantic vistas widened. She was coming into her own, realised she was good-looking – though convinced she trailed behind the true beauty, Mary, and even the still awkward Regina. All shared their mother's high-cheek-boned, delicate-featured face, although Fannie had inherited her father's longer nose. But Fannie had style, studied from her mother's pattern books.

In her new world, a textile-factory office, she shone. Her stenography was good, she took dictation fast and well, and she excelled at figures. She was dating Irving, a Russian-born skilled cutter in the factory. He was sophisticated, polite, reserved and perfectly groomed. Regina, who shyly, then more comfortably, chatted with him in the front room while Fannie got ready for their dates, shared Fannie's admiration. Or Fannie thought she did.

One day shortly after she'd begun seeing Irving, as Fannie was folding away a cashmere sweater Regina had borrowed, the bond between them was threatened, Irving being the cause. Fourteen-year-old Regina languidly watched Fannie perform the ritual of tidying. Regina had falteringly entered adolescence: her thin legs and arms pushed out of too-tight clothing, her short, wide nose spread out of proportion to her eyes and mouth, and small spots sprayed her forehead. Fannie tried to summon the spontaneous adoration she'd felt formerly, tried to put together this sprouting girl-woman with the delicate child of only months before. Lately, with the onset of her adolescence, both recoiled from cuddles and hugs. And lately Regina had been questioning everything, from Fannie's taste in clothes to their parents' hard-line socialism. She'd become prickly, hard to adore. Unlike Fannie, Mary accepted everything about Regina – and about Fannie, and their parents, for that matter. The adolescent Regina, who pulled away from embraces and who was full of tactless criticism, however honest, was as wonderful to her as the baby Regina had been.

As Fannie laid the sweater in the drawer, Regina idly asked, 'Doesn't it bother you he speaks badly?'

Avoiding Regina's gaze, Fannie pretended airiness. 'Not at all,' she replied. Protective loyalty to Irving welled up, but also in that instant she was, internally, defending Regina, despite her gauche snobbery. The horrible question festered. Over the following days Fannie was uncomfortably aware of Irving's cadences. But only Regina – not Mary, not Fannie – would have questioned them. Regina had been taught – by Fannie as much as anyone – to push boundaries back; even then it was clear to Fannie that Regina would leave the immigrants behind.

The incident passed, the potential crack sealed. Today Fannie luxuriated in the bath, planning what she'd wear on her date with Irving, celebrating her recovery and return to work. Once her dodgy health had been a simple annoyance, a mystery why her body worked less reliably than others', though her mother attributed it to fussy eating. Now it posed a risk: if she were off work too long, any of a queue of hopefuls might snatch her job – they were living through what the papers called a Depression. Indeed, her stolen bath was made possible by her mother's daytime job at S and W, Isidore's mill. Fannie took expensive soapy baths on the recommendation of Dr Jolson, their family doctor and her parents' patron saint. She understood the beatification: Jolson had saved her as a small child from diphtheria, now he delivered her from possible pneumonia. Regina, offended at her parents' subservience, bordered on rudeness to him. Fannie did not like to think what her sister's life would become when she, Fannie, married, and left Regina alone with their parents. The Smiths would never countenance the university education Regina's teachers were urging. Regina would have to work, like the rest of them. Their parents would be offended by Regina's hopes, Regina hurt by her parents' dashing of them.

In the bath Fannie scraped the black stubble on her legs till they emerged white and delicate from the thick bubbles of the Lux flakes her mother used for washing stockings. Like all the women's legs in the Smith family hers were skinny and misshapen. 'Look at that girl's legs,' some rube once cackled after her in the Port Authority Terminal in New York, 'bow-legged as a heifer.'

Her soak over, she daintily alighted on to a faded yellow cotton mat. She wrapped herself in a towel marked 'Belmar', a New Jersey Shore resort where they'd all once gone overnight. With her mother's pink muff she slapped talcum powder against her back, her stomach, under her arms, releasing clouds of fragrant dust. In her room, she slipped into a spotted black silk dress with a floppy scalloped white collar. She slicked red lipstick across her wide mouth, draped faux pearls round her neck, and slid on silk stockings and red pumps. She surveyed herself in the standing mirror, licking a stray spot of lipstick off her white teeth: Joan Crawford. Well, almost. She glanced about for her perfume bottle and spotted it, fallen into Regina's open top dresser drawer. Regina's side of the room was a mess – drawers out, bed unmade, dirty clothes strewn about. Out of habit Fannie began to tidy up, but she stopped herself. Her bathtime thoughts flitted back like a warning: she and Irving had begun to make allusions to the future, to discuss shared plans. She would have to prepare herself to let go of Regina, and Regina to let go of her. Regina could start by tidying up after herself. Turning her back on the mess, Fannie dotted perfume on her neck. She and Irving would never leave Paterson; they would never want to. But Regina would need to go; Fannie would have to help her leave.

2

Separations

Paterson, November 1935: Mary

Mary struggled with a large bundle, shifting it on her hip: her perfect son, with his golden curls and plump pink cheeks. People – perfect strangers – stopped her in the street to coo, to peer more closely, to exclaim over his beauty. Mary was amazed she had produced something so perfect. If heavy. The baby buggy her parents had given her didn't fit on the buses she took from the Bronx to Washington Heights, across the George Washington Bridge to Paterson, so Mary carried him. She passed her old shops, her cinema, the big white houses Regina admired, singing softly to him. She hardly noticed the comforting old sights, for while she sang she pictured herself, dancing in a silver dress, crooning into a microphone.

Her family always knew when Murray mistreated her. She hoped this time she'd avoid the tired battle: in one corner Mary, insisting it would work out, in the other her mother and Fannie, with Regina in support, urging her to stay right there in Paterson. Fannie would be vocal. 'Why did you marry him? I could have fixed you up with a hundred men a million times better.' Their father stayed silent, but later would cajole, too: 'You make mistakes, you correct. Your family – we help.' She used Paterson as a punctuation mark, a break from marital strife. Early this morning, after a heady day spent together on a Young Communist protest march, she'd tiptoed round a drunken Murray, crashed out on the floor, mattress amid distressed bedclothes, bedframe still to be purchased, delicately stepping round – and leaving – shards of a glass lamp smashed on the floor next to him. She'd pocketed the lighter he'd thrown at her, gathered what she and the baby needed, snatched all the small change she could find – he'd obviously been to the track that week – and left. Now she pushed through her parents' front gate and made her way up the steps. She still had her key.

Fannie and Irving had married a few months earlier. They were about to move to their own place from Irving's small rented rooms, but then Fannie was hospitalised with a persistent infection to a leg wound. She lost her job; they moved into her parents' house. In shifts Regina, when home from school, and their mother, when home from work, fed and nursed Fannie. The couple were given the girls' room. They pushed beds together, swept the cosmetics off Mary's old dresser top, and installed Irving's cologne and shaving kit in their place. Voilà: a married couple's room. Regina was removed to the sewing room, which she proceeded to claim by strewing her clothes about the floor and cluttering the Singer with her books.

Mary crept in and settled the sleeping baby in a corner of Regina's room. She peeked gingerly in on Fannie. She sighed in relief; alone in the house with a sleeping Fannie and napping baby; peace at last. Downstairs again, she made a cup of tea and flopped heavily on to a kitchen chair. Grateful for the quiet, she lit a Lucky Strike. Behind her came footsteps. She hoped it wouldn't be her mother, or even Regina, both of whom, in different ways, would require energetic conversation.

Instead a sleepy voice crackled, 'Mary?' Fannie was propped against the door to the kitchen. She clutched a blue chenille robe around her. Her hair stuck up in front like a toilet brush, her skin was a pallid yellow.

Mary jumped up, stubbing out the cigarette on the saucer. 'Fannie! Here, let me help you.' Mary grabbed her arm.

Fannie crossly shook her off. 'Mary! For God's sake, I'm not paralysed.' She cracked a wan smile to soften her testiness.

Mary kissed her cheek; poor Fannie, fed up with that stupid leg. 'Tea?' she offered, and she put the kettle on and got out a cup and saucer from the cupboard.

Fannie was at the table, lighting her own Lucky. She nodded, inhaling. 'Thanks,' she said, the smoke trailing the words through her mouth.

Mary put the sugary tea in front of her sister and joined her to smoke. Fannie sat silent; something was awry. Mary did not speak, in case Fannie's silence stemmed from the – correct – idea that Mary was here because Murray's behaviour had once again driven her to leave. They sat and smoked for a whole cigarette, until Mary cracked.

'You OK?' She looked deep into her sister's faded eyes – even in illness Fannie remained chic, her chenille robe drooping lazily over her shoulders like a stole – for evidence of decline or improvement. Fannie nodded. 'When does Irving get back?' Mary asked, changing tack.

'Six' was Fannie's response.

Even though Mary was impervious to Fannie's moodiness, the mounting silence was becoming uncomfortable. So Mary tried the safest question she knew. 'Where's Regina? Shouldn't she be home?'

Fannie stiffened. She affected a shrug.

'Is she OK?' Now anxious, Mary lit another cigarette, offering Fannie one in encouragement. Slowly Fannie dragged, then looked away, as if she couldn't bear to see Mary's reaction to what she was about to say.

'There's been a . . . I don't know what you'd call it. At the moment we're not speaking.' Fannie paused, and fixed a cold stare on the white enamelled cabinets. 'A rift,' she finally decided. 'To tell the truth, the problem's between Irving and Regina.' She drew on her cigarette. Mary waited. Only smoke emerged. Mary was now truly alarmed.

'What are you saying?' she demanded. 'They get on beautifully. Regina loves him. He loves her.' There was an infinitesimal shift through Fannie's shoulders. Mary ploughed on. 'Look, you should have seen them. They missed you. OK, you might have minded she took your riding lessons, but what was he to do? I think it was kind of him to take her . . . they were . . . comforting each other.'

As Mary was expostulating to the back of Fannie's unyielding head, Fannie half turned towards her. On her face was such anguish that in a flash Mary wished she could swallow her words. Fannie was not one to weep. She was stoic during illness, heroic in the hospital, and now she was trying to stop her lip quivering. Mary closed her eyes against conflicting loyalties. She was sure Fannie had it all wrong. Or at least had lost sight of the fact that Regina, only fifteen, might be unaware of her crush, that Irving's attention was paternal. But Fannie's pain closed off reasoning. Clearly she felt Regina's feelings about her husband during her own incapacitation, whether conscious or not, were a betrayal. 'I see,' Mary conceded.

If Murray and Regina had behaved similarly – impossible though that was – would she feel bitter? she wondered. She ached for poor Regina, who'd probably been convinced Fannie wouldn't notice her infatuation, was surely embarrassed by it, and certainly shamed by its discovery. To be treated with respect by the urbanely charming Irving must have thrilled the still gawky Regina. Falling in love did happen willy-nilly, Mary ruefully observed. She took Fannie's hand, and let her rest against her and weep.

'We're moving out next week,' said Fannie, tears spent. 'Irving's cousin is letting us stay with her.'

Mary tried one last time. 'Fannie, she's a kid. Plus I'm sure he intended nothing.'

Restored, Fannie flashed, 'Of course he meant nothing. *Irving* did no wrong. You realise, of course, Ma and Pop are furious.'

Mary's heart heaved for her little sister. She figured her parents knew only what they'd witnessed: Regina's silly flirting. But she'd driven Fannie out. Regina, wronged, stood alone in that Paterson house, and Mary, out in the Bronx with a baby of her own, could do little to help. Regina's perceived betrayal left her defenceless against their parents' incomprehension. Perhaps, thought Mary, searching for something good out of the mess, her resources would grow without sister-guides.

1936–1942: Regina

It was quiet after Fannie moved out. Regina's gramophone sang out, lonely, through the closed door, accompanying her through her homework or when she lay on her bed and dreamed of college. Each day after-school she returned to a silent house, both parents at the office. But by the end of 1936 they were grimly packing papers and discarding inventory as her parents closed down S and W. The Depression had hit the Smiths like a hurricane. They were due to move from Paterson to Belleville, a small town near Newark, in March. They would sell groceries in a small shop and live above it.

In January 1937 Regina graduated, six months early, and took a factory job. In the evenings and at weekends the close-knit group of school friends who had replaced her sisters used to meet. If they'd saved up enough from their after-school jobs – Regina's was at a factory – they might ride the bus into Manhattan and see a play or go down to Market Street in Paterson for a film. They clung to each other, knowing that by September each would be far away at college. Because her career adviser at school had suggested she'd be a shoo-in for a scholarship, Regina had her heart set on the University of Chicago. Her adviser had said it was the most intellectual college in the country. Her parents hadn't known she'd applied.

One morning in early March, while in the kitchen her mother filled cardboard boxes with kitchen utensils, and in the sitting room her father emptied bookshelves, Regina heard the plop of the post and scooped it up before they noticed. Her heart began to pound at the postmark, Chicago. Delicately, as if it were a piece of prized porcelain, she opened the envelope. She raced through the formal 'Thank you for your application' bit and landed on the part that began, 'We would like to offer you a full scholarship.' She'd done it! She glanced around her at the rooms becoming bleakly naked, heard the thud of books in boxes and the clatter of cutlery in her mother's hands. Her jubilation tumbled into despondency. They'd never consent.

'Chicago!' her mother exploded, when Regina awkwardly began

to explain. Her father nodded in vehement agreement with her mother's every outraged splutter. 'Vere did this come from, young lady? Vot haf you been doing behind our backs? And vere did you tink ve'd get money for you to come home?'

Her friends were bound for Smith College, Cornell University, University of Michigan. She was smarter; she was the one who was salutatorian of her class. She'd been voted 'Most Intellectual' and 'Most Likely to Succeed'. How could she not take up this offer? But every tear, every protest, sank her case further, confirming her parents' view: she was an ingrate, a dreamer.

Later that day she sat waiting to see the principal at East Side High, hated tears streaming. The principal, almost as revered by her parents as Dr Jolson, was heroic. Through him a deal was reached. Night school in Manhattan, in the first instance, along with a job. If the store in Belleville became solvent, she would switch to day classes. New Jersey then lacked a good state university system. Like many bright students in eastern New Jersey, Regina applied to the private New York University. In the 1930s, particularly at its grim Manhattan campus, NYU played a poor second fiddle to its northern neighbour, City College, which was free to New York City residents and a magnet for the brilliant and talented. After a year she became a day student at NYU.

Almost immediately on moving out, and still barely recovered from her hospitalisation, Fannie became pregnant – with triplets, to boot. The harsh pregnancy took its toll. Irving took two jobs to support his suddenly large family and, unsurprisingly, shortly after the triplet girls were born Fannie contracted pneumonia. But the triplets, adored by Regina, did heal the rift between her and Fannie, and even worked their magic at New York University.

At NYU Regina's Paterson gang was replaced by Phyllis and Evelyn, and with them Evelyn's writer brother, Irvin, Phyllis's fiancé. On the bus between New Jersey and New York they dissected books and politics – their parents were also committed socialists; arguments about the greatness or otherwise of Clifford Odets, the Studs Lonigan novels and W. H. Auden were undercut by Phyllis's off-centre humour (she dubbed herself and Regina 'Phallus' and 'Vagina'). The triplets were minor New Jersey celebrities. 'Paterson's Pomerances Turn One [or Two, or Three, or Four]!' cried the captions under the yearly photos in northern New Jersey's newspapers, while the same little girl in triplicate, with golden ringlets and large light eyes, stared back. Glamorous Fannie, in a rakish hat, black curls arranged to float around her jawline and waft softly down her neck, would stand behind them, as if displaying her wares. 'Want to come to my nieces' second birthday party?' had been Regina's shy calling card to Phyllis.

Regina picked the triplets' fifth birthday party in February 1942 to announce she would be taking a job in Intelligence for the State Department after graduation, down in Red Bank on the southern Jersey coast, at Fort Monmouth. Her parents expected her to come home, settle down like her sisters, find a nice Jewish boy from Paterson. But her college friends were joining up, the boys in the armed forces, the girls working for the government. Evelyn would do translating, Phyllis and Irvin, now married, were moving to an army base down south. Regina's job would allow her to gather data, simultaneously, for a master's thesis under one of her NYU professors. Surely, because it was part of the war effort, her parents would understand.

So after cake and crêpe-paper streamers were cleared, when the crabby girls had been put to bed and the grown-ups were sitting round the table, she began by gushing about her patriotic duty. She'd calculated wrongly. Her mother rose, went to the sink, set her jaw grimly and turned her back, pretending to be engrossed in scrubbing a pan. She addressed the pan: 'I don't know,' she chanted, shaking her head in disgust.

'It's the war effort,' Regina angrily repeated, as if deafness were the stumbling block. If only she could be like her sisters, and not yearn to leave. Mary glanced at Fannie, who looked away. Instead they watched the crumbling grey ashes of their cigarettes fly up, then settle into their ashtrays. 'Ma,' Mary tried, out of habit. She tried to catch Regina's eye, to beseech her wordlessly to understand, not to wish for the impossible, her mother's blessing. Her mother carried on scrubbing. Fannie rose, hesitantly, shooting Regina a look of pained sympathy, and hugged Ma, who began to sob. Watching Fannie comfort her mother made Regina want to scream.

At least her sisters did not feel rejected like their mother, she reflected later, in her cupboard of a bedroom in Belleville. At least her sisters knew their parents were being unjust. Despite herself, though, she yearned for their cheers. They'd stopped their applause and she missed it.

Her house in Red Bank had a large porch decked with flowerpots. On balmy summer nights the five roommates sat on the steps, smoking, drinking Coke, munching pretzels. They worked at the base. Men swarmed, like drones, around them – the queen bees.

One day she waited at the club on base to meet Edgar-from-Yale. Men eyed her. She stole practised glances back but the dull newspaper she read was more interesting. As she glanced through a dismissive film review – OK, she'd give that one a miss – she noticed a dark-haired man approaching. He looked like someone. The bandleader Artie Shaw? The film star Ray Milland?

He was almost at her table. His black hair was slicked back, his manner confident. She began to shrink into her seat and return to her paper. Still, she was drawn – she noted his chiselled nose and good profile. Then he smiled. He had straight-to-the-heart dimples and even white teeth, and at that point her newspaper became history. He slid into the seat opposite her. She didn't object. Gesturing to the name tag she wore which allowed her on base, he grinned, 'Hello, Miss – ahem – Smith. Smith? Somehow you don't look like a Smith.' His read 'Sgt Reibstein'.

How did he know? She looked as though she might be Italian, or French, she'd been told. Off guard, she blushed and stammered, 'It was originally "Schmidt". Anyway, what makes you ask?'

He looked at her. He was close enough for her to catch his fresh, soapy fragrance. 'Don't know. Just a guess. Just an opener. Hope you didn't take offence.' He smiled – those dimples! She was hooked.

Her family, at first awed by Lou's worldliness, now relaxed in his easy presence. He had her father's jokiness and Mary's sweet temperament. Evelyn, visiting Fort Monmouth the week Regina and Lou met, had appraised him early. 'She's fallen,' she reported to Phyllis and Irvin, after observing them on the dance floor. She was right. Within six months they were engaged.

Lou was seven years older than Regina and an only child. They shared a few biographical features, but with radically different twists. He had also gone to NYU, but to the uptown, academically superior College of Liberal Arts, with a well endowed country-club campus in the then suburban Bronx. His parents had also been immigrants, from Russia. But they had been wealthy and well educated and had come to America in an earlier wave, his grandfather settling his family comfortably, his mother's generation becoming businessmen or professionals. Lou's graduation from college symbolised the difference between the two families. Thrilled at his college degree, his parents had bought him a car. Rather than get a job immediately, he'd driven cross-country with college friends. Like Regina, he loved books and writing. He had casually sent off stories to magazines, selling one to a cheap action collection, then stopped, bored, with no apparent regret. He had drifted into teaching history at a girls' high school. He didn't know what he wanted to be, but he knew he didn't want to go into business – though that, in the end, is what he did. Lou's easy confidence and lazy lack of direction were as foreign to Regina as her ambition was to him.

Lou's family were thrilled about the wedding. Regina could not have felt more adored. She thoroughly enjoyed their vivid family gossip (for example, concerning Blanche, Uncle Arthur's married girlfriend, with her dyed red hair and ample bosom; or the larcenous, divorced, fake Countess Maritza from Greenwich Village, Uncle Jack's ex-wife, who had absconded with his money but left him with their child), their high spirits and their worldly sophistication. But she found their eager involvement in planning her wedding a new and somewhat uncomfortable phenomenon. They brimmed over with helpful suggestions about getting things wholesale, about caterers, dress shops and more, and were full of excitement and kindness. Lou's mother, Rae, even offered to lend Regina her cherished pearls to wear on the big day.

The wedding took place in Manhattan on January 9. Regina wore a blue-white silk gown with square-cut neck and long, tight sleeves, and Rae's pearls. The families and friends trudged through the slush to the temple. Mary and Fannie again wore red. Fannie had made the triplets yellow organdie dresses with big sash bows. Now beautiful baby sister Regina, pretty Aunt Genie, as the triplets called her, had stepped into a world of impossible glamour: a college degree, a handsome, sophisticated husband, a prosperous family. They were proud.

Instead of wedding photos Lou and Regina had a studio portrait at their engagement. It sits above the mantel today, in my study, next to a newspaper photo of Ava Gardner and Artie Shaw taken in the same era for their engagement, or so I presume. It's a joke: look fast and they look the same people – anyone without an eye for detail usually assumes they are. In fact, my mother looks more like a dark-haired Joan Fontaine, and my father is better-looking, more finely wrought, than Ava's Artie Shaw. Their features shimmer. They stare out, three-quarters view, cheeks almost touching. My father's beauty – his aquiline features, his slicked-back, straight black hair, and long hazel eyes – is matched by my mother's. Her skin looks milky-satin. Her prominent, high cheekbones lend her delicacy, her full lips smile slightly, her dark, almond eyes, with their arched brows, shine, her dark hair falls in soft waves to her shoulders.

Aunt Mary and my grandmother used to reminisce to me about the wedding, possibly the last formal family gathering when everyone was happy. Everyone threw rice and shouted good wishes. Mary and Murray were having fun – she hadn't yet tried to throw him out, and they used to do well at parties. As Fannie waved my mother away, any reserve remaining from their rift melted in joy for her sister. Whether they felt sadness at knowing she was lost to Paterson, my relatives never said, though I imagine some twinge, however momentary, arose in them at the different paths chosen.

What the three sisters had become by that day was what they

would each be in the face of illness, each facing it (or not), each battling (or not), in her own fashion. They'd been shaped differently but also strongly by their sisterhood.

In 1944 no one knew anyone with breast cancer. Or, if they did, the victims were old women – people's grandmothers. Everyone at the wedding knew something of death in war – the 'lost in action' telegrams that arrived, the news of distant horror and persecutions. People lost, now assumed dead, loomed large in their emotional landscapes. In America in 1944, people died of tuberculosis, pneumonia, blood poisoning or, in childhood, polio. Abroad – like the ghosts who hovered over that wedding in Manhattan, the Polish Schmidt girls who never came to America, the sisters and cousins of my grandfather, who by then had died in the gas chambers – people died from hate. Perhaps without Hitler the Schmidt girls might have lived, and Fannie, Mary, my mother and their daughters might have been warned what our bodies had in store. At my parents' wedding there wasn't a hint. The bad fairy did not dance at the celebrations, delivering her cancer curse.

3
Fannie's Story

Paterson, 1945: Fannie

Fannie had moved into a new house, divided into a flat upstairs and one downstairs, near her childhood home on East 33rd Street bought by her parents. They'd saved during the prosperous war years and moved back to Paterson. The Smiths lived in the downstairs flat, Fannie, Irving and the girls in the top one. 'Jack's' candy and paper shop was next door, the butcher and deli within a short walk. The triplets were at a primary school which backed on to the back garden. Most days the house was noisy with little girls – everyone wanted to be the celebrity triplets' best friend.

Irving worked six and a half days a week, counting overtime. He dipped into the world of domesticity whirling around him, exhausted and distracted. Mary remained in the Bronx in her embattled marriage. Norman, her first child, was nine, obstreperous and undisciplined; Nina, her younger one, quiet and sweet. But Norman's mistrustful eyes and Nina's frightened ones were distressing. Mary had once confessed that Murray beat Norman, though she gave no details; reluctantly she'd also admitted that she'd once found him hammering tiny Nina as well. That was a bridge too far. 'Leave him! Don't do this to them! To yourself!' Fannie begged. 'He wouldn't dare do it again,' was Mary's stubborn response. Mary's capacity for foolishness or forgiveness was amazing. She dug in. Grumbles about Murray went underground. Sometimes she brought the children and stayed for weeks, no questions asked.

Meanwhile, Regina and Lou had moved to an apartment on New York's Lower East Side, in a new complex, part of the post-war housing boom. Regina worked as a research assistant for her professor at NYU and on her master's thesis. Lou returned to teaching. Once a month they crossed the Hudson for a weekend in Paterson.

When the war ended the Smiths latched on to rumours flying across the ocean from Displaced Persons' Camps, scrabbling through the gossip for hints of a brother, an uncle, a sister, a niece, finding only an unconfirmed sighting of a second cousin. At last they found a cousin and his new wife, and sponsored their emigration. Temporarily, the relatives squeezed into the bottom flat of East 33rd Street.

Refugees camped out all over Paterson's East Side. The newly found cousins had all once had families. How many children had died? How old? What sex? These were the spectral questions. The cousins might have survived but nightmares haunted them. They cried out in the night. They spoke no English. The Smiths jabbered to them in Yiddish, this time shutting two generations out; the triplets could only smile and gesture to the new arrivals. The cousins had dull eyes, grey complexions, sagging skin over thin frames, and an over-eagerness to please the triplets, which stabbed Fannie's heart. When they smiled their gold teeth caught the light.

Everyone was shell-shocked in the aftermath of the war. On East 33rd Street it brought back a past left in Poland, embodied by the refugees who had miraculously evaded death and who now lived in their front room. Sometimes Fannie shivered, realising that if her parents' misfortune in Poland hadn't driven them out, if she had been the daughter of Pop's sister or brother, she would not be alive today. It was a sliver of luck that gave her, her sisters and her daughters life.

Her father restarted his old firm, S and W, now a small wholesaler. Paterson enjoyed halting prosperity; the war had wiped out the Depression. But the mills were gone for ever, with no strong industry to replace them, so the more ambitious of Fannie's generation had moved out, as Regina had done. A new wave of immigrants moved in – relatives of the old ones, like her mother's cousins, the only-half-here 'survivors' of the war – taking over the large houses and turning them into small apartments. They would take any job, no matter what they had been in the Old Country. By 1945 the mansions had deteriorated; they were now two-family homes like the Smiths'.

On Wednesdays Fannie played mah-jong with friends she'd known most of her life. Shirley, her coarse and voluble best friend, would collect her. Most mornings after chores Shirley showed up for coffee. The triplets wilted in her vast presence. 'She's horrible,' they wailed. 'She calls her daughter "Fatso".' Fannie knew they were right. Shirley had an acid wit Fannie loved, and an edge she guiltily recognised in herself. It was what had driven her to shun Regina over the foolishness with Irving, grow impatient with Mary's hapless domesticity, and, in her weariness, snap bad-temperedly at her daughters: 'Clean this.' 'Stop that.' Such admonishments left her lips too quickly; she wished for greater tolerance. The girls were only little, and they tried hard to please. She did not want to bequeath them the disapproval her mother had showed Regina or Mary, or the task of comforting each other like miniature mothers. So far she was, mostly, succeeding. Unlike Mary and Regina she ran a tidy, orderly household, and in it her children were safe and happy, in contrast, sadly, to Mary and her children.

The first shadow of the Smith girls' fate was cast on a mah-jong morning. Fannie dusted the blonde wood coffee table, polished each wax orange, apple and pear in the large pottery bowl till they shone. She straightened the stacks of the *Sunday Daily News* which Irving hadn't yet read – weeks' worth piled up until she chucked them out, anyway. She wiped the brown wood surrounding the green upholstered armchairs that flanked the coffee table and plumped up cushions on the modern sectional sofa, removing hairpins and popcorn as she did. She unravelled the hose to her new vacuum cleaner, which recently had displaced the weedy, inept carpet sweeper that always left her exhausted and frustrated, and worked the carpet nap, pushing against it till the nasty dirt disappeared, then smoothing it down again. Fannie, unlike Mary, pushed deep into corners.

When she had finished, she stored her miracle vacuum cleaner with its various heads and snaky hose in the cleaning cupboard, and sank into a chair with a cup of tea and a Lucky Strike. She was sweating. Checking the time, she thought, 'I'll take a bath.' In 1945 this was no longer the indulgence of a decade before. She finished her tea, washed her cup and saucer, and started her bath, pouring in bath oil – Lux flakes irritated her skin.

The water was hot and silky. She closed her eyes, reached for the bar of Ivory soap and her razor. She slid the bar over her arms, shoulders, legs; zipped her razor up and down till her legs were as smooth as the soap; she rubbed the bar under her, then up over her navel and on to the rounded bulk of her breasts. Replacing the Ivory in its dish, she worked the suds over her breasts, around their soft curves, closing her eyes, lying back. Then suddenly she was startled into sitting upright. Gingerly she felt again. Yes, there was something there, on the side, near the bottom of her breast, just by her armpit. She sloshed suds around, nobbled the thing. It wasn't a pimple – too large for that. It didn't hurt when pressed. Curiously, it moved slightly, under the skin, back and forth. Like a swollen gland. Fannie didn't know anatomy but was pretty sure there weren't any glands there. Occasionally in the past she had felt nodules in her armpits, but those were tender when touched. And there were glands in your armpits. She pressed again. It was still there. It still moved and it still didn't hurt. Disturbed, she quickly finished her bath.

She dried herself, patting the thing in her breast, pushing it around gently, worrying it. Some type of pimple, she decided. She promised herself she'd buy new bras – she hadn't changed her bra size after the triplets' birth, but had simply gone back to her pre-maternity bras and she had to confess they were a bit tight. She was not really worried, just puzzled. If that body of hers hadn't been so unreliable she'd have forgotten all about it. As it was, she figured she'd call Dr Jolson. Just in case.

Two days later she was sitting in his office, staring at him across his desk.

'Look,' he told her, 'there's probably nothing to worry about, but I'd feel better if we removed this thing and had a look.'

Fannie was on her own because she hadn't expected this – she'd thought he'd either wave her away or give her some ointment. What was he implying? She continued to stare at him.

'I mean, I think I'd like to admit you to the hospital just to make sure.'

Oh boy. The hospital again. She closed her eyes, resigned. What about her children?

'What could it be?' she asked softly.

'It's probably nothing. It's likely to be a benign cyst. Women your age get them all the time. You may be thinking cancer – but get that right out of your head,' he admonished, with a throaty laugh – ho, ho, ho, never that, of course, that would be ridiculous. Fannie felt as if her nerves had been ignited. She hadn't thought cancer at all, actually, but now, well, she had no choice. He had shoved it right under her nose. 'As a doctor,' Jolson continued, 'I would be unprofessional not to take it out and have it looked at properly. OK?'

It had to be OK. She had no notion of how to think about what Jolson implied. In a daze she compliantly followed his orders and arranged for admission to hospital. She mentioned the C-word to no one. Mary and Regina would help their mother, staying downstairs. Her girls would think it was a treat.

'It's a growth,' she told Irving, who held her tenderly and said little. 'Like a wart they just need to check,' she told her parents and sisters. Her sisters, concerned, saw her closed face and asked little; her mother was tearful, her father calming – 'It vill be all right' – and reassuring, because to be otherwise was unthinkable.

She entered hospital. She knew the routine. She was a good patient, polite to the nurses, happy to be obliging. She stayed briefly and left hardly feeling she'd been away.

In 1945 there were no mammograms or breast checks. No one discussed diseased breasts. Breasts were good. Jane Russell was soon to be number one at the box office solely because of them. Breasts were for sex, were wholly desirable, wholly healthy, and absolutely not something to discuss openly. Except among friends, to complain about their size.

Fannie waited a few terrible days until the biopsy was done: it was benign. She felt normal again.

Paterson, 1947: Fannie

The lump, though, made her vigilant. She thought about her breasts, knew their possible disease. But she felt lucky – she'd defeated illness – so she checked them casually, without fear.

And then, in 1947, in the bath again, feeling her breasts, her fingers found a thickened, rounded something protruding under her skin, a creepy foreignness. The water at once felt icy, her fingers rigid: because of her first lump, the worst had been named; she was no longer shielded by innocence. The word began to clang in her brain: 'cancer'. She reassured herself: 'It's another cyst.' She rose, shaking, from the bath, wrapped a towel round her shoulders, and tried to stay calm while she made her way to the phone to call Jolson.

This time her daughters were almost ten, with a memory of the earlier episode. She had described the lump in the following way: 'It could have been a bad thing which could have made me very ill, but when the doctors removed it they saw it wasn't bad after all. It was like a wart you don't really want on your body but which won't hurt you.'

'It could have been a bad thing,' she had said. So they would worry, too. But the benign result of the first lump would reassure them, as it would Irving, her parents and her sisters. It did Fannie. After all, as Jolson had told her, 'Breast cancer's a disease of old women.'

Unlike women diagnosed with breast cancer today, Fannie was offered no choice of treatment. Before her first surgery, Dr Jolson and the oncologist Dr Heyman had painted for her the gruesome picture of what they would do should the unexpected occur. Breast cancer at that time had not yet formed the industry which helps and guides the Fannies of today: the specialist nursing, the counselling, the tips for coping, the support groups for advice. If the worst happened, the doctors informed her, their tone pooh-poohing the possibility, she would have the only thing on offer then, straightforward 'medical' intervention: surgery – radical mastectomy (the Halstead mastectomy, unchanged since the end of the nineteenth century), in which the breast is sliced away and all the surrounding muscles cut out – then strong radiation to destroy stray cancer cells lurking in what would remain underneath her sunken chest; thereafter, check-ups and physiotherapy.

Fannie was unlucky enough to be diagnosed before a key advance in understanding breast cancer. In 1947 oncologists still believed, as Halstead did, that breast cancer took a well-defined route, spreading centrifugally from the breast, progressively infiltrating tissues leading off from the original cancerous site. In other words, they thought it was a local disease; removing the whole breast and surrounding muscle and tissue therefore made sense. The change in understanding finally came about in the 1970s. We now know that breast cancer is a systemic, not local, disease. That means that, unless it is stopped, the pattern of spread in breast cancer is wide and scattered, for the tumour sheds its cells into the bloodstream. Now we have methods for stopping the spread without removing the entire breast. Now most women know the importance of early diagnosis and in many early cases the cancer can be excised when the site is very small. Only a small part of the breast needs to be removed. If it's caught early enough, it could well be before cells have entered the bloodstream. We also have better targeted radiation to kill the local cells. But if the cells have begun to travel, we now can kill them with chemotherapy, which will meet them in the bloodstream. We also can send hormones into the bloodstream which will prevent the cells from colonising other parts of the body. None of this was available to Fannie, whose harsh treatment stemmed from a well-intended but cruel ignorance.

Fannie did not at first enunciate the shock she felt. A breast removed? How would she live with that? How does anyone live knowing they've been given a death sentence, which cancer then certainly was? Her children . . . Her husband . . . She was not stoic. As she wailed Dr Jolson patted her kindly, urging, 'Don't worry!'

Fannie was under the surgeon's knife for hours. Whole chunks of her – a breast and then muscle – were gouged out. For this time

Fannie's lump was not a cyst. She was indeed that freakish thing, a young woman with breast cancer.

She was left alone in her hospital bed in the days while the anaesthesia and morphine from the surgery subsided. When she was fully conscious again she refused to look down at her oozing bandages; she propped her head with pillows till her neck ached, to prevent an accidental downward glance. She was nursed, dressings sorted, food brought, and nurses and doctors were kind and efficient, but no nurse, no medic, asked how she felt inside. Her mother wailed, her sisters cried; Irving and her father took their tears elsewhere, but she knew they, too, wept. Her daughters were told only that her recovery this time would take a long time.

Fannie's vigilance in fact had made her relatively lucky: her treatment had been speedy and early, before the lump could turn more lethal and nasty – in other words, she would not be likely to die soon. But she didn't know she was lucky because she had no comparisons. Fannie was one of breast cancer's lonely victims. Women then didn't know that others like them were also fighting in isolation. Young women in particular were hidden – to have a breast full of poison was unspeakable. Fannie would not be able to 'come out' after leaving the hospital. Even big-mouth Shirley would know she must keep silent. It was just too shocking and shameful. So Fannie remained mute about how it felt, even to her sisters. And they themselves had no words with which to ask. Inside Fannie the unspoken thoughts swirled, 'I am deformed . . . Something which gives life and pleasure to other women is killing me . . . I am no longer a complete woman . . . I won't touch the other breast or look at it ever again – sneaky betrayers.' She was not yet thirty-two.

She left hospital exhausted, bedridden, emaciated. She'd been through this ritual before, her return heralded with flowers, her sisters fussing, her mother bustling but with tears running down her face, her daughters showering her with handmade paper cards and colourful paintings in thick poster paint on white paper that curled up at the edges. Last time she had been cheered by this show of love and loyalty. This time she had to put on a show, with fake smiles to soothe the worried relatives gathered around her bed. She was way beyond soothing herself. For this time, unlike her leg wound, her diphtheria, even her pneumonia, she did not return waiting to mend. This time she entered home waiting to die. Cancer equalled death. She vowed inside she'd live as long as she could.

Fannie tried to scoop up a doll she found under a daughter's bed. She cried out in pain, as she often did. Not a day went by when something did not hurt – with the muscles she'd been accustomed to using in her chest removed, she often began movements, found she could no longer complete them, then tried again, using another muscle, and strained something else. Moreover, she suffered from lymphoedema – water in her upper arm – which was a common, painful side effect of her operation: it, too, limited arm movement. Her house was no longer pin-neat. This piqued her. She could no longer look at her reflection below her neck without sadness: she trained her gaze to flit over the middle part of her body. Her upper arm was so filled with water that it looked misshapen, especially next to the hollowed-out section where her breast had been. Her shoulder, once straight and proud, was now rounded and sloped forward. First she lost her breast, then her beauty.

'I am a patient,' she thought repeatedly. Circumstances made it so. She had appointments with Dr Heyman, her oncologist, with Dr Jolson and at the hospital. She offered her body for examination over and over again, determinedly looking away as they viewed her deformed chest. Her life was punctuated by treatments, examinations and frequent, unwelcome reminders of her condition, as pain shot through her arm at each impossible movement. The mah-jong games continued but she had to miss many for medical appointments or because she was too tired. She submitted to doctors, to the silence, to impotence as a woman and a patient because she had no choice. Except to succumb, and she would not do that.

Class and gender were themes running through her treatment. Her doctors were by definition middle-class, highly educated men. Older, male versions of Regina, they had left the working and lower-middle classes, the immigrants, behind. Fannie, on the one side, and Dr Jolson and Dr Heyman, on the other, were, respectively, products of their time. She, and they, did not know how to ask questions about her treatment – especially about how she might feel, what she ought to expect, how she might mentally prepare herself for all these after-effects. They did not even know that they should.

After her operation life carried on, for the most part, as if it would carry on and on. After their initial tears, disbelief, anger at her diagnosis and shock at her breast removal, her family said little directly to her about her condition. Besides, they'd heard of miracle recoveries. Perhaps that would be Fannie's story. Regina and Mary shied from discussions of the physical, which were not invited by Fannie. She never mentioned what it felt like to have a flat, hard, scarred surface where a breast used to be. Her parents believed blindly that doctors knew best – with touching faith they thought she was in Dr Jolson's hands rather than in those of a God in whom they did not believe. Irving went silent, but gazed at her sometimes with tears in his eyes, then grabbed her hand and kissed it tenderly. The girls were told she was ill, but recovering. Which she seemed to be. Unwittingly, Fannie's behaviour and that of her family helped her survive: believing you will live can help you live. And they were right: she did not die. She lived in apparent normality, going to school meetings, shopping, cleaning, playing mah-jong, even with one breast.

No one knew then about the genetics of breast cancer; if the first breast was cancerous, there was no reason to think the second would be, too. Indeed, we now know that unless the cancer is genetic, there is no heightened risk of developing it in the second breast. But there is if a woman has inherited a faulty gene. Two years after her operation, the normal life Fannie had begun to resume and tentatively believe in was shattered anew. She found a lump, hard and springy to the touch, in her other breast and recognised its texture. So did Jolson. Back in Barnert Hospital she endured it all again – the days of discomfort and oozing bandages, the burns of radiation, then afterwards, more hunching, and swelling in the other arm. The cancer this time spread faster, was more advanced. This time her doctors offered her additional, new treatment.

After her surgery, strong beams of radition to her ovaries shrank and destroyed them in order to cut off the oestrogen supply (oestrogen is thought to stimulate the growth of cancerous tumours). Fannie went into early menopause. But there was more.

To back up the radiation, androgens – masculinising hormones which counteract the production of oestrogen – were injected. Coarse sprays of tough black hair formed above her upper lip and jutted from her chin, while a thick dark down spread over her cheeks. Her arms and legs bristled. Touching her shoulders, she recoiled from the wiry shoots there; soon they appeared on her knuckles, then on her toes.

Her life as a lovely young woman was finished; she was thirty-three. Her moods swung rapidly and deeply, darkening the world around her and her daughters. She tried to control her temper, but the hormones coursing through her were too powerful. Her normally curly hair lost its lustre and became dry and wiry; her breastless upper body stiffened and swelled, twisting so that it aged decades in a matter of months. Fannie had now lost both the body she knew and her pretty face with its smooth, soft skin. She recoiled from any discussion of either her feelings or her condition, so in her presence her mother grew grim but affected false cheer, and her sisters were tentative, sniffing out her moods.

On good days she was fine, fun and easy, back in the world of her daughters, of TV, of books, of heated discussions excoriating the dread Senator McCarthy. Her family overlooked her temper, her gloom, and held out for days like these. Regina, now with two small children and living on Long Island, came out to Paterson at first every other weekend and then more frequently. Mary came every weekend. Indeed, for six months just after Fannie's second operation, Mary, having gathered suitcases and children, left Murray in the tenement – and to his just discovered girlfriend – and moved in with the Smiths. A temporary separation, it turned out, but fortuitous and a balm to the sisters. They spent days playing cards, seeing old school friends who dropped in on Fannie, even shopping together when Fannie felt well, sisters in a shared house, with their parents, again.

On really good days, in the summer following her second surgery, Fannie even drove her daughters in her grey Buick across two bridges and over to Regina's new house. Sometimes Mary followed in her black Chevy, with Nina, and more occasionally the teenaged Norman, in tow. Irving stayed in Paterson. They'd have a respite, Regina happy to serve them meals on her pretty dishes, delighted to be able to offer a lazy afternoon, in the cooling shade of the trees in her garden, with vodka tonics and noisy children playing on the swing, back and forth, soothing and comforting.

For a few years, from the discovery of the cancer in her second breast until the end of 1951, that is how Fannie lived. Even so, her sentence was final.

Great Neck, NY, 1952: Regina

Regina, my mother, was now comfortably ensconced in a pretty, detached house. There were birch trees on the front lawn, which was bordered by hedges and the azalea and rhododendron bushes she'd recently planted, and groups of dogwoods, oaks and lilac bushes in our spacious back garden, a luxury after the concrete playgrounds of Manhattan. In 1950 my father's parents had bought them the house in Great Neck – the commuter village on Long Island Sound famously disguised as *The Great Gatsby*'s West Egg – where my brothers and I grew up. There were three of us by 1952 – me, aged five, and my two little brothers, Gene, almost three, and Ricky, born that June. We lived in a world in which people, including my mother, believed anything was possible. There had to be better medical treatment, more for Fannie than Barnert Hospital – a medical backwater – offered. My mother would have wanted to give to Fannie, to Mary, to her parents, something wonderful – like saving Fannie's life – from the world she'd entered. Urged by her friends and my father's family, she phoned Jolson. He bristled at her questions: Fannie's treatment was sound. It was standard.

Soon afterwards he off-handedly mentioned her sister's intervention as he pressed his fingers into Fannie's scars during a routine check-up, adding that she had the 'college girl's disease' – uppity behaviour, he meant. Poor Fannie was mortified. 'Darling,' she said to my mother when she phoned later, 'there's nothing they're not doing.' My mother took that to mean 'Back off. I've chosen Jolson and Paterson. Let me be.' I think my mother would have pushed the issue if the truth had been different, if she hadn't found out from her Great Neck friends that no better treatment existed. Jolson was right.

Great Neck, NY: Janet

Aunt Fannie's diagnosis had come in August 1947, a few months after I was born. One of my earliest memories is the smell of hospitals and with it a picture of myself, bored, looking up at the legs of older relatives hovering around her hospital bed. For a time most Sundays were spent like this: I saw my aunts, cousins and grandparents around a hospital bed, then went out for Sunday lunch. My father's mother, ill with a heart condition, was often in a different hospital then, so sometimes we visited her, too, and there we saw the other side of the family. Through the years no one commented on the oddness of having conducted so much of our family social life around illness. I remember Aunt Fannie's visits when she was well. She had an easy, joking manner, but wasn't effusive like Aunt Mary. Mary was soft and cheerful; she would get down on the floor with me and play, sing me songs, hold me on her knee and tell magical stories. I'd make up dances and she'd join in. But in one striking way Aunt Fannie, when well, was easier: Aunt Mary used to be whisked off by my grandmother behind closed doors while she preached at her, Mary emerging with an embarrassed, tense laugh, pretending a lightheartedness which, it has to be said, soon became real as our play, in a twinkling, melted the tension.

In contrast, the well Aunt Fannie was just *there*, chatting with my mother. She smoked Lucky Strikes. That feels shocking now, but the link in the public mind between smoking and cancer – or any disease, for that matter – was years away from being made. Smoking made my mother and her sisters sophisticated. When they lit up together

I watched them unbend, relax and settle down to gossip. They were affectionate with each other, my mother proudly displaying her new furniture and gadgets, prompting us – usually me – to perform. Or she'd shoo us off to bring out the childish scrawls we'd created that year at school or more recently, at the kitchen table while she was preparing potato salad and coleslaw for the barbecue we'd have later on. I picture them, golden-skinned, red-lipped, in white piqué dresses or pale cotton shorts and blouses, on deckchairs in the garden in Great Neck in sunny summers, smoking and laughing.

I waited patiently for my mother one Wednesday lunchtime in 1954 outside my gleaming glass-walled first-grade classroom at Clover Drive School. I crunched crisp leaves at my feet, crushing a big, doubled-up dried maple leaf with gusto while I gazed at the sprawling red-brick house across the street with its giant oak like a flagpole on its front lawn.

On Wednesdays I had only a half-day of school. My mother, with my two young pre-school brothers in the back seat, swung the car past the school entrance. I jumped in, and we began the hour-and-a-half drive to Paterson. I used to like going to Paterson to see my grandparents, aunts and cousins. During the autumn of my first-grade year we went every Sunday and every Wednesday – no playing with friends on Sundays, no after-school dates on long Wednesdays. On Wednesdays in particular, visits were hurried and unpleasant, with nothing to do until the triplets' school was over, and then they had homework and couldn't play anyway. My grandmother unvaryingly cooked dull boiled chicken. In the dark we'd climb back in the car, and make our way home, we children asleep, crushed against each other in the back.

During the few hours there I would pay my respects to the focus of the journey, and it never ceased to upset me. I tried to avoid going into the front room, with its hospital bed, its single chair, and its chest of drawers, whose top was littered with bottles of tablets. There was no TV in the room to distract me. And always my aunt, thin and ashen, her hair a tangled mess, lay on the bed. Sometimes she was asleep. Sometimes she'd talk to me, her voice slurred, and I never found anything to say in return except to reply to her questions: 'Yes, I like school.' 'Yes, I'm the best reader in my class.' 'Yes, I'm the oldest in my class.' Every week she asked the same questions and heard the same answers. She didn't seem to remember.

On rare occasions the bed was propped to a sitting position, and my aunt was fully awake, smiling and joking. She'd ask for a hug. When she was like this she was momentarily restored to the aunt I'd loved, not sick, just my mother's sister, her daughters' mother – normal. But whenever I hugged her that sense vanished smartly, for she smelled stale, of illness, and I'd be ashamed that I noticed. I knew I was supposed to feel sorry for her. Mostly, I did – she'd been sick a terribly long time, and I knew being sick was horrible, bad enough for a mere few days, and she'd been ill, off and on, for as long as I'd been alive. I recognised her pain and her sadness, and I knew my mother's as well: I'd heard her crying with my father and Aunt Mary, and talking anxiously to her mother on the phone. I saw her pained concern when she entered the sickroom. On some visits we children were kept downstairs, or in the back of my aunt's top-floor apartment, far away from the sickroom. Aunt Fannie's moans through the rooms were muffled then, but they were long and frightening, even so.

I could not understand why she'd been sick for so long. She wasn't old, like my invalid grandmother, who lived with us on the ground floor of our house. I used to be impatient with my grandmother – wished she would get out of bed and be lively like my adored grandfather, who still commuted with my father into the city. Then both Grandpa and Grandma Reibstein died, a week apart. My shame at my ungenerous feelings deepened – look what happened to Grandma! I was also guilty of yearning for my cousins' return. For at least when the door was flung open and they ran to my grandmother's kitchen for their after-school snack the focus shifted from the sickroom. From the moment I set foot in that Paterson house, I used to hope my aunt would remain asleep. Then I wouldn't have to go in and see her. I hated myself for that and for what it would do to my mother if she knew.

Even so, I never questioned that we went. Nor did I think it strange that on our visits we ate separately from my cousins and that I only ever glimpsed their father. For even as my aunt lay dying Irving came in one door and my mother went out the other; my grandmother fed one set of grandchildren and their parents separately from the other.

On this particular Wednesday in 1954 Aunt Fannie was perky and sitting up. I was summoned to the sickroom. As usual she asked about school and, now, my friends. 'Are Patty and Sukie in your class?' Oh boy, was that the wrong thing to say! How could she think Sukie, the shrimp, who still sucked her thumb in public, was my age? I mustered my dignity. 'Just Patty.' The awkward silence of spent topics descended. I waited politely for her to speak. 'And where is Gene?' she asked. I bristled. *I* was here. Wasn't I entertaining enough? Why would anyone want to see Gene-the-pain? Then came the bombshell: 'Where is he, my favourite?' I was stunned. Angry and baffled, I blurted out – so much for my careful courtesy! – 'Why is *he* your favourite? Why do you want to see *him*?' 'Because he's the second child, just like me,' she answered sweetly. That halted me – why on earth should that matter? Let him have her! I hustled off to find the little brat. Let him stand there and make conversation – and his conversation would be pretty dull, she'd see, with him being only three years old.

Years later my mother and I sat in her bedroom, she reminiscing. She remembered how effortlessly she'd been the 'good' little girl, adored by her sisters, protected by them. She rarely talked about them – they were like a closed book, a private, precious one. But in these moments she opened up, and the days of our twice-weekly Paterson visits came back. Fannie by then wasn't Fannie to her any more. A shadow remained in her wasted body, and that was to whom my mother pleaded, as Fannie spoke of defeat. 'I want to go, Regina,' Fannie announced. 'It's enough.' My mother, who at the time still knew nothing of insurmountable pain, couldn't properly understand. Passionate to keep her sister alive, she argued with her. 'You can't give in. You have to fight. Your girls need you,' she cried. She left an exhausted Fannie, resistant to her pleas, to sleep.

That was the day Fannie sent for Gene. My mother, now unwrapping the pain of years before, went on. She'd been downstairs, but returned a short time later to check on Fannie. Creeping upstairs to peek in, she saw Gene toddling into the sickroom. Puzzled, she tiptoed behind. From just outside the door, she watched in growing horror as Gene padded over to the low dresser, just out of Fannie's reach, and groped among the bottles of pills. 'Yes, sweetie, that one. Bring me those, that's a good boy,' Aunt Fannie prompted. He managed to grab a bottle, and proudly handed it over. At that point my mother lunged, swooped her son into her arms, grabbing the bottle from Fannie, and hissed 'No!' at her sister. Startled, Gene began to cry. She rushed him downstairs to his grandmother, then, heart still pounding, ran back upstairs and faced Fannie. She was stony with rage, Fannie shrivelled with shame.

My mother sobbed as she told me, 'We held each other. "I can't take any more," Fannie wept. "He wouldn't have known what he was doing. Who could I ask?"' My mother went silent, then turned her sad face to me. 'I couldn't let her do that. Not to my son. I didn't understand then, you know. My God; it came so close.'

Paterson, October 1954: Fannie

In the last two years Fannie's cancer grew vigorous. She underwent further surgery to slice out more tumours, again lay under strong, burning radiation. Her patience ebbed, her tongue grew acid, as pain unremittingly chopped away at her. She came to realise she would never again feel the sweetness of relief – not till the end, when she'd get morphine, the final solution.

Irving had engaged a nurse, Helen, a thin red-haired woman. She frightened the girls and when once she airily mentioned a daughter to the girls they recoiled in sympathy for the unseen child who had to suffer this hard, chilly woman for a mother. Every day Helen entered the enclosed top porch, now heated and turned into a sickroom, closed the door, and in private injected Fannie. Then she sat next to the bed and read her *Journal American* and *Confidential.*

Sometimes one of the girls, missing her mother, forlornly wandered in during this operation, and would find Helen herself nodding off; it seemed she was sharing Fannie's morphine. When Helen was sure Fannie was safely in a morphine stupor, she'd go into the kitchen, cook herself some lunch, and spend the rest of the afternoon painting her nails, smoking, watching soap operas and laconically, coldly, telling the girls off if they interrupted her.

Fannie lay in bed in the sickroom. Resting atop the neighbouring small table were *McCall's*, *Life* and *Look*, a recent visitor's goodwill gift. Fannie could no longer read, but sometimes kindness still touched her. The rest of the table was covered with a small towel to protect against the drippings of medicine. Next to it stood the infamous chest of drawers, with the myriad medications, a loudly ticking clock and a silent radio. Noise had become painful. A kitchen chair, aluminium, with a red leatherette seat and back, was pulled up next to the bed for visitors. She was glad to be in this room with its wrap-around windows and their views of Paterson life. Sometimes, if she felt up to it, the hospital bed was cranked up so she could stare into the distance. Eventually she could see the far-off factories that formed the boundary to her East Side neighbourhood, the only one she'd ever lived in. Looking to the right, she could see into the houses across the street. New people had moved in. She had never met them. She never would. They didn't interest her; she gazed on them because they were there. And that was the biggest change. She'd lost interest. Most of the time she slept. She'd be wakened for a jab from Helen and then doze off. She lived in a half-world of sleep, dream and hazy awakening. The constant in it was the thin, white-sheathed form of Helen with her topping of orange hair. Her daughters floated in and out. Sometimes she was aware of Irving's hatchet-like face, most of the time giving nothing away. Occasionally she felt him holding her hand and, through the blur of images, knew he was weeping. Others, like Shirley, her parents and sisters, drifted in and out; there were even whole hours when she felt almost connected to life again, and had conversations. She never thought of her appearance. She couldn't have cared less what others thought.

At first the pain had been terrifying. She was desperate to live, but living in such pain was insupportable. Now she'd stopped fighting. It had won. The big difference was that for the past year – or, since she had been in that sort of pain, more often than not – since she had not been able to do the necessary things that defined any mother, wife, sister or friend, others had replaced her. Most pertinently her parents had looked after the girls, as had Mary when she and her children lived downstairs. Her daughters came upstairs to glance in at her, to give her kisses, to report the headlines of their lives, to change their clothes, and to sleep. The rest of their lives they conducted below, in their grandparents' domain. Fannie knew they would survive; the past year had been evidence of that, and it had given her the permission she'd needed to go. Soon her hours of wakefulness, of engaging with people – with her sisters when they popped in, and their children – would diminish. She would finally disengage wholly as the pain deepened and no longer ebbed, as pain and morphine consumed what was left of her. She would stop. And it wouldn't be so bad; this kind of dying was gradual. Everyone, even Fannie, herself, had become used to it.

Helen found her. Helen had seen a lot of death. She covered Fannie's face, then went downstairs to my grandparents and told them.

The death certificate was signed by Jolson. 'Cause of death: Metastasis to spine and lungs.'

Paterson, October 1954: Janet

We spent a week at my grandmother's when my Aunt Fannie died. All the grown-ups cried, my mother, my aunt – even my father, when he held my mother, her shoulders shaking with grief. Everything about that period up to her death – all the visits, and then the week in Paterson after she died – feels dark, as if it was always night in New Jersey. Breast cancer, I was told, had killed her. Breast cancer meant a drawn-out, grey and painful death. It meant leaving three children motherless. It meant ageing and draining my distant but till then energetic grandmother. She hadn't been fun before, like my teasing, playful grandfather, or my once sparky if bedridden other grandmother, or my fabulous, vibrant and sorely missed other grandfather. But she bustled with purpose, and was joyful for our presence. After Fannie died she was never the same – she became preoccupied, not quite there, and occasionally she'd hug me to her, suddenly, baffling me by her intensity.

Within the grey walls of the house on East 33rd Street, the curtains drawn, I listened to my grandmother's wails, witnessed my normally comical grandfather's stoniness, my glamorous teenage triplet cousins' blank looks and red eyes, and my mother's and Aunt Mary's sobbing during our stay, the ritual week of sitting shiva, a ritual my mother's atheist family performed without question.

My mother, though I didn't understand this then, had lost a sister to whom she needed to make amends, one she felt guilt over leaving behind. Aunt Mary had lost an anchor, a confidante. The triumvirate, the three who looked alike, who were shaped alike, who formed the American Smith girls like a barricade against my grandparents' shadowy Polishness, had been smashed. Each sister had had a different role in the family. My mother had been the ambitious, brainy one, Aunt Mary the sweet, careless one; Fannie had been the sharp-witted, steady, but puzzlingly frail one. So it might have made macabre sense that a crazy, unseen illness should claim her: her, but never them. When Aunt Fannie died my mother and Aunt Mary were left with grief. Not, at that point, fear.

PART II

LEARNING

4
Regina's Long Story Begins

After Fannie's death our trips to Paterson became less frequent. We children were busy with friends, birthday parties, Scouts, dancing and music lessons, and, in the summers, camp, Little League and swimming lessons. Going to Paterson held few attractions. Aunt Mary and Nina, the triplets and my grandparents now more typically came to us.

By then Paterson had become a town of old people, with East Side Park and its scrappy little patch of old-fashioned swings, slide and sandbox. In this quiet period of my middle childhood many of my father's vast, energetic family of uncles and aunts died, mostly from heart disease: periodic weekend treks to hospitals ensued – and it felt normal, a continuation of the past, to watch them grow whiter and thinner – until finally the phone call came saying they'd died. But none, apart from the death of my father's parents, exploded home life the way Fannie's illness and death had done.

In 1955 my father left his job as sales director of a medium-sized luxury watch company. He had given up teaching for financial reasons as soon as I was born, and had joined the hated jewellery business. Our staple game over dinner became seeing who could come up with the most outlandish answer to 'What mind-bendingly stupid thing do you think that jerk Warnock [the chief executive] did today?' Not to mention the nightly instalment of the machinations of Warnock's scheming secretary, wily Mae. My father began his own business, manufacturing gold jewellery. My mother stayed home.

Doing so suited her then. Couples with young children like us occupied most of our neighbourhood. My mother joined a Temple Sisterhood, although neither my father's family nor hers were practising Jews. The Sisterhood was the centre of neighbourhood social life, and my mother had a tropism for both friends and sisterhoods, so, although our family did not join the synagogue, as a newcomer she was allowed to take part in the Sisterhood's Purim play. I was thrilled watching her speak her single line, thought her beautiful in her pale green organza toga. That was the last time we attended the temple, organised religion being abhorrent to both sides of the family. Her performance had been an introductory offer: we had to join or she was out of the Sisterhood. She'd made the friends anyway. Instead, on Sisterhood mornings she and I and my two tiny brothers went to the library, and she would take us into a corner to read. Later, when I was in school, she and I went every Thursday afternoon. We savoured our library jaunts – nothing got in their way. I could choose one book and she three for me. I would read my one, she the three others to me, in bed. As I got older I chose them all. I loved it that she loved my choices.

Once a week she and my father met in Manhattan, often joining either Max, my father's best friend and his wife Horty, or Phyllis and Irvin – until Phyllis and Irvin moved, first to England for a year, then later to Florida, and finally to Boston. Evelyn had married and moved to Mexico, though we saw her each summer when she brought her daughters to visit. Either in a group or alone they'd go to a show. The next night, when she put me to bed, my bedtime story would be an edited version of the play they'd seen (I'm sure she drastically modified *The Crucible*, and cut and mauled *The Rose Tattoo*). My favourites were the musicals. Not only did she tell the stories, but she sang some of the songs in a small, unsteady voice. I thought her voice as pure and sweet as those of the singers on my collection of Little Golden records, though she laughed at my praise.

I requested favourites again and again: *South Pacific* was number one. She told a shortened, moving tale of Nellie Forbush, and her prejudice then redemption through war and Emile de Becque's love.

I studied the shape of my mother's lips as they moved, memorised their arches and curves, drank in the even shapes of her teeth. I felt a comforting thrill as the rush of her voice signalled the happy denouement. But I loved best the punctuation marks – the few scanty bars of her handful of songs: 'Happy talk, keep talkin' happy talk, Talk about things you'd like to do. You gotta have a dream; If you don't have a dream, How you gonna have a dream come true?'

Lying next to me in my narrow bed, her body warm, her graceful fingers running gently along my arm, she'd croon to the ceiling, while my eyes closed, as she repeated bars of the requested song. 'Bali Ha'i may call you, any night, any day.' She sang; that and the rhythmic, silky strokes sent me drifting off to sleep.

My mother was patently happy. Only at odd moments would I see her face change, her brows knit, eyes go unfocused, and a soft tear spill out of one eye. As soon as she felt my frightened eyes on her, her face would regain its shiny sweetness. With a kiss and a hug the sadness vanished. That was the remainder of Fannie for me.

We lived near Allenwood Park, and in the summer my mother would assemble her brood – baby Mark, born in 1957, in a stroller, we older ones following in a straggly line – and we'd walk down the hill and over the next few streets to spend our days there, picnicking under the great oak near the swings. There was a paddling pool, and a duckpond. Friends would be there, all seeking relief from the soggy heat. In 1957 a neighbourhood swimming club was built on derelict land nearby, and became the focus of our summers.

My mother was a graceful, strong swimmer, and when I was five she tried to teach me. That was the single sustained sour note between us in my early childhood. She hated to witness – and saw it in a flash, even before I'd start my protests – the fear pinging like a rubber band through me at the mere thought of discarding my inflatable tube. I was miserable about it. I hated to fail her – and I did. Of course she hated to fail me, too, and she did. I was sure I'd drown: it seemed illogical that any heavy, upright body should float. She would lift my rigid body atop the water, place it like a horizontal board. As I screamed she'd grip me more tightly and viciously, her voice more shrill and imperious: 'Relax! Stop it this minute!' She could not fathom my fear, was insulted by my mistrust. I wasn't used to her cold dismissal. She tried to teach me again the next summer, when I was six, and again when I was seven. The lessons made me phobic, and I learned to swim way after my school friends did, through a series of private lessons.

But normally my mother was cheerful, proud of me and her beautiful, black-haired, precocious son Gene, happy with her sunshine boy, the dimpled, gorgeous Ricky – according to her 'the easiest child in the world' – and delighted with Mark, who was 'the funniest', and, later, 'wise beyond his years'. At first, displaced by Gene, my nose was out of joint; it may have been then that I began to perform, to try to capture her attention and claim back my rightful place at the centre of her world.

It worked to a large degree: she screamed with laughter at my made-up songs and ballets performed to a Little Golden record accompaniment. She encouraged me to perform at family get-togethers, which I did with no hesitation. When Gene was old enough I found a use for him: he was the token small male part in the plays I produced in our garage. The plots were inspired by costumes handed down from my mother's cousins and stuffed into a dresser in my room; mostly Gene was a prince or a dragon and I a princess or a queen. Later, in school, I grabbed the best parts in the class plays, and danced my own creations in the school hall. She looked pretty and glowing as she watched me: Queen Mommy of the Queen Little Girl. I thrived, as she had done, on my teachers' encouragement, loved finishing my school work and getting '100 per cent' or 'Excellent work!' scrawled across the top. As she had done, I wrote stories, and made books. Before I could write she was my scribe and helped me staple the pages and put my scribbles on the cover. When I was older she found scraps of fabric for me to paste on to cardboard, to make real covers. As her sisters had done to her, she applauded me with love.

Ricky was born when I was five. I happily took the role of mother's helper. He could be my baby, too. I could hold him for her, prop his bottle to free her up, hand her diaper pins while she bathed him, fetch his baby towels, lay out his pyjamas, and I could show him off to friends. With Mark's birth when I was ten, I went further; I took over whole feedings, bathed him and even changed his diaper. We made a good team in the sea of males, my mother and I. Such feminine teamwork must have felt familiar and consoling. Maybe she felt her own childhood echoing through mine. But this time the mother and daughter would understand each other. This time they'd feel as one. This time the parents would offer paradise, in the guise of Great Neck. This time there would be no reason to reject it, as in her time she'd rejected Paterson. Our being so in tune must have soothed her old wounds. In those years she *was* Queen Mommy: she passed on to me – and my brothers, too – the secret she'd learned in childhood from her sisters: the magic of reciprocal adoration.

As, over the years, my parents' social circle and community involvement grew, so the noise and bustle of our house grew, too. My mother entertained frequently. Suburban America in the fifties meant people dropping in without notice. The doorbell and phone rang repeatedly. Our friends crashed in and out of both back and front doors, sometimes shattering the glass outer doors, or, in summer, smashing the mosquito screens that replaced them. The house often tipped into unruliness; few rules governed privacy. Anyone could storm into anyone else's room, and often even the bathroom door-locks didn't work. But when 'company' was expected the appearance of order was required. At those anxious points my mother showed her rare harsh side: 'Clean up the mess right away!' she'd bark, mainly to Gene and me.

A few years after she'd tried and rejected the Sisterhood, when Rick was in nursery and Gene and I in primary school, my mother joined the League of Women Voters, whose members were women who in a later generation would have been professionals. She became their vice-president and, briefly, president. The months when she wrote *This is Great Neck*, a comprehensive guide to our town, for the League consumed too much of her for me. She wasn't readily available and I resented her preoccupation, the hours it took her focus off us. I would lurk about her bedroom as she sat at her makeshift desk – the top of the sewing machine – glimpsing her slim fingers flying – she hadn't taken typing at East Side High for nothing – across the old green Smith-Corona, and impatiently long for her to be finished and back with us, finished with that stupid old typewriter. I resented the Wednesdays she had League meetings because they prevented her from being at home when I burst through the front door, eager to recount my day at school. But I was deeply proud when *This is Great Neck* became the history text for my third-grade class. 'My mother did this,' I bragged, pointing to her name, oblivious of the other children's reaction to my boasting.

Unlike my father, whose Saturdays seemed to be for napping, my mother didn't need much sleep. She relished our early years. Perhaps in manic overdrive to compensate for lack of sleep, she fired on all cylinders. When a magazine writer came to interview her about the discovery she'd made while writing *This is Great Neck*, that double water taxes had been levied in a section of town over twenty years, we children crept around quietly, trying to do her proud as model children – and be noted as such in his article. (Not a mention!) Perhaps he'd make her famous.

I think she was truly happy in those years. She'd at last got the admiration and adoration she'd craved since her sisters had left her to lead their own lives. She'd at last got on to a wider stage than Paterson. But she still tried to get her parents to notice. She bought copies of the article for them. 'Wery nice,' they said, and they meant it, too. But they didn't understand. Her life stood as an implicit criticism of their own. Mary bragged to her neighbours in East Paterson, where she lived now, again with Murray, and Nina, Norman now in the Army. But for my mother Mary's pride was bittersweet, mixed as it was with awe. During her visits vibrant Aunt Mary faded, saying little, but laughing in admiration as the conversation swirled around her, when my mother's pretty, stylish friends came to call.

Through my early and middle childhood, even I could see my father was in love with my mother, though I wouldn't have known that's what I saw. My parents weren't like my friends' parents. They openly kissed and hugged, and my father was obviously happier when my mother was around than when she wasn't. It didn't bother him that she had more time for her children and friends than for him. He enjoyed her vivacity and energy. He had his own, slower pace. He adored her much as he adored us: he chortled in delight over her as he did over us, gazed at her with the same fond gleam. He had pet names for all of us, including her, though no one had one for him. His role in our family, it seemed to me, was to admire and cherish. No one took his temper outbursts seriously – they didn't seem in character, though Mom's did, and we never ignored her sudden, though infrequent, eruptions.

A few times a month they had dinner parties, when she changed from familiar Mom to Hollywood Mom, as she did whenever they went out. Her hair, often unkempt during a week spent ferrying four children, cooking, driving back and forth to the supermarket and to League of Women Voters meetings, was professionally 'done' that day. Her make-up – during the week she wore only a light red or pink lipstick and then only when leaving the house – was light but skilful. I sat on the toilet lid and studied her as she applied it in front of her bathroom mirror. For her lips she used a bright, compelling red lipstick. For her eyes, boring black mascara. No eyeshadow. I wished in vain for little pots of pretty blues, greens or purples. Using a gold pencil with a dark brown point she tidied her brows and lined the top of her lids. Finally, either sliding her fingers over a sticky red cream in a pink pot (difficult to remove when I surreptitiously tried gliding it on to my childish cheeks), or dipping them into a peachy-red liquid in a little black pot (a muted but smeary look in my attempts), she blended in circles of rouge on her cheekbones.

By party time the normally untidy rooms were spare and elegant in gold-hued light. There were flowers and beautiful food on sparkling china from my father's family, normally stored away in a glass cabinet. The scent of 'Calèche' or 'L'Air du Temps' or 'Arpège' wafted as she wandered past. A half-hour before the guests arrived she would race into her room and prise her prettiest clothes from her overstuffed cupboard: a thick green brocade dress, a black Italian knit, a white piqué hand-painted with pink roses and matching stole. Out would tumble boxes of shoes and she'd step into high, pointy-toed heels. From its hiding place she'd extract a bunch of fine jewellery and try each piece against the chosen dress. When the bell rang she went calm and regal, and as she greeted her guests – pow! – her charm flashed. We watched, sitting on the top step, peering into the foyer, in our pyjamas. When we were older we passed around hors d'oeuvres and offered cigarettes from a Persian mosaic cigarette box.

My father's job was to tend the bar. He did Martinis, Manhattans, Tom Collinses, gin and tonics, whiskey sours and daiquiris (from mixes), Bloody Marys, and a whole roster of 'women's drinks', such as 'Seven and Sevens' (Seagram's 7 whiskey and 7-Up), rye and ginger (rye whiskey and ginger ale), rum and Cokes, and vodka and orange juice. He stood in the background, at the far end of the living room, mixing and handing out drinks from his trolley, while my mother managed the foreground.

I studied my mother, 'the hostess': she listened intently to each person. If someone was boring or not socially skilled she worked harder: she grabbed strands of conversation, and kept up a flow. This was not an effort for her. Some of our most delicious moments were when I talked to her about my friends or the people in my class or my teachers, or asked her about her friends, their children, what she liked or didn't about them. She found me interesting. She took my observations, even when I was only seven, eight, or nine, seriously, and without condescension shared her own. I loved to listen to her talk to her friends, lingered near the phone as she chatted. I knew how she talked to grown-ups. That was how she talked in those moments to me. Together we speculated about why people did things, or had certain tastes, or had been cruel or even particularly kind. We'd sit at the rickety round white kitchen table, after I got home from school, and while I scoffed Oreo cookies and milk and she sat down and stopped whatever she'd been doing, we'd talk. She found people intrinsically interesting.

Apart from arguments about money, which flared up especially while my father's business was being established, my parents seemed extremely happy. When my father came home from his daily commute to New York City, we children would race down the front hallway to jump into his arms, and then, shrugging us off gently, he would enter the kitchen, where my mother was, and they would kiss on the lips. It was both toe-curling and riveting.

But there were dark sides to life, even then. I can't be sure that my aunt's death was their source, but I can say that my mother had something her friends did not: a sense that something tragic had occurred. Not that I could define this quality then.

Her temper could be short. Maybe that had nothing to do with Fannie, but maybe grief limited her patience. When I panicked during swimming lessons, earning her displeasure, I had to find ways to make amends, but it always required total capitulation, which I resisted more, I think, than my brothers did. She never seemed as cross with them and forgave them more easily, perhaps because they were younger, or boys. Though sometimes Gene, resisting anything new or different, drove her to the edge, and she'd lose her temper and be short with him, too. My mother hardly ever lost her temper with Rick, who was born shortly before Aunt Fannie died. Perhaps because he gave her special hope and comfort, a warm, wonderful bundle to hold and cherish in the face of her loss. Later, with Mark, she was similarly patient and forgiving, almost never harsh; perhaps towards her youngest maternal protectiveness couldn't waver.

I think I came in for criticism, in general, because of our intense identification with each other. Her legacy of sisterhood continued through me. I reminded her of herself, the good little girl, the model, ambitious student. Being like her, I ought to have known better; being like her, I shouldn't have made mistakes, or should have been braver facing challenges. I should have behaved as she'd have wanted herself to have behaved. I did myself no favours in our incipient struggle. Even before adolescence, when resistance was normal, I resisted our fusion. I resented her criticism: it felt like an infringement of who I was, a misreading of me. At the same time, I was confused by my resistance: I admired and wanted to be like her more than anyone in the world. But saying I was wrong even then felt as if I'd lost something of myself to her. To re-establish harmony I had to apologise, even when I didn't mean it. Reunions were sweet, with tears, hugs, stories at bedtime, and a shared belief that discord would never cleave us again. And, truly, through most of my early and middle childhood, it rarely did.

During this period, before Mark's birth and after Fannie's death, my parents had only one terrible fight. It happened soon after Fannie had died and not long after my father's parents' deaths. Both were grieving, I now see. It was after dinner, just before bedtime, the time of the day when the tempers of parents of small children are most frayed. Ricky, the baby, was asleep. Playing in our bedroom after dinner, Gene and I were startled by angry shouts from below. We played on, casting uneasy glances at each other, trying to pretend we weren't frightened.

An eerie silence descended. My mother, grim-faced, dutifully mounted the stairs to bath us. As she reached the top she turned and, almost as an afterthought, yelled one final recrimination down at my father, who was at the bottom of the stairs. He turned on his heel and stormed out, slamming the front door behind him. My mother's face was contorted and purple with rage. She shouted after him, at the shut front door. We wailed, Gene and I, afraid of the anger, and terrified Daddy wouldn't return. 'Divorce' came to mind; it was like a curse word. We'd never before witnessed a rift of this magnitude between them. The breach shocked us both: it exposed how secure we had felt till then, despite deaths, and how easily security could fail. The triplets had lost it, after all. Nina and Norman had never had it. My mother had lost Fannie. Could she have been perversely testing, pushing her boundaries to see if she'd lose my father, now her anchor and best fan, too?

Great Neck, June 1962

On a brilliantly sunny Sunday in early June, my mother, as usual, had risen earlier than anyone else, and had unloaded the dishwasher. Through the clatter of silverware and crockery we slept on. My two little brothers, four and nine, were asleep in the room they shared, the largest of the three bedrooms upstairs. Gene, almost twelve, was out for the count in his messy, pine-panelled one, and I, fourteen, slept deeply in my larger room with twin beds – for when friends slept over – with their jungle-printed bedspreads. My father, in their downstairs bedroom, also slept peacefully, though the clatter was close by. He had a talent for sleep.

We would be up soon enough though, because that was the day my mother was to march in graduation from NYU's Graduate School of Public Administration. Sixteen years after laying it aside, my mother finished her MA, and her thesis had been passed with gratifying comments. Her discovery, years earlier, of Great Neck citizens' payment of double taxes formed the data for her research, and she was to be awarded an MA in Public Administration. She was ahead of her friends. In a few years' time they would be returning to finish their degrees, or polishing their CVs and taking up part-time work. Our mother was the first. We were proud.

In the luxury of quiet and calm she let herself imagine what she'd look like up there on the stage, receiving her degree. She thought first about what to wear. She opened her double closet doors. A pokey, inadequate, full-length mirror was nailed to one, the lighting for it so poor that she was startled whenever she saw her reflection in a well-lit, proper full-length mirror: 'Oh, so that's what I look like.' Recently we children had heard her increasingly put critical words to slight discontents and irritations she'd endured, like pesky neighbours, since moving into our house eleven years earlier. 'This doesn't work. We need a new one of that,' she would complain. Then the wait would begin, in which my father was expected to act. She had not yet got to the point at which she realised he never would. He could live with a sundeck door that didn't close properly, and was happy to sit in a broken garden chair under the dogwood trees and read his paper while we kids swarmed around. My mother had once loved it that he was so easily pleased. Now we noticed shards of resentment. She had become resentful of the devotion that had followed him through his childhood and which we kids continued. She felt soiled by her envy, alone with the thrusting ambition he had never shared.

Our devotion to her had till recently magicked away the restlessness of her Paterson years. But now my mother felt the veil of adoration dropping from my newly critical adolescent gaze. Till then I had exalted her beauty, knowledge and competence. Till recently her advice and opinions had been final, like the Bible. Only she could provide solace for my wounds. And I'd basked in her adoration, as well. I would catch her watching us, pie-eyed with love, when she thought we weren't looking. Now even that, with its implied expectations, was becoming burdensome.

She could not bear me to lie around lazily and sullenly locked in my bedroom, listening for hours to my tinny radio. She found it hard to allow me to reject what she *knew* I needed for 'success in the world', whatever that was. I interpreted it to mean she wanted me to be the First Woman President, or a Great Writer, or a Doctor, all the while being a Perfect Wife and Mother. She could not bear to watch a stranger – who looked and behaved like other young girls, who chewed gum loudly in public and spoke in an unrefined Brooklyn accent, who rejected books, and wouldn't be caught dead going to a ballet – inhabit my body. She began to scorn me. 'You will be *ordinary*' was her curse, shouted at the angry tears I shed over her vetoes and condemnation.

I had become adolescent. I didn't know that she had once looked as awkward and unappealing as I did. I didn't know that, as I both ached for and recoiled from her embrace – she hardly touched me now – I was echoing her own adolescent feelings toward Fannie, her maternal sister. I knew only that I hated her in sudden bursts and myself much more consistently: my flat-chested figure, mocked by the scary, cocky boys who in groups called out 'BB!' which referred not to Brigitte Bardot but to a basketball backboard. My too-wide nose taking over my face. The spray of blackheads suddenly joining the hated freckles around and on that nose. My curly hair, which misbehaved in a frizzy mop.

It seemed entirely unfair that she should react so badly to the scorn I felt she deserved in retaliation for her criticisms. My voice would swell with contempt. I would hear a request – 'Janet, please set the table' – and an automatic twist of revolt would begin in the pit of my stomach. I'd pretend not to hear; *maybe* I would do it in my own time. I stayed out late at my friend Cheryl's; her ineffectual mother was also at a loss to handle us. 'So what if I'm late?' I would yell when I got home, flounce up the stairs and slam *my* door, to *my* bedroom.

The boys still revered her but perfection was no longer reflected back to her through my eyes, nor my father's. Sometimes he took my side. 'Couldn't you let her go?' he suggested tentatively when she refused to let me go to a dance at Cheryl's temple (we were not members, of course). 'Aren't you being a little harsh?' That loss – and becoming bored with the League of Women Voters and the smallish stage of Great Neck – may have motivated her to pick up her MA studies again.

When she received her diploma later that day my mother would be only a speck in the distance. She should look perfect, though; she should be allowed perfection, by all of us – my father and me included. Dimly she felt my father had let her down, that he should have said, 'Hey, let's buy you a new outfit.' But that was not my father – he wouldn't himself have needed icing on any cake and would never understand her need for it. She wore a navy short-sleeved sheath dress and navy pumps. The day before she'd gone to the hairdresser's, where the spectral Jeremy with the green mascara had set and teased her hair. She pushed it into place, and drew Cherries in the Snow deep-red lipstick over her lips. It cheered her up.

In the kitchen she filled a mug with Nescafé and lit a Salem, though she rarely smoked now. The weather was shaping up well. A coffee and cigarette, alone, in the quiet of a sleeping house, with the birds singing in the trees, the cat lazing in a pool of sunshine on the back-door step, and bees and butterflies darting in and out of the lilac bushes, felt wonderful. She leafed through the *New York Times* and treated herself to the image of herself on stage, waiting for her name to be called, her black gown swaying in time with the others in front and behind as the line snaked past the university president, who would shake her hand and hand her her diploma.

A few moments later the first of us woke – the little ones in their flimsy summer pyjamas asking to be fed, then Gene and I, lumpy and silent, refusing breakfast. We dressed, and piled into the car for the city. That afternoon we saw her just as she'd imagined. She was the best, I thought, superfluously. She was, indeed, restored to perfection, again Queen Mommy.

Her MA graduation marked the end of early childhood for me, the era when all was encapsulated, predictable, until recently harmonious, in the house in Great Neck. In September, when we three older ones had returned from summer camp, when school had started and Mark had begun his first year, she would start work as a research assistant at the National Bureau of Economic Research three days a week. She wouldn't be the mommy at home who sat at the table with me after school, even though by then I often bypassed the kitchen and went straight to my room. The Manhattan of that afternoon would soon be hers again.

November 1962

When she began her job housekeepers and babysitters filled in at home. She would call out instructions to me as she raced down the front path to my father, waiting in the car: 'Don't forget to put the chicken in the oven. Set the table in time. Back at six thirty.'

I didn't like it, no matter how proud I was of her. The only other mothers who worked did so because they had to: divorcees who lived in rented apartments, or poorer women who needed their income beefed up from part-time jobs. Why did she have to change everything? The routine had been just fine as it was. I liked to know she was behind the door when I walked up our front steps, even if I didn't talk to her. I didn't like the sullen housekeepers who didn't know what to do with me – whether to boss or ignore me. I didn't like having to cook, and often got it wrong, chatting with friends on the phone too long and then putting the meat in much too late, making dinner late, everyone crabby, and my mother furious. I lorded it over Gene, making him do my tasks – 'Set the table', 'Put out the napkins' – which led to arguments.

Probably I'd have been out of sorts anyway, given my adolescence and the already ensuing battles between my mother and me for control over my time, tastes and ambitions. She and I would have argued more and perhaps Gene and I less. 'Don't you have homework?' she'd bark while I chatted on the phone. My bile would rise and I'd resolve not to do my homework, then or at any other time. It didn't help that work and commuting tired her. Her temper was shorter on those days, and her efforts at control on her days at home fuelled my rebelliousness. My adolescence was not easy for either of us.

My mother was an anomaly at work. The other research assistants were graduate students, their jobs part of doctoral research, which meant that they were typically in their mid-twenties. Her work split her into two people: Regina of Great Neck and Regina of Manhattan. Three days a week my father drove her to East 39th Street, a few blocks from his office. He didn't like her using public transport and, unusually for a commuter, he enjoyed driving to work. She read in the car, working her way through the *New York Times Book Review* and the *New Yorker*. As soon as he dropped her off, she shed him and us, the house in Great Neck and her wealthy friends, and became one of the National Bureau girls. They lived on the Upper West Side or in Greenwich Village with too many roommates in horrid apartments: filthy kitchens, dirty floors and old, stained toilets. They seemed oblivious. They had sex with their boyfriends, and, stunningly, were not compelled to marry them. She was not innocent – she read Iris Murdoch and Muriel Spark, watched arthouse films – but she grappled with how, just exactly how, these new friends did it. How did they leave the yearning for respect and predictability at the door to the bedroom? How did they rid themselves of visions of a house and kids when they woke up next to men they didn't love? She didn't condemn them; she was curious.

My mother and I were still able to indulge in our deepest pleasure, the easy talk about people, our interested speculation about their motives. We still discussed books. Instead of our library trips she lent me books she'd read which she thought I'd like. I read Murdoch and Spark, too. And soon I started on Roth and Bellow. She talked to me about the Bureau girls. I met them – some of them came out for Sunday lunch in Great Neck. They were about the same age as the triplets. One, Lynne, was particularly nice to me, treating me as if I were at least sixteen. She took me to see *Who's Afraid of Virginia Woolf?*. Afterwards we went out for dinner and she told me how much the Bureau girls admired my mother: she was so beautiful, so easy to talk to, such a clear and sensible thinker. What a lucky girl I was, in other words, to have that kind of mother. I knew she was right; I *was* lucky. And I yearned to be best friends with her again, all the time, not just now and again as it had become.

But I wasn't the only one who became different with her. My father and she no longer kissed when he returned home on the days she didn't work. At weekends he took naps, while she raced around shopping, taking us to tennis or to the dentist, and meeting her friends. Then, exhausted, she would pick a fight. 'For God's sake,' she'd gripe, sounding tight and harsh, 'I asked you to get that vacuum cleaner fixed two weeks ago.' At first my father was hurt and bemused. Then he grew grumpy. On weeknights she went to bed first and read, while he fell asleep, snoring, in front of the 11:00 p.m. news, the melted remains of his chocolate ice cream in a bowl on the floor in front of him.

After a year at the Bureau my mother left for a better job, more prestigious, more responsibility. She was the only woman working on a transportation study for the Port Authority. When she told me, jubilant, I was discomfited, though my father was proud. For her new job she began to buy smarter, more glamorous clothes: suits, Italian knitted dresses, which she got wholesale in the garment district, where Aunt Mary now worked as a bookkeeper. She changed hairdressers, from Great Neck to 57th Street in Manhattan.

She grew both jauntier and more forgiving, and it seemed as if we were on our way to repair. I was growing up, too. I wanted to go to exhibitions, concerts and ballets with her in Manhattan on Saturdays – no longer did it embarrass me to be seen with my mother, as if that declared to the world I was such a loser I couldn't get a friend to go out with me. She and my father sometimes stayed after work in the city, meeting Max and Horty for shows again. My father used to joke with the guys at the car park who brought him the car late in the evening. The skinny brown young men floored the sedate Chrysler, whipping it round bends, pretending they were racing. They lit up when they saw my father: 'Hey, how you doin', Mr R?' My mother warmed to his easy manner again. Happier in herself, she found she could draw comfort once more from his comfortableness.

December 1963

On our Christmas vacation in 1963, when I was in my penultimate year of high school, I went with ten of my nearest and dearest friends – the Girl Scout Troop, the boys called us – to Stowe, Vermont, to ski for ten days. My mother's work allowed her, too, to enjoy a holiday. Sweet languor set in during school breaks. There'd been a snowstorm during this one; my little brothers sledged and flying-saucered down the steep hill near our house, and then down the tiny but gentler one of our front garden; even Gene, now fourteen, and his big-boy friends were enchanted by the crystal snow. Children once more, they pulled their beige and red American Fliers out of garages and joined the little ones, sliding fast and gloriously on their bellies.

While we children were each in our snowy heavens, the disaster that was to change our lives was unfolding behind the curtains of my parents' bedroom. The slow healing of my adolescent breach with my mother and my father's renewed ease with her were about to take sharp U-turns. Our family was to take a new and painful route.

I deduced how it must have happened from the bits my mother told me later, in a blank voice, throwing in details randomly, like

'Your father found it.' Or 'Your brothers were making a snowman.' Free of children my parents remained that morning, luxuriously, in bed. 'What's this?' my father apparently wondered. He pressed a spot on her left breast. My mother sat up sharply. Passion and pleasure immediately dispersed and a bell sounded in her brain. Breast. Lump. What's that? She pushed his hand away and felt it herself. They did not speak. She imagined my father to be searching for words. What she wanted him to say was 'Oh, that's just a pimple, like I've had myself.' Or something as ordinary as that. When he did speak he was unconvincing, which angered her. He told her it must be something to do with her periods. When he reached for her she pushed him away.

She rose, grabbed her dressing gown and phoned Dr Blum, our family doctor, who rather alarmingly asked to see her immediately. My father went with her. Dr Blum examined her breast. Afterwards he asked them to wait in the reception area while he had a word with an associate, then he beckoned them in. He'd arranged for them to see a specialist in Manhattan, and he advised them to make an early appointment. They went the following day.

My father held my mother's hand as they sat across from the specialist. She suddenly looked a vulnerable child, not a capable, stylish forty-three-year-old. They both hung on the doctor's words as if those words themselves were her fate. He recommended immediate surgery. My father watched him form the words, their meaning taking a few seconds to register. Immediate? My parents felt their reactions slow down as shock spread through them. If it hadn't been for Fannie, perhaps ignorance would have protected them. My father clutched my mother's white, slim hand wearing his platinum wedding band, the one his mother had chosen for them. Her nails were always perfect. Now, unaware, she dug them into his hand.

She would be a patient at Gracie Square Hospital in Manhattan under a specialist, the very best in the field, Dr Blum had assured them. They began thinking fast: whom do we know who might know about breast cancer now? But the specialist recommended the same operation Fannie had had, with the same consequent radiation. Had nothing changed in over a decade? The doctor went to consult his secretary about the earliest possible surgery date, and my parents were left starkly alone with the echo of his words. The doctor returned. 'January 2,' he said. She'd register the afternoon of New Year's Day. In less than a week.

As if life had been reduced to slow motion they rose, shook the doctor's hand, put on their coats, and silently left his office. Out in the white, glittery sunshine of the snowy street my father put his arm round my mother as they went to the car. Inside, my mother folded into herself and sobs shook her body. My father touched her lightly on the shoulder, and then he, too, began to cry.

My parents picked me up at Great Neck station when I returned from skiing, bursting with tales and plans for another trip during the next break. I babbled happily in the car. Suddenly, my mother snapped, 'Don't make any plans.' Her voice almost cracked it was so brittle. I was stunned and hurt. Where did that come from? My father and she exchanged meaningful glances. My father didn't try to soothe ruffled feathers as he usually did. Instead, he was silent. I shut up. Something scary was happening.

Over the kitchen table I heard her, as if through an echo chamber, tell me that while I'd been away my father had felt a lump on her breast. I knew – and my parents reassured me – that it might be benign. But we'd seen Fannie. No one who had could find easy solace in hope. My brothers didn't yet know: my parents were trying to decide how much to tell each one, according to his age. This made me special in a grim way: I could carry the burden of my own special panic, but it would have to be silent, hidden from my brothers. I looked across at her, my eyes filling with tears. We both knew the bell was tolling for her, too. She, like Fannie, would end up in bed, grey and grizzled, moaning in pain; years of hospitals beckoned and we were all, my small brothers, my father and I, entering a tethered state of painful attendance while cancer played out its gruesome dance. The immigrant humour in which we were steeped suggested that this was a grim joke played by fate, something which simply could not be right: two young women from the same, ordinary family marked by the same silent killer?

But dimly – so dimly we weren't conscious of it – at the moment my mother became the next in line and she told me about it, we shared, across that kitchen table, a glimpse of the shadow of my possible fate.

My experience of the family story has always set me apart from my three brothers, not in the amount of love or grief or pain it has engendered but in its reverberations for my mother and myself. I think she became more anxious for me in general, more demanding of me, driven by an unconscious anxiety that I, too, would be struck. Perhaps. I think our relationship became unavoidably distorted by the spectre of the family illness. We had no idea then of breast cancer genes. Even so, her story might have prefigured mine.

5

Regina: Living with the Enemy

Great Neck: New Year's Eve, 1963–4

It was New Year's Eve; my mother was to be operated on in less than forty-eight hours. Before I knew about her surgery I had planned a Sophisticated Evening with Cheryl and my great friend David, who was conveniently Cheryl's boyfriend, plus a date of my own, Jonathan. To my surprised gratitude my mother joined in the spirit of the thing and altered for me a beautiful turquoise silk designer dress she'd worn only twice. I had sneaked into her room earlier and sprayed myself liberally with L'Air du Temps. So one worry was how by that evening I would stop reminding people of a beauty salon: 'Peee yooooo!' my brothers shouted in my pungent wake.

After my mother's bombshell exploded I phoned Cheryl and David. How could I go through with our well-plotted New Year's Eve? How could it be right to party the night before my mother was sliced open? I didn't expect my friends to be helpful. When I called it was in supplication and they answered accordingly: 'Of course you should still come. Your mother would be horrified if you didn't.' So we went out for New Year's Eve – and my parents did, too.

I read the menu at the Swan Club, the swanky steak house we had chosen on the North Shore of Long Island Sound. There wasn't a single thing on it which tempted me. My friends were patient and kind, though still chatting excitedly, whizzing their glances up and down the menu with its curlicued script and heavy, embossed cream pages. None of my friends had weathered divorce, financial instability, or deaths; none had seen a young aunt or uncle die. They watched me faltering over the menu, and out came a rush of what they imagined was encouragement: 'Your mother's young and strong, she'll be fine . . . It'll probably be nothing . . . You'll see, next New Year's Eve you'll be sitting here with us, laughing about how scared you were.' 'But my aunt had this and died,' I replied. After a moment's flustered silence, logic took over. They said, 'But that doesn't mean anything.'

They eventually cajoled me into celebrating, which was, after all, what we were meant to be doing. I started to worry that I had spoiled New Year's Eve for them, but in the end courtesy saved the evening. I managed to divert the conversation and in so doing I fooled myself as well – as if I'd whistled a happy tune, as recommended in the song from *The King and I*. Superficially it worked; I turned my thoughts elsewhere and they went. But my stomach was no dummy. What a waste of my father's good money, I thought, sickened by the rich food (steak in thick Béarnaise sauce, served on heavy white china). Of course, they were right: my aunt's illness had nothing to do with my mother's.

January 1964

We managed, with false cheer, to endure New Year's Day. In the morning my mother cooked us a New Year's breakfast of bacon, eggs and pancakes. Ricky and Mark, aged eleven and six, had been given a gentle form of the truth: 'Mom's going into the hospital for an investigation; they have to remove a growth.' Gene had been told a story intermediate between mine and the little ones, that she might require more surgery, though what for was left unstated. My parents were able to fudge it: seeming not to be scared themselves, I think they made it seem to the boys that it was something cosmetic or gynaecological – not, in any case, serious. Ricky didn't remember Fannie. Mark hadn't been born. They were easy to fool.

My grandparents and Mary were to be told only if and when necessary; that is, only if my mother had cancer. And the fact that the New Jersey relatives weren't involved helped bolster my parents' claim to their sons that there was nothing to fear. If there had been, Mary, the triplets, and certainly our grandparents would have become involved. After my parents left for the city, many of their friends looked in to check on us. That evening a tired Dad let us order pizza – one of the few meals on which we could all agree. Mom's operation was to be 9:00 the next morning.

My father left for the hospital around 8:00, to talk to the doctors, to wait for news, to be there when she came around. Before he went, he came into my room. His comforting scent helped a bit, as did his kiss of solidarity on my cheek: you and I are in this together, it said. He tried to be reassuring: 'She'll be fine!'

I had set the alarm to wake before he left. I had to be up with her, imagining myself in her place. I wanted to be somehow *with* her. I kept looking at the clock, trying to imagine what she was doing or feeling. Around 8:20 I decided she would be being wheeled down. At that point I couldn't swallow and it occurred to me, desperately, how much more scared she would be. I fixed my eyes on the clock; I could not miss 9 a.m. When the minute hand landed on the twelve my heart began pounding, as if set off by an alarm. I made myself concentrate, think about what was happening in the hospital room. My mental screen went blank. I seized a pillow and stuffed my head under it. I sobbed, then I prayed. 'Please, God, please. Please make her be all right. Please make her not have what Aunt Fannie had. I'll be good. I'll never fight with her again. I'll always love her, be kind and helpful. Let her come home well.'

Downstairs I had to be normal. I cleared away my brothers' cereal bowls, snapped at Gene for making a mess with his Frosted Flakes, and left them all sitting in front of the TV, filling the den with their messy games. Friends rang all day, the doorbell, too, as people appeared with bowls of soup or stew, or boxes of cookies and cake. My father phoned mid-afternoon and said, 'She's fine. She's recovering.' But when I asked if they'd found anything, he was evasive: 'They don't know yet. It's too early. Tell the boys she's fine. I'm sure she'll be fine.'

Early that evening he came home ashen. He told the boys

Mommy was still sleeping and missed them; she'd talk to them tomorrow. To me he said they didn't know yet. They had operated but nothing was clear. He hugged me and told me not to worry. In the end, I decided probably she was at least cancer-free: something about the fact that he was home, rather than staying over in Manhattan, comforted me, though there was no logic in it. If she'd had cancer he'd know: her breast would already be gone. In fact, he'd lied. The effort of containing his own grief was too much: he'd handle mine in the morning. I went to bed anxious, puzzled, but hopeful.

The next day he told me the truth: they'd removed the whole of her left breast. I was too shocked to be angry with him for keeping me innocent the previous night, but I cursed the God I'd prayed to – whom I'd never believed in, anyway. I knew it, I thought bitterly: I knew my friends had been wrong to jolly me along, because of Aunt Fannie. I couldn't justify my conviction. It just felt correct. I drove with my father to the hospital. Gene would come another day, after my father had dealt with me, after he figured out what to tell his fourteen-year-old son, and then the others, in good time.

We entered the green-halled hospital. My mother had her own room. The sight of her rooted me to the floor. My father tried to nudge me gently forward. He had misjudged the stunning effect on me. There was my mother, yet not. My mother, who was rarely still, lay asleep, her skin white, with yellow bruises on slim arms which lay lifelessly on the bedclothes. IVs streamed out of her, their aluminium posts hovering over her like guards. I wanted her home, as if being there would cure her and restore normality.

Like most men of his generation, my father had no notion how to look after a house. He was deeply proud that he could cook himself lunch: he cut up a sausage of liverwurst and fried the slices in butter, then arranged them between two slabs of sliced bread. He made tea at the end of meals: a tea bag dipped into a cup of water he'd boiled. And he ostentatiously pushed the carpet sweeper under and round the table after dinner – defining himself as a helpful husband. There was no question but that he needed help while my mother was incapacitated, so he hired a nurse for us.

Poor Hennie. The full force of my anger at my mother's illness and abrupt removal fell on this dim, dumpy interloper, who was a bad cook, to boot. I was horrible, and my brothers took their cue from me: Gene refused to eat her food. I made snide remarks, I couldn't bear to meet her gaze. Her smell, because it came from her, offended: I ostentatiously gave her a wide berth. She was a fraud, a sham mommy in a white uniform. Lumbering, clueless, she fought us, missing the point that we were children whose mother's life was under threat. By then Gene had been told the truth; Ricky and Mark knew she was very ill and would need to recover at home for a long time. While what she had wasn't named, they knew enough to be worried. They saw her friends' concerned faces when they called to check on us, understood my father was stretched thin and haggard with anxiety. But Hennie neither noticed the little ones' pinched looks nor forgave my nastiness for the distress it was. Instead, she harrumphed pointedly and complained to my father. After a week she handed in her notice. It is to my parents' credit that they understood and never blamed me. 'She was an idiot,' my father said. And that became the official story.

I took over, gratefully, what I could. I made hamburgers and spaghetti. My father shopped. Friends invited us to dinner or left home-cooked casseroles and chicken soup on the doorstep. I aimed to be extra-best, super-special, the perfect daughter. A teacher who lived in the neighbourhood awarded me 'O' for outstanding attitude on my report card that quarter. I had not shown 'outstanding' attitude in her class. The mark was for being a model daughter, just as I'd promised God I'd be if my mother came back whole and well.

She came back neither, of course. After a round of radiation to her left armpit, which was still raw and sore, my mother called her friend Leona, an anaesthetist who worked in oncology, for an interpretation of the medical reports from Gracie Square and Long Island Jewish Hospital, where she went for radiation. The medical profession behaved like Brahmins, as if the patients were of the lowest caste. Leona – that special treasure of the time, a woman doctor – talked straight. She assured my mother that her prognosis was good: 'stage' and 'aggressiveness' are the two characteristics of a cancerous tumour that predict prognosis and my mother's was a 'good' stage – stage two (of four) – and a 'good' aggressiveness – mild. We could not determine Fannie's; presumably, though, her first one had also been 'good', her second not.

According to Leona it wasn't known whether, how or in what way my mother's cancer might be related to her sister's. Her mother, her mother's sisters and their daughters had not had breast cancer, though my mother thought of the cousins she never knew, some of whom did not reach adulthood. But it was likely that she and Fannie, both, were victims of grim things dubbed 'sporadic' cancers, cancers that occur spontaneously within a population. 'Sporadic' hardly described what my mother felt. It was with her always. Her radical mastectomy had, like her sister's, left her without muscles near the breast, as well as with lymphoedema.

By this time Mary and my grandparents had been told. Their grief, shock and incomprehension augmented my mother's. They anxiously, dutifully came each week. Her parents' visits were healing, reassurances of their love. Mary brought more: consolation, as she had in childhood. She rocked my mother as she had in Paterson in their rose-patterned bedroom. But my mother's diagnosis recalled Fannie's death, and it also suggested that Mary might be vulnerable. Would she fall, too? Would she be the only daughter left standing, an unsafe support for their frail and elderly parents? Those questions were unvoiced.

For my mother, recovering over the next two months, thoughts of Fannie were constant. During the days in hospital, awaking to the immediate knowledge that her left breast was gone, that she now had a label, 'cancer patient', she'd felt twinned with her dead sister. She ached doubly in her wounds, knowing that Fannie had ached alone. Each time my mother rose and strained to avoid peering at her newly flattened, asymmetrical chest came the realisation that Fannie had done this, too. My mother knew how alone she felt in trying to avoid the empty site. She cried, knowing Fannie had also felt that way. Even more painfully, she realised that she herself had been part of the world of whole women, a world from which Fannie had been excluded. With the realisation came guilt. Now, too late, my mother understood the loneliness of Fannie's struggle.

In the hospital the nurses were kind. But they nursed only her physical wounds. On the fifth day her thoughts turned, unbidden, to clothing. Bras. She had no information about bras. While still foggy from shock and anaesthesia, she had heard a nurse mention 'aftercare', and vaguely recalled leaflets. In the drawer with the Bible she found a slim, slick brochure. Smiling, fully clothed models, arms round children, perfect husbands standing firmly behind them, grinned from the top of a mail-order form, with coyly worded phrases: 'Look your feminine best'. She stashed them angrily behind the Bible. How had Fannie learned about bras?

Before she left hospital a nurse gave her what looked like a floppy white cotton falsie stuffed with cotton wool to put in her bra, to tide her over, the nurse explained, until, following surgical check-ups and radiation, she could be fitted for a 'prosthesis'. Like a person with a false leg. Would she now be a client of those medical supply stores, with their comically depressing – especially at Christmas – window displays of wheelchairs and crutches ('And for the holidays, brighten up her life with this elegant, tinsel-covered oxygen tank')? A soft prosthesis. She sagged compliantly – yeah, fine, just stick one on me – in reply. Inwardly she was repelled. What's it going to feel like? Will it itch? What will it look like? She needed Fannie – the thought of asking at the hospital was distasteful. Only other sufferers could help. She was troubled by whether to tell or not. Especially friends. In shame and confusion she wished for silence, but her friendships were founded on intimacy and revelation. She'd told friends she was going to hospital; obviously they'd asked why. Surprisingly, revelation produced a serendipitous bounty: whispered names of a few older women, still alive, most of them happy to talk.

Days after her return, Lee, a neighbour from across the street, came to visit her. Ten years older, a woman whose country club was her life's pivot, Lee was barely more than a nodding acquaintance. But she took my mother's hand and said, 'I had this, too, you know.' An image of Lee hulking her golf clubs into her car, waving distractedly as my mother struggled with a pushchair down our front path, flitted through my mother's head. Suddenly the image was recast: the woman with the golf clubs was one-breasted, carrying a breast cancer label. It was unbelievable.

'Yeah, about eight years ago,' Lee smiled. 'You know what that means, don't you?'

It meant 'cured' – or at least that the doctors considered you so. She'd made it through the magic 'five-year' mark, which my mother had recently learned was the benchmark signalling 'cure'. The thinking was that if you made it that long without a recurrence you were likely to have beaten the cancer – at least, that was what the statistics indicated. Lee was living, breathing proof that a relatively young woman could survive breast cancer. And so the miraculous Lee became my mother's guide through her new world.

Rhoda's, in the centre of town, was where to buy prostheses, bras and bathing suits. Even calling Rhoda's for an appointment felt a giant step. 'I'd like to make an appointment to be fitted for a prosthesis and mastectomy bra,' she'd rehearsed. But when she got there, 'mastectomy' gave her particular trouble. Eventually she found herself whispering to a young shop assistant that she'd made an appointment, glancing around as if doing something illegal, praying that no one she knew would pop in for a browse through the tennis wear or the lingerie. Please let no one discover she'd become a freak: she'd lost a breast; needed special bras; had the Big C. An elderly woman in a fussy blouse approached with a measuring tape. Stifling the urge to escape, my mother followed her into a dressing room.

The prosthesis was squashy, a disembodied fantasy breast, smooth, pink and shiny, wrinkle-free and pliable. Creepily unskinlike, it was cold and rubbery. She wondered if the woman herself had had a mastectomy, or whether she'd had a special course to fit mastectomy bras.

'Um, does it, itch . . . you know, when it gets, well, really hot? Because it's kind of, well, heavy, you know,' she fumbled. 'I mean, in your experience, um, selling, have you heard anything? I mean, do you know?' My mother looked away, tried not to catch the woman's eye.

The saleswoman, briskly measuring her, dropped her tape and made my mother meet her gaze. 'Well,' she began, 'it's in a pocket in your bra. You slip it in like this,' she took the bra, with its sewn-in pocket, and slipped the model prosthesis in and out, watching to see if my mother understood. 'OK?' My mother nodded. The woman continued, 'It sometimes does get sticky. It's heavier than your own breast would be. You notice that at first, and then you'll find you get used to it. Here's a tip: you dust a little talcum powder on the pocket, and that helps. You'll adapt, I'm sure.' She smiled gently.

'Thank you,' said my mother in a small voice.

Later that day I found her sorting through clothes in her room, high-necked tops to the right on the bed, deep-arm-holed, halter-necked and skimpy ones in the discard pile to the left. 'Here,' she said, holding up a pink knitted sleeveless V-neck. 'You can have this. Go through that pile' – she gestured to the discards – 'and pick what you'd like.'

I hesitated. I felt like a vulture, picking over her clothes – some of them I'd coveted. She watched impassively. I held the pink V-neck against me and looked in the mirror. Behind me I caught her smiling approvingly. Then the smile crumpled and she turned away. 'One of the worst things about this is you don't feel like a woman,' she said to the opposite wall.

I wanted to comfort her. Her completeness as a woman was finished. At sixteen mine was just starting. Guilt over my own body, sadness over hers – what could I say? As I sat on her marital bed, the sexual undertones of what she'd said were discomfiting, and I recoiled from the complex issues she and my father faced. Before awkwardness grew, she hugged me and laughed it away.

April 1964

My mother looked terrific as she prepared to go back to work after her long recuperation and then a final week in Puerto Rico in the sun. But appearances were deceptive.

I hadn't gone – I'd returned to Vermont to ski instead, with my mother's blessing: she knew how much more fun I'd have there than on the beach with them. But, judging by my mother's mood on their return, their trip had not been a satisfying end to post-operative purgatory. My brothers had been fractious, my parents had argued. Each related a slightly different version, but all agreed on one thing: it hadn't been an easy break. My mother said my father was stingy and lazy. He allowed hotel staff to treat them shoddily, accepted, uncomplainingly, nasty rooms with thin walls and inadequate plumbing, and was unperturbed by inedible food and foul weather. She returned exhausted, tired of battling without the support she demanded from him, and at the same time ashamed of her demands.

Because I knew how prickly she could be when I upset her, my sympathies veered towards my father. But I also shared her impatience. His easy tolerance was not enough for the present demands: I wanted him to take charge. The direction the family was moving in was scary. Mom should have come back better, not worse. Like me, like my brothers, my father was now behaving as if she was alive and would remain alive. Instead of treating her as fragile, we tried to behave, as frequently as possible, normally.

I suppose images of Fannie could have dominated us, but there in front of us was my mother, tanned, pretty, lucid, doing Mom-things like cooking and seeing friends. Alive. But our apparent belief in such normality bothered her. My father didn't join her in her struggle against death; he didn't draw out her fear that she might not survive, didn't voice his own fear, so she concluded he was deaf and blind to the possibility. Treating her normally increased her misery.

When my father had turned fifty, about two years earlier, my mother threw him a surprise party. About fifty friends had turned up, a boisterous, affectionate group. Stunned at the yell of 'Surprise!' my father had scooped her up, shrieking with laughter, and cameras flashed. That moment and that surprise party became an ember in my memory of their once abundant affection. The shock of discovering that she had cancer, that she'd taken the first step her sister had towards death was, of course, terrible. But we were beginning to understand that living with it was terrible in other ways, too, ways that crept up on us insidiously, twisting our relationships with her and darkening her mind.

Until Puerto Rico, all of us had behaved with delicacy, the physical evidence of Mom's recuperation – Mom in her sickbed, Mom not at work – spread before us. I did homework dutifully and shortened my phone calls. I sat on her bed to talk each day after school. Skiing, I'd met a boy from New Jersey: we wrote poetic letters every day. I was in love. Did Mom think it was possible to be in love at only sixteen? Yes, she assured me, she did. She seemed delighted by my helpfulness, her harsh side left behind at the hospital. But just before Puerto Rico, as her return to work loomed, her energies surged, jerkily and anxiously. She had to start travelling: first she'd go to the Caribbean for spring vacation, then Europe in the summer. The subtext was obvious: see the world now, before you die. Until then Cape Cod, Vermont, New Hampshire, upstate New York, Montauk and the Hamptons had served her well. Why travel anywhere else when you have it all practically in your own backyard? was my father's philosophy, and she had complied. I think we expected the sun of Puerto Rico would heal her. As if she'd had pneumonia.

Her harsh self – the self I'd come into conflict with in my earlier adolescence – took up residence. I became caught again in the web of trying and too often failing to please her. The impatience with the girl who chewed gum and sounded common returned. I was no longer that girl, but I had new flaws: my lack of organisation, my forgetfulness, my temper, my surliness and, once again, my contrariness in the face of her attempts at control. Since her operation her expectations had acquired a sharper edge: I needed to be on the right track – the successful one – not just for myself but for her. She was impelled to ensure I was on it – and faster now – before she died. I might think I had time to waste. She knew better. If time was short, it had better be good.

No longer was my mother patient with my father's shortcomings. Where once she had laughed affectionately at his silly jokes, now she gazed distractedly, tapping her fingers till he'd finished. Once upon a time in my youth his procrastinations had met with rueful affection, now they provoked harangues and slammed doors. His incompetence with home repairs became a serious fault.

Mom's return to work brought relief for her, and therefore for us. In Manhattan, as she left Great Neck Regina behind to become Professional Regina, she also shed Cancer Regina. The familiar routine begun on her first day back lulled us into thinking we'd turned a corner: there we were, back at pre-operation life. The little ones were already at the table, dutifully eating. There was my mother applying her familiar pink lipstick – which accentuated her tan – at the bathroom mirror. Outside in the car my father was waiting again, drumming his fingers on the steering wheel impatiently. And there I was once again grumpily making my way down the stairs while Sue, with whom I walked to school, was at the front door with her usual look of anxiety: was I going to make us late again? Gene was already downstairs, hiding under his pile of books a pair of too-tight trousers which Mom would have banned and which he would put on at his friend Kit's on the way to school.

My mother ran a comb through her hair, then brushed her teeth again. She adjusted her prosthesis, the only variation in the old routine. She yelled at my back, as I departed, 'Bye. Wish me luck. I'll be back about six thirty. And don't forget to put the pot roast on – I've left instructions in the kitchen.' She waited for my grunted response and then she left the house and slid into the Buick next to my father. I waved as the car pulled out. So normal.

6

Mary's Story/Regina's Story

Aunt Mary was always happy, always laughing, yet I felt sorry for her. Even when I was a small child there was something forlorn about her, something very hard about her life. It had to do with the creepy Murray. It had to do with Norman's waywardness in high school – though later he was calmed first by the army, then by college and accountancy training, and finally by marriage and the birth of two children. It had to do with the fighting between father and son. And it had to do with Nina's nervous eyes when we were small. Even when I was little, I disliked Uncle Murray. I didn't like him touching me, and he had a cackle, a missing tooth, and an unsettling, leering eye. On the plus side he was not often home.

It also had to do with where Aunt Mary lived. Why didn't she have a house? If my mother could have one, why couldn't she? Since she'd been married Aunt Mary had always lived in apartments, the first being the cramped, dark one in the Bronx. When she and her husband separated in the early 1950s, she moved back in with my grandparents in Paterson on East 33rd Street. After that she decided to try living with Murray again, believing he'd given up 'the other woman', and they moved into a garden apartment in East Paterson.

The garden apartment was nicer than the dark one in the Bronx, and it was closer to my grandparents. It was one of a tract of apartment developments which in the early 1950s changed the face of rural routes from northern New Jersey into New York City – Route 4, Route 17, Paramus Boulevard. At their entrances the developments bore signs – 'The Regency' or 'The Ambassador' or 'Four Gates' or

'Rolling Acres' – as if a cursive script and fancy name lent class to the ordinary red and white brick boxes. Aunt Mary's building lay handily across from a Food Fair supermarket in the middle of a little mall with squiggly scripted signs which lit up at night in pink neon: 'Lobell's for Children's Clothes' and 'Two Guys from Harrison: Everything you Need' next to a flashing red 'Liquor' sign. Garden apartments were in single-storey blocks built around a common courtyard. Each dwelling had its own, street level, entrance. 'Garden' must have sprung from some developer's mordant wit: walkways spun outwards from a worn-out central plot of grass towards the apartments, the whole fronted by sparse bushes and a few sad plantings. The entire time they lived there – about ten years – Aunt Mary had intended to plant red, yellow and purple petunias in front of hers, but she never got around to it. Surroundings, like possessions, didn't matter much to her.

Aunt Mary worked as a bookkeeper. With Senator McCarthy discredited she became employable after years of trouble: she had joined the Communist Party in her late teens. The marches in the thirties had been heady; she still felt communism had a simple, moral superiority.

I once stayed overnight with her. I was ambivalent beforehand – it was messy, with unmade beds, dishes in the sink, and old magazines strewn over the tables – but I adored Aunt Mary and, having decided I would, I stayed the night. Magically, she imposed no rules and, unlike my mother, had no discernible routine. I dropped my clothes where they landed, had candy on request, and could go to bed or not. In fact, I fell asleep on the floor in front of the TV, though she must have moved me into bed, for I woke up in one. Most charming of all was breakfast. I'd always found breakfast an ordeal, with tension hanging over the table – would I eat or would I not? My aunt didn't care. More remarkably, she transformed the meal: she offered me spaghetti, cold chicken, an éclair – anything and everything she pulled out of her fridge. With great enthusiasm I reported back to my mother: the way to solve the breakfast problem was to cook me spaghetti or hamburgers. I never stayed at my aunt's again – I suspect because her bohemian style made my mother nervous.

Fair Lawn, New Jersey, June 1964

By spring 1964 Aunt Mary had saved up enough to put a deposit down on a house. She chose Fair Lawn, a developing community of modest detached houses, next to East Paterson. Her new house was a white wood-frame split-level, its door and shutters dark red. It boasted both a front and a back garden; the latter backed on to a wooded section not yet bulldozed for development. It had three upstairs bedrooms, a middle section with a kitchen and dining/living room, and downstairs, on the bottom level, a utility area and large sitting room. She planted flowers in front. Her Chevy sat in a sloping driveway which led to the garage. She was over fifty, but now, like her parents before her, she had her own, private slice of New Jersey.

We drove the familiar route from the George Washington Bridge out towards Paterson, but left the highway at a different point, and entered unfamiliar territory. Neither my father nor my mother had a good sense of direction. 'Entering Fair Lawn', a sign eventually stated encouragingly. We were packed, all six of us, in our not quite blue, not quite green Buick, recently sprayed this curious colour by my father, a trick he had of lengthening the life of the family car so that it looked newer than it was, and the colour was always deeply, embarrassingly eccentric. My father, trying to follow the directions my mother read from a wrinkled scrap of paper – 'There, turn there. That must be the Italian restaurant. There's the gas station. It must be coming up right now' – snatched the offending paper from her hand: 'Give me that!'

We arrived late and frazzled, but Aunt Mary didn't mind. My grandparents, Nina, the triplets, Norman and his family had already begun the celebratory feast. She hugged and kissed us with extra gusto. She had laid on platters of chicken salad, cold meats, delicious rye bread from the bakery near my grandparents' house – 'Paterson Bread' we called it – potato salad and coleslaw. On a separate sideboard, in the dining/living room sat a seven-layer chocolate cake and a Boston cream pie, my father's favourite dessert.

By the time I knew her, Aunt Mary had ceased to dress up, wear lipstick, or go to the hairdresser's: she had neither to remember appointments nor to scrimp and save for something special. If she had been a reflective woman she would have had to admit that this was a consequence of life with Murray – it didn't matter how she looked, he didn't pay attention. In any case, unlike my mother and Aunt Fannie, she had never been vain. She'd come to prefer old, beat-up shoes to prissy, shiny ones. She was relieved not to have to waste time choosing clothes; she wore virtually the same thing each day. Similarly, she wasn't bothered about the state of her apartment, although she was hurt that my mother disapproved.

I found it hard to reconcile my mother's account of her glamorous older sister with the aunt I knew, until I found Aunt Mary's high school yearbook, smelly with mould. Mary stared out from her photo in the sepia-tinged album, stunning despite the dated hairdo, with a sly, expectant smile. The girl in the photo, in her proper velvet and lace dress, was quite evidently flirting with the photographer. Under the photo her hobbies were listed as 'dancing and going to Passaic', the next mill town to Paterson, rough and poor, where boys who had left school early, like Uncle Murray, lived. 'Ambition,' it went on, 'Live, learn, and be lazy.'

She was always late, sometimes by hours. My grandmother never learned: she'd pace, her blood pressure rising, imagining disasters. Eventually Mary would wander in, bubbly and unconcerned, kiss her mother affectionately, assuming that her trilling laugh would dissipate my grandmother's anger. Meanwhile, my grandfather would be playing solitaire while his wife stewed; soon Aunt Mary would drift over to join him, and later my brothers, in a round of cards and my grandmother was left on her own to calm down.

Indeed, keeping turmoil at bay was the unsolved mystery of Aunt Mary's life; problems always took her unawares. She fought constant small battles – with Murray over money, women, gambling or drinking; with the badgering vice-principals in charge of discipline at her children's schools. She found it almost impossible to push her sleeping children out of bed in time, and when they complained of upset stomachs she hadn't the steeliness to cast them, grouchy and heavy-hearted, out of the house. Yet after each squall died down

Aunt Mary returned comfortably to her resting state – a serene belief that life is fine – thus remaining perpetually unprepared for the next, inevitable one.

But now her life was changing. The party celebrated that just as much as it toasted her new house.

The day was a success. That evening, after we had left, the flowers, trees and dead calm of her suburban street underscored the sense that she was entering a peaceful new chapter of life. She even did the dishes immediately, wiped the kitchen surfaces thoroughly, then stood back and viewed her new kitchen with pride. Then she went outside, pulled out the white-painted iron filigree garden chair she had bought at the hardware and gardening store, and sat out on the back patio, with the radio going softly behind her until her eyelids became heavy and it was time to go in to bed. She touched the small bump in her chest, the only shadow over her new life.

It had appeared a few years earlier, even before Regina's. She'd felt it, alone, at home. In a daze she'd automatically phoned Jolson. Medicine offered nothing new, it seemed, since Fannie's illness. So Mary decided to do nothing. She would hope for the best. She wouldn't put herself or her family, certainly not her children, through an ordeal such as Fannie's. If she had cancer, she'd gamble on dying slowly. This was her secret. And that night, in her quiet back garden, she knew she'd been right. The lump had neither disappeared nor enlarged. She was alive. So was Regina.

Mary believed my mother was fine. She believed it because my mother looked fine. After the first week, when my mother was too shocked to contain her fear, and Mary, protecting their parents, had absorbed my mother's distress and comforted her, my mother took care not to let Mary see it again. Mary never heard my mother's doubts about her womanliness, her struggle with the ugliness of her wound, her terror at the idea she would soon enter the hell she'd seen Fannie endure, or her panic at the Big C diagnosis itself. My mother wanted to spare both Mary and her parents – the whole of the Paterson contingent, in fact.

Her strategy worked. It fitted in with Mary's blithe optimism. Apart from that first week, the two sisters did not cry together. Mary visited frequently. Fannie was almost conjured into being through reminiscence: they talked about her more than they had for years. My mother did not describe how Fannie's suffering influenced her own. Perhaps Mary understood. The unwritten rule was: don't mention pain. Nevertheless, the fact that her visits were frequent made it plain that Mary knew. As my mother sprang back to apparent normality, so Mary's belief in her recovery did, too: after all, Regina pushed boundaries back. *Somebody* beats cancer. She might be the one.

Intermittently over the years Mary's small bump had, of course, niggled at her. But in her wrought-iron chair in the sublime, darkened peace at the end of her first party in her new house, she made herself stop thinking about her bump, and pretended it had gone away.

Great Neck, July 1964

In the summer before my senior year of high school I had to think about universities. In contrast to my mother's story, mine involved a struggle to keep her away. We'd been talking about colleges for a long time, deciding which ones to consider. At that point I didn't know how and why she'd ended up at NYU. All I knew was that she'd gone there because it was all her parents would allow. Through discussions with my teachers, friends and parents, my choice was narrowed to small, prestigious women's colleges on the East Coast. By the summer before my senior year I was more eager to apply to colleges so that I could stop serious schoolwork sooner rather than later: as soon as you were accepted you could stop working. I decided, therefore, to apply for early acceptance. That way I'd hear by December, not such a long time ahead. My other major motivation was eagerness to leave home, to escape the troubled atmosphere. It wasn't the lure of Great Ideas or New Vistas that drew me; I only thought of getting out. As I'd done in my early adolescence, I shut myself in my room, or surrounded myself with friends.

One of those friends had an interview at the all-male Amherst College near all-female Smith College. His mother would be driving him up to western Massachusetts. I could go along. Just getting away for a couple of days appealed. I agreed and arranged an interview at Smith. It never crossed my mind that doing so could seem anything but virtuous.

But I was wrong. I knocked on Mom's bedroom door to tell her I'd made arrangements to leave early the following week; I'd be gone overnight, and the admissions office at Smith had arranged an interview. My mother was reading in bed, resting on a day off as she often did. Her face tightened and turned white. She looked as if I'd just slapped her. Then her lip jutted angrily. I was baffled. She gathered herself, stiffening up against her pillows, taking measured breaths. Icily she began, enunciating her words clearly. 'I see. Well. You just go. You, of course, must do whatever you think is right. If you'd prefer to go with Steve and his mother, I'm pleased for you that you are doing so. Surprised, but pleased for you. I have to say I never would have expected this of you, Janet, but, then, perhaps I should have.' I was shocked. How had I disappointed her?

Apparently my crime was to arrange to go on my own and then, to crown it all, to see Smith with another mother. Callously, selfishly, I'd put a different mother in Mom's rightful place. I left, a few long, strained days later, my optimism about Smith College curdled to an amorphous guilt: I hadn't realised what these college interviews meant to her. I'd thought she'd be proud of my initiative.

I tried, when at Smith, to think of ways to mollify her. I bought little trinkets, mementoes of Smith College – a mug, a postcard, a frilly yellow and black garter, all labelled 'Smith College'. I liked Smith, and pictured myself a student striding around its red-brick, ivy-covered buildings. I warmed to the nice blonde lady who encouraged me to apply. But I realised that it would be impossible to go there. Smith had been tainted for ever by my unconscionable error.

When I got home my mother was in bed, still poleaxed, apparently, by my cruelty. If she stayed in bed more than a few hours it often meant something had upset her: a flippant, rude response from me that had escalated to a row; new evidence of my father's lack of initiative; Gene's haphazard homework. I handed over my peace offerings. She chuckled at the fripperies. She rose, casting off the bedsheets, hugged me, and cried. Tears meant the ice was broken and we were on our ritual way to repair. Then her story, pent up all those years, came tumbling out: I should have known that she had dreamed of wonderful times exploring colleges together, of contemplating together my university years. Doing so would heal her wounds. I'd had no idea. I realised that subconsciously I'd known that my grandparents had never understood her, that, though the most successful, she was their least appreciated child. Her parents' relative emotional distance from us, their palpably closer ties to the others, took on another layer of meaning: it wasn't just geographical distance that set us apart.

As she hugged me and wept I caught both the depth of her vulnerability and my power over her. But as soon as she pulled away and restored her composure my mother became supreme again. Her painful past receded into silence. Years later I read a poem she wrote some years after the Smith College episode, which hinted at it.

I Was Good

Such an angel, the neighbours agreed,
I cleaned up after supper,
hung my clothes in compartments,
got an A in Deportment.
Being good was a habit
bred in shyness and fear,
an escape from reproach.

Disapproval,
no dessert or the use
of the car were reserved for the ones who excelled,
for the fragile,
for those who unwatched
would disgrace,
and if watched
would bring honour.

My children are sceptics,
half-amused, unconvinced

I was once certifiably good.
Though they listen politely.

The ritual healing ended with my 'I'm sorry', then hers, then tears, hugs and declarations of love and determination to be better, on both our parts.

Maybe it would have happened if she hadn't had cancer. But I think cancer gave her a manic desire to set her children into secure moulds, to ensure our success, to make what little might remain of her life as full as possible. Because of cancer, the ambition her sisters had spotted and helped to kick-start was packed with a pernicious anxiety. And the cancer exploded that anxious, manic activity, its debris falling all over our family life.

As I've said, I think it fell on me as much as it did because she saw me as herself, with a second chance, and, perhaps, also a shortened life. And because I fought back. I didn't want her to be sick. I was angry at her for being un-whole, vulnerable. Cancer: it was like moral blackmail; I should have been a good person and always borne it in mind. But I couldn't. In fact, I refused to, because when I did think of it I was not just angry but sad and frightened. I hadn't forgotten Fannie.

It was easy to forget, because most of the time my mother behaved as if she were well: she refused to make sickness her main identity. That was clear in her public image, still charming, vibrant, full of plans and energy. But naturally she wanted me to remember her vulnerability. And so I should have been extra-vigilant, extra-understanding, should have seen that her resilience was limited. But against this she wanted to remain a whole mother, who was still the protector not the protected. Instead of being gallantly mature, I became stupidly childish. I was like a jack-in-the-box popping up in her face each time I had a problem, craving sympathy and comfort. But my problems made her gloomy. They showed I'd been stupid, thoughtless. She had no time for such ignorance. That I continued to rely on her strength rather than give her my own may have been my key failing as her daughter at this point. Understandable, but still, in the end, a failure. Cancer, we were discovering, was stronger than we were.

Cancer made my mother impatient – either to die, or to get on with dreams. Life was short, death might come any time now. In all these ways cancer, without actually claiming her body, took hold of her mind and subverted our lives.

In September 1965 I entered Sarah Lawrence College, which at that time was especially selective, a large proportion of its students coming from wealthy and privileged backgrounds; it was the second most expensive college in the country. It was also, however, subversively progressive, with no required courses, no formal grades, and an emphasis on the creative arts – these were the things that had attracted me. My mother was thrilled to deliver me to the graceful mansion where I'd be living, set behind a long lawn and arbour covered in wisteria, where well-known writers and performers taught and which was made famous in novels by Randall Jarell and J. D. Salinger. Meanwhile, words like 'pampered' and 'hothouse' occurred to my father as he glanced around at well-dressed young women pushing into the dormitory.

When my parents left me in my room I felt momentarily empty, even guilty, as if I'd abandoned them. I'd left my father to cope with a wife he seemed bewildered by, and my mother miserable with a man from whom she wanted more and more. I think my father was relieved that, at least while college was in session, he would be released from running up and down the stairs between our slammed bedroom doors, trying to make peace between Mom and me without taking sides. He'd coax me to make the first move, to end the stand-off, to show kindness. Perhaps if he or I had said the word 'cancer', I would have been more ready to make the first move. But perhaps not.

Still, on the day they delivered me to Sarah Lawrence I'd made her proud. We'd felt great that day. So maybe everything would be different now.

A few weeks into the first term, I went home for a weekend. I proudly wore the uniform of Sarah Lawrence: brightly coloured mini-skirt, black tights, knee-high crocodile-print boots, a multi-coloured 'poor-boy sweater' and gold hoop earrings. 'Do you like the way you look in that?' Mom greeted me, and immediately I was a five-year-old, lip quivering, ridiculous in a silly costume I had no right to wear. She appeared ignorant of why I turned surly and retreated to my room for much of the rest of the weekend. My father again ran up and down the stairs, trying to get me to apologise for my rudeness. 'Rude to *her*?' I challenged him. 'Why should *I* say sorry?' He begged, 'Don't expect her to say sorry. Just say it to her, Janet, don't be silly about it.'

Apologies made – we had only two days together so the whole process had to be speeded up – she reverted to being my best friend: there was a whole host of new people to dissect with her. We swapped books; when I called home we'd discuss them. Sarah Lawrence was just the other side of Manhattan from Great Neck. We'd meet in the city some Saturdays. We'd go to films or to the Museum of Modern Art; sometimes after class I'd ride the train into Grand Central and my parents would treat me to a meal and the theatre. And then, again as if out of nowhere, I'd say something I meant – at least I think I did – in innocence and she'd go mute, fold into herself, and, then, like a coiled snake, suddenly strike and hiss at me.

So university didn't save us. It just made the scenes less frequent.

November 1965

My mother had always written. She kept a diary now and again, and she and my father wrote poetry for birthdays, Valentine's Day and their anniversary. My father's poems were always clever, funny ditties, hers serious, 'real' poems. Around six months after her operation she began to write – mostly poetry – in bursts on yellow legal pads stashed in the next drawer down from her sewing kit. Phyllis and Irvin had moved away, and Evelyn had been in Mexico since the early 1950s, so her relationship with them had been mainly through letters. Besides, they were literary themselves; Irvin was a playwright and professor of English. They were the ones she sent her poetry to, implicitly asking: was she any good, and should she keep at it? They encouraged her – I have seen scraps of their replies, Irvin's writing illegible and big, the women's neater and prettier like my mother's. Her friend Muriel, a playwright, and she began to read their work to each other. Her surge of writing stemmed from her 'now or never' mindset. My mother honoured writers; if she was going to be one she had to try *then*. She submitted a poem for publication just around the time I left for Sarah Lawrence. In October it was accepted, in November published in the *New York Herald Tribune*.

Prayer

To hope is unstylish. I stifle
with firmness intractable wishes
which surface in stealth and,
I know, with derision not wholly concealed.
I will hold to my compact:
Not hope and not tender the question.
I petition for vagueness;
Leave endings open.
Permit me the privilege
of unconscious postponement.

I kept it pasted on the wall over my bed at college.

December 1966

Six months after her operation Mom began the standard medical check-up regime: consultation every three months. Then she went only every six months. She didn't report on her appointments – we children did not even know when they were. This was a failed strategy of protection: if she made no allusions to cancer we wouldn't suffer. In two years, if she'd had no recurrence, she would watch her specialist write 'CURED!' across her chart. Her check-ups would be reduced then to once a year for five further years. After that . . . Well, she would never let herself think that far. She had found little written about breast cancer for the layman. She knew no other woman under fifty who had lost a breast and who was still alive. And Lee was over fifty. Mom had heard of only one other woman her age in Great Neck who'd had breast cancer, the mother of a child Gene knew. She'd died.

My father accompanied her when she went for a check-up. Usually they argued on the way, anxiety short-fusing their tempers. Mom wanted my father to draw her out, to enquire tenderly how she was. She wanted him to declare his desire for her – perhaps that would have offset the ugliness of her chest – but he never did. She now undressed in the bathroom or behind closet doors. In bed she never took off her nightgown, even on the infrequent occasions when they made love. He never touched her chest. Nor did she touch herself. It had come between them, this loss of her breast. But they did not talk about it.

Years later she told me what cancer had done to their intimacy. It was uncomfortable – I felt disloyal to my father, listening – but I think she wanted me to understand her anger at him. At the time, though, she kept it all inside. To her parents she appeared fine: she was the lucky one, she'd caught it early, she'd pleased her doctors. To their daughter my grandparents appeared reassured. Perhaps behind their own doors they spoke in their own language about their fears.

My parents did not talk directly or sensibly then about my mother's conviction that she was alive only on sufferance of some God or fate. Instead, it erupted in arguments, vengeful, sad declarations made: 'I won't be around long. Why must it be like this while I am?' Once, exploding, she cried, 'What will you do when I'm gone?' and my father was shocked and devastated. She was astonished. 'What planet is he on?' He seemed unable to fathom her conviction that she was living out her sister's fate. Maybe he did understand, but did not know what to do about it.

Their relationship had faltered during the period, a few years before her cancer, when my mother was growing bored in Great Neck, when I'd begun to withdraw from our mutual admiration society, and my father got caught up in our subsequent discord. But, like my mother's and my relationship, before her cancer it had begun to spiral slowly upwards, particularly when, in her second job, the buzz of work and life in Manhattan restored her verve and energy.

But cancer zapped their upward spiral. They were trapped in the same house, same bed, behind the same door.

By December 1966 she had been free of cancer, though obviously not of its horror, for almost three years. Her battle might have gone haywire at times, but at least it had passion. What she did while she was still alive – and what we did – mattered terribly. Moreover, she had never passively accepted what was on offer medically; she'd always made sure she was an informed consumer of any medical expertise available, with Leona a particular ally. Most days she worked, entertained, played tennis, often exhausting herself. But such vibrant moments alternated inescapably with recurring fury and fear. She never had a rest.

That month she had a check-up. As her oncologist examined her she stared at a fixed point on the wall, letting her thoughts drift far from the clinical examining table to a set of to-dos she would attack as soon as she left the doctor's rooms. It helped her forget she was exposing her disgusting wound and deformed left side to his gaze. Finished, he motioned for her to get dressed. She went back into his consulting room, where my father was, and, holding hands, they waited for his verdict. Each of them had prepared a set of questions, something they always did before a consultation. The doctor sat opposite them across a wide walnut desk with the obligatory black-and-white framed photos of his family and tastefully arranged flowers on either side of the leather-bound blotting pad.

He grinned. 'Fine,' he said. My mother thought how nice it must be for an oncologist to be able to say 'Fine' to a patient.

They could go home now, to another Christmas break, this time with a special gift, optimism. She would coast on 'Fine' for a while. Looking back over her three years with cancer, my mother conceded that each good check-up bought more belief in survival. She found herself putting her arm through my father's as they walked towards the car, and as she did, like magic he kissed her. Sometimes life was very simple, but she forgot that. For the moment she remembered, and she looked forward with tentative optimism to 1967.

7
The Curse

Manhattan, January 1967

Aunt Mary and my mother were meeting for lunch at a luncheonette in the garment district. Mary had been working for a few years at a leather-coat and -jacket manufacturers, a perk for us: she could 'get it for us wholesale'. She herself had had a lovely brown full-length suede coat made.

Mary got there first, and sat down at a Formica table in the back, flipping through the *New York Post* to Murray Kempton's and Max Lerner's columns. Down the long aisle of swivel seats against a soda-fountain counter on one side and tables on the other in the front section of the restaurant, she caught sight of her pretty younger sister, her fair skin pink from the damp cold outside, removing her scarf and gloves, peeling off her black wool coat, and waving to her as she made her way to the back tables. This was a day Aunt Mary had tried to put off. She glanced at the menu: pastrami, corned beef, chopped liver, Hebrew National salami – ugh! Everything turned her off, though she supposed she would have to order something. She hadn't a speck of appetite. Still, she had to hold herself together. She was not at all sure how her sister would react to what she was about to hear.

My mother kissed Mary hello and settled into the seat opposite. She looked wonderful. No one would have guessed that she had undergone disfiguring surgery. She was smart in a black turtle-neck sweater, with a charcoal-grey Chanel-style cardigan piped in black, and a grey pleated skirt. They made small talk for a bit – how were the kids, the triplets, friends, jobs?

My mother was no fool: she knew Mary had summoned her for a reason. She felt the unsettled undercurrent. She spoke first: 'What is it, Mary? Something's not right.' She peered intently, with kind concern, into Mary's eyes, while Mary's gaze wandered.

Well, here it is, thought Mary. The turmoil again. Please, she hoped, shaking, please make me not cry here; make Regina be calm. She took a deep breath. 'I've been trying not to believe that there's been anything wrong,' she started.

My mother nodded.

Mary started again. 'For the past few years there's been something. Now, please, promise me you won't yell. Promise me you won't say anything about what I did or didn't do. We do things differently, OK?' She waited, watching my mother grow tense, her sympathetic expression replaced by wariness. Eventually, my mother nodded reluctantly.

'I'm not like you, right? A few years ago I felt something.' My mother was dumbstruck. She knew what was coming next; her body slumped. 'I felt,' Mary resumed, 'yes, I felt a thing, a bump. I didn't want to think about it. I really could not face telling the kids or Ma, getting them worried again. And then Ma and Pop were deciding to move to Florida; I didn't want them to feel they couldn't go, or be worried about me. And, in fact, it didn't change for a very long time.'

My mother, horrified, ploughed in, breaking her promise: 'You just let it go? I just – I don't understand. I cannot fathom it: why weren't you extra-scared, super-vigilant because of me, and Fannie. How could you not be?'

Firm for once, Mary stopped her. 'You promised, Regina. If you go on like this, I'm leaving. I'm sorry. I'll leave if you don't stop.'

My mother, who had tears rolling down her cheeks, was silent. Mary tried again, but at first the words wouldn't come. 'It didn't go away,' she declared at last. My mother half choked on a sob, then grabbed Mary's hand. They sat in silence. Mary tried not to cry. She swallowed hard, gulped her iced water. 'I didn't want to upset you, most of all. And the timing's not bad now, as it turned out: Ma and Pop moving to Florida, to sunshine. They can go in blessed ignorance, maybe never having to know. You never can tell, can you, 'cause who knows? Maybe I'll be fine. Oh, I've told the triplets this week, I talked to them. I wanted to know something about Fannie, so I had to tell them. And of course I've had to tell you. Oh, how I wish I hadn't had to. Oh God, how I wish it had gone away.'

They both stared down at the table. The waitress made her way towards them, but when she saw them hunched over as if bowed by some terrible weight, holding hands, and staring at the table, she turned abruptly away.

After a while my mother asked huskily, 'What doctor have you seen?'

Mary braced herself. 'Jolson's partner, the one who's taken over from him, at first,' she said, and watched her sister sigh in exasperation. 'He's referred me out. But it's bad, Regina. It was suppurating by the time I got to him. That's why I went. It even scared me.' My mother winced as she absorbed this shocking detail, floored by the inescapable conclusion that Mary was now probably beyond help. Finally, in a measured voice which concealed her anger, she asked, 'And so? So what have they told you? What's next?'

'I go into the hospital next week. Then they'll see what's next. Listen, Regina, what will be will be. I'll take whatever comes. I'm not scared.'

They held hands for a while. What could be said next? Mary broke the silence. 'I know what this means for you. I do. Sweetie, I do know.' And then she did cry, though soundlessly, and my mother, who had been crying more or less all along, tried looking away, to control herself. Other diners had noticed by now. Oh, screw it, Aunt Mary thought, this is a matter of life and death and I'll cry if I want to – and that song by that girl from New Jersey, though she could not recall her name, got stuck in her head. Lesley. Lesley Gore – Gore, like the people who used to live across the street. And that restored her, and she stopped.

Westchester County, NY, March 1968

Aunt Mary lay on her sickbed in the Catholic nursing home that Medicaid was paying for. My mother and father had helped find it. It was in a pleasant setting, a large former estate in rolling, well-tended acres, in a village called Valhalla, no less. The nuns were kind. The fact that it was Catholic was an oddity, something of a joke – here lies Mary Kaufmann, née Miriam Schmidt – but a Jewish one would have been almost as inappropriate, given her Marxist atheism. There weren't many nursing homes that took in the dying, and she was grateful that she was not causing problems for anyone, was not asking her children, nieces or sister to tend to her – she would have taken an overdose rather than let that happen. Murray was out of the equation, though she caught him weeping when he came up to visit. Crap, she felt. Crap. Let him suffer. She was glad her relatives had no sympathy for him. When she died he'd play the victim, but they'd give him nothing; which was exactly what he deserved.

She'd been a fool, she knew. They'd all taken what they needed from her. All of them. Everyone close to her. She'd never had a chance. Just when she thought she might have one – the house, the car, the job, the peace, the clean kitchen, the space – this happened. She would have kicked Murray out in the end. If she'd lived.

She'd said all this to her sister, who was shocked. No one was prepared for the change in Mary. They thought she'd always be sweet Mary, kind Mary, complacent Mary. She'd soon be making her exit. Was this the way she should go? With black hairs sticking out of her chin? With a man's voice? With acned, scaly skin? This was how Fannie got, only she, Mary, was worse. Uglier, more mannish. Because of the operation, she noted bitterly. Great advances those doctors had made in the past twenty years. Now they removed your pituitary gland, which made you properly ugly.

Properly robbed of any dignified femininity you might have clung to before you kissed this world goodbye.

Yes, she'd changed. She was nothing like the Mary she had been for fifty-five years. It was as if she'd been unaware that behind her sweetness lay enormous reserves of cynicism and resentment. The androgens, the hormone treatments, literally went to her head. She remembered Fannie's huge mood swings and bitter outbursts. And now, years later, there she was: Mary in Fannie's place. Was this some grim joke of the Catholic nuns' God? Here she was, if there was ever proof her atheism was the only feasible position. There had been Fannie too. Please, she pleaded, to whatever – not God, that's for sure – please, spare her little sister from becoming such ugly proof, as well.

Shortly after seeing Dr Jolson's partner Mary had gone into Barnert Hospital for her first operation, a radical mastectomy, still the standard treatment. It was pretty demoralising, but that was that. She'd had extensive radiation, because her disease was diagnosed at a much more advanced stage than either of her sisters. For a while she'd felt better, had even gone back to work. But there was a recurrence. Her ovaries were removed, just as Fannie's had been.

But the cancer spread. Another procedure for advanced cancer had been added since Fannie's day: Mary's pituitary gland was removed, to prevent the production of oestrogen. Even then she'd been the Mary of old, grateful they were taking care of her, bearing her fate with as good humour as possible, quietly, trying not to impose. Questions went unasked – she believed the doctors would give her whatever treatment they thought best, of course! – unlike my mother who chased them and questioned them. But for advanced cancer there was only this; research in the field of breast cancer was meagre. And finally she became angry.

In the end Mary became a Fannie, though in a prettier setting and with a flock of Catholic nuns who were kinder nurses than Helen had been. Her family visited at weekends, and sat, as they had with Fannie, at her bedside. She had clear, sharp moments when her anger pierced the fuzziness of her drugged stupor. She came to slowly and vaguely wondered where she was. She was in Valhalla. How funny. She'd never liked Wagner.

April 1968

In February 1967 my parents had driven my grandparents from the apartment they'd moved to in Paterson a few years earlier to Pennsylvania Station in Newark. They put them on the train for their first winter out of Paterson since they'd arrived in America. They looked small and old, frightened of the long journey – the longest each had taken since the ship almost sixty years earlier – but they wanted nothing to do with airplanes. In Florida there was a housing complex owned by the Workmen's Circle, a socialist organisation to which they and their friends belonged; they'd rented an apartment there. Most of their surviving Paterson friends were there already. They planned to return home briefly in the summer, when it got too hot in Florida, then go back south in the autumn. In fact, they came back to Paterson later and left for Florida earlier than they'd thought, which hurt my mother. Paterson was quiet and boring. The Paterson grandchildren were all working, Norman and one of the triplets already married. Irving had died. Mary was commuting to New York from Fair Lawn. And my mother was in Great Neck, of course, which was both far away and boring for my grandparents.

By then my grandmother had a heart condition and was so deaf she appeared more remote than ever – Yiddish as well as English eluded her now. They were aware of Mary's diagnosis, but were led to believe her prognosis was much better than it was. They left for Florida with cautious optimism. In April, as Mary lay in Valhalla, my grandmother died suddenly, her heart simply stopping one day. Her body was carried back North by train, and we met my grandfather at Newark's Pennsylvania Station. The funeral was in Paterson, and after my grandfather had sat shiva, he came to stay with my mother, where they tried to comfort each other, my mother thrilled to have him with her. She hoped he might move in but after a week he got restless – no friends, no Yiddish-speakers, no easy access to his Yiddish newspaper. He moved in with two of the triplets back in Paterson, and never returned to Florida.

May 1968

My college roommate phoned me at my boyfriend's on West 94th Street: 'Call your parents, it's urgent.' I knew even as I dialled that Aunt Mary had died. I'm ashamed to admit that at that moment my prime concern, though of course I grieved at the loss of my sweet, big-hearted aunt, was my mother. She was only a little over six months away from her 'free and clear', 'cured' consultation with her oncologist. Boy, did that seem unfair!

We buried Mary next to Fannie and next to my grandmother in New Jersey.

After the burial, as she was about to open the car door, my mother heard a shrill babbling of women behind her. She glanced briefly over her shoulder. The women, intent on their gossip, didn't notice her. 'Damaged goods, those Smith girls, you know. Must be. Poor Murray, marrying into that.' The ugly words were spoken through hard-edged fuschia lips; the woman's eyes and brows were pencilled with thick, black lines, her hair sculpted into a stiff, lacquered black beehive.

My mother had to catch her breath. Her grip on the door handle tightened. These women were Murray's relatives. The rest of us – except me – innocently waited to get into the car behind Mom. I, too, had heard and I, too, was shocked, then seized with an urge to smash their brittle faces into shards with the sharp little heels of my shoes. Mom laid her cool hand on mine. No one spoke as we slid into the car. I watched my mother, her back rigid, shifting in the seat in front of me as she tried to compose herself. Then, turning to me, she whispered, 'They're ignorant. They're hateful. Don't think about it.'

But those women had spotted something, in spite of their

ignorance, something that the whole of the surviving Smith family, their partners and offspring also suspected. As did the medical establishment. In 1968, breast cancer was still a relative backwater of medicine. Men still comprised most of the medical task force fighting this women's disease. Women whispered about it – and, as in my mother's case, those whispers sometimes unearthed a few fellow sufferers. There were no demands from the sufferers that their doctors give them better treatments than the horrid ones Fannie and Mary had endured, or help them over their self-doubts, self-loathing and uncertainty. No one had yet publicly asked, 'Is there any way we can make sense of this experience?' Or 'Are my responses normal?' Or 'Am I getting the best treatment possible, and how do I find out if I am?' Or, the question the ugly, lacquered woman had inadvertently posed: 'Is this just a fluke, or is there a reason why three sisters have been struck?' In 1968, breast cancer was still only a private concern.

I was angry as I watched Mary's decline, remembered Fannie's and worried about my mother. But it was a diffuse anger, like anger at fate or God. I didn't know I could be angry at a whole profession. That was to take a few years – till the questions women with breast cancer were asking individually were framed collectively. Till others who had watched women die found common cause, and all of us connected the lack of progress in fighting a women's disease with the fact that it was men who held the key to treating and understanding it.

By the time we buried Mary in 1968, a number of well-educated, articulate women had been diagnosed, and, unlike Mary but like my mother, they'd been asking their doctors those questions. In the next decade the wonderings of women like these joined and became a groundswell of discontent.

8

Regina's Story: Attempted Life

My fears were justified. As my mother approached the five-year mark her emotional state worsened. As it moved into sight her sister died. How could she feel free? Instead of her spirits rising as the months turned into cancer-free years, the legacy of Mary's death turned her grief into depression. It was a tenacious and intense one, and it darkened her life for most of the following two years. In the space of two short months three profound losses – her mother's death, with its unhealed, unspoken hurt; Mary's death, with its ghost of grief over Fannie; and her father's decision to return to Paterson instead of living with her – had pummelled her energy, her optimism, her belief in life till they practically died inside her.

The depression increased her anxiety about me. It focused on two things: I was aimless, and I drifted into relationships with unsuitable boys, boys who seemed even more aimless than I was. I agreed. Their very aimlessness frustrated me. But at least I looked better put together than they and, besides, my struggles with them provided a focus for my life. College did not. College demanded that I think seriously about what I wanted to be. I'd inherited none of my father's insouciance. I looked at his life and saw disappointment. Not from his family, even if at that point his marriage was a source of pain, but in his work, which had been nothing but a tedious slog. 'Work stinks,' he'd report to Max on their twice-weekly catch-up phone calls. I never heard otherwise. As for my mother, she was discontented about her work, too: she should have gone back to work earlier; she'd wasted time; illness had retarded her progress and so had motherhood; she should have been running whatever show she was in, and she wasn't. That meant work was something which a) would almost surely disappoint, and b) was a choice loaded with dynamite. What do you want to be? What's worth doing? What if you choose wrongly?

And I was exhausted. I'd picked Sarah Lawrence College because I thought I'd be free to study what I wanted. But that begged the question that stalled me: what did I want to be? Underneath my lethargy, my democratic nihilism – nothing was better than anything else – was what later, when I trained as a psychologist, I realised was depression, paralleling my mother's. Getting up was difficult: often I didn't manage it. I almost stopped eating one summer – not to lose weight, but because I'd lost my appetite and nothing restored it, not hot-fudge sundaes, cookies, strawberries, nor steak. The thought of food made me ill. I became self-conscious and insecure. Underlying my depression was the omnipresent theme of my mother. Would she survive? Would I please her before she died? Indeed, it wasn't till towards the end of my penultimate year at Sarah Lawrence, when perhaps I was galvanised by the thought of my studies soon being finished, that I could claim I felt engaged with studying more rather than less of the time.

The summer following my aunt's and grandmother's deaths I worked in one of Lyndon Johnson's Great Society 'enrichment' school programmes for kids in the Bronx and lived on the Upper West Side, just as my mother's National Bureau friends had done. My best friend at college, also called Janet – whose mother, coincidentally, had been a friend of my mother in Paterson – worked in Manhattan.

One humid summer evening, at an outside table at the Riviera on lower 7th Avenue in Greenwich Village, I waited for her. When she arrived, the normally cool Janet was flustered.

'Something weird just happened,' she declared. I knew at once she had proof – of betrayal by Marc, my boyfriend – again.

But no, it wasn't Marc. It was my mother. They'd met at a bus stop in midtown. By the time they'd reached my mother's stop at 34th Street she'd done with pleasantries and was grilling a squirming Janet about my love life. My mother was tense and anxious. What Janet reported was completely uncharacteristic. My mother was punctilious to a fault about appearances – do not show the world your problems – and just as respectful of boundaries – while welcoming to my friends, she'd never invite friendship. These were sacred rules and she had broken them. She was out of control.

We ordered our drinks. Why was my mother so obsessed? Yes, I was directionless, and yes, Marc wasn't making me happy at all. But I wasn't hooked on heroin as some of her friends' kids were. I wasn't pregnant – one of my childhood friends was already a mother. However tenuously, I'd stayed in university, not dropped out to 'find myself' as many others had.

I was due home that weekend and I went, judging it would be worse to stay away. My father, antennae honed by her gloom, heard me walking up the front path and ran out to head me off, scooping up my overnight bag and whisking me into the car. 'She's in bad shape. It's best you don't stay tonight.' He drove me to my friend Patti's, where I remained that weekend.

A day later my father reported she was better. Why? He didn't know. It had just passed.

To the world she displayed a brave face: she rarely spoke about her cancer or directly about her worries. But this very reticence – her unreported check-ups, for instance – blinded me to the fact that she was trying to protect her children from her illness. I came to hate the silence: 'Don't take your bitterness at cancer out on me in this roundabout way.' I could only complain to Janet or Roni, my friend whose mother had died swifly of cancer, to my roommates or to Marc.

Now that I'm a mother I recognise that she was fighting to remain mother, not victim, trying not to let her own terror frighten her daughter.

In January 1969 my mother's doctor stamped 'Cured' on her medical chart. We drank a toast at dinner, in a whoosh of elation, but for my mother the word on the chart wasn't sufficient to dispel the fear of Mary's and Fannie's legacy. Since Mary's burial she had taken to heart the fuschia-lipped curse: 'Damaged goods, those Smith girls.'

I was at that point finishing Sarah Lawrence College and off to do my last six months in Florence on a college programme. It was also a failed attempt to end my bumpy relationship with Marc. Gene was in his second year at university and Rick in his next to last year of high school; Mark would soon enter secondary school. No small children left. Perhaps this loss, coupled with what it signalled about my parents' relationship – more time for each other, time to rattle around angrily together in a roomier, emptier house – helped depress her. 'Cured' was a false final mark: she'd flunked optimism.

And so, when her spirits did not lift, despite our celebrations, my sympathy shrivelled further. I wanted to leave for Italy with a clear conscience. She was, indeed, generously thrilled, sending me off on the liner *Rafaello* with a party at the pier. But I knew this was a brief weekend off from misery. My father slowly withdrew emotionally from her. Pushing sixty by then, he had symptoms of his own and was treated for heart arhythmia and ankylosing spondylitis. He unabashedly complained of back pains, retired from tennis games when his breath was short, took to his bed. He did the very things my mother refused to do – he bowed to pain, allowed his body's frailty to prevail. A new battle was joined, an emotional tug of war. On his side, 'Now I'm the patient. Attend to me,' on hers, resistance. She compromised by catering to him grudgingly. And she exhausted herself further, trying to set him an example: frenetic writing, hectic socialising, regular tennis games, frequent travel.

In summer 1969 my parents spent a month in Europe, partly to visit me in Italy. Rick and Gene were left to care for the house, and understandably it was a hub of teenage activity in Great Neck, a social centre free of parental control for a whole idyllic month. When my parents returned the house was in disarray and this was Mom's breaking point. Perhaps we should have seen it coming, but the decline had been gradual, a simple upping of the foul moods and heightened anxiety we'd seen in the five previous years. Her sleep became disordered and running the house a crushing burden. I learned from her years later that thoughts of death and how to cheat it, on the one hand, and welcome it, on the other, increased. Only at work and with friends did she pull herself together. At home she collapsed from the effort: she either snapped or withdrew. On my father's insistence she saw a psychiatrist, who told her that she was fine – it was her family who needed changing. But she never stopped writing. More poems were published in increasingly prestigious journals. It became a lifeline: writing soothed her and brought her out of the cloud of misery to a more balanced place.

I graduated from Sarah Lawrence College. Marc persuaded me to come back from Italy, where I'd thought about staying, to New York, where I thought perhaps I'd try to become a journalist, possibly on the *New York Times* with my own byline, the youngest person ever to . . . That might make her happy.

Instead, I was hired as a secretary on a local children's television show, even though at the interview I told the producer I couldn't type. On my first day at work his hiring priorities became clear. My team, in addition to the producer/director and the show's child-hating host – a big gold star, with his photo in the middle, hung without irony on his door – comprised three women, all under twenty-five, in very brief mini-skirts, with glossy hair and thick black eyeliner. I'd seen the cult film, *A Thousand Clowns*, which I can attest was a sharp satire on kids' television, and in which the Jason Robards character commits spiritual suicide every day by working there. I'd joined him.

A few months later the production crew quite reasonably demanded my dismissal. 'What does "Stqgel3ft chulr3n enter" mean?' the stage manager yelled, throwing down the working script I'd typed in what might as well have been Ukranian. I sent my sparse résumé ('Member, National Honour Society; Copy-editor, High School Yearbook') to every magazine I could find, and was offered a job interview at *Dance Magazine*, which I'd read as a teenager. Throughout my childhood and into college I'd studied modern dance. For years I'd leaped and stretched in a dark studio under a hairdresser's in Great Neck, a pupil of the celebrated modern 'interpretive' choreographer, Anna Sokolow. When I was six, Max's wife Horty, an ex-dancer, convinced my mother to send me to Anna rather than ballet ('Anna Sokolow in Great Neck! Don't miss the chance'). So, to my distress, I got no glittery tutus or pink toe shoes; dance meant black leotards, black footless tights, black soft shoes, and black, doomy choreography, but I did love the lessons. I'd also danced at Sarah Lawrence, till depression made me doubt my performance and I'd stopped, just as I'd stopped studying.

In a twist of fate the entire editorial staff of *Dance*, including the editor, had walked out the day my letter arrived. Within a month, with a skeleton staff, I was practically running the magazine – though I did not realise how exploitative that was. It was just a bit more high-pressured than copy-editing my high-school yearbook, and I was being paid for it. I was twenty-two and managing editor of *Dance*. For a while I felt sure I was Mommy's golden girl. We'd be back to the closeness of my childhood *and* her misery would begin to dissipate.

One evening, as I worked late to a deadline, my father rang. 'Have you heard from Mom?' he asked. It seemed she had stormed out that morning, gone to work, and had neither returned nor left word. My two youngest brothers, still at home, were frightened, my father agitated. I slumped in my chair in the familiar gloom. My father was close to panic, so it fell to me to think straight. I guessed she might have run to the solace of Phyllis in Boston, but he'd already phoned and she wasn't there. I forced myself to believe what I said: 'She's fine, Dad. She'll turn up. She's punishing us. Don't let her win.'

I was right. She'd gone to a film. The incident passed silently into the frayed fabric of family life.

The punishment she dealt, even though it was driven by unseen forces, turned me cynical. Probably we hit the nadir of our relationship a bit later. It was a shameful scene, for both of us. Perhaps it shocked us into improvement, because soon afterwards my mother began, slowly, to seem more robust.

* * *

It was July 1971. My father had belatedly acknowledged, if not shared, my mother's desire to travel. No more cheap, last-minute, end-of-the-range deals – he'd learned at last. On this occasion they came back, tanned and well-fed, from St John, Virgin Islands. Their return from vacations remained stubbornly problematic: inevitably there was a blow-up, between my parents, the children, or both. My mother seemed to believe the outbursts were out of her control, perhaps a punishment for taking a break from suffering. But as soon as she set foot in the door – as if her very footstep sparked the row – she began sniffing for evidence of something awry. By 1971 we'd come to expect it – in fact, I think we came to believe that it was part of the Smith girls' 'curse'.

I'd come back to Great Neck from my tiny, hot apartment in New York, to look after the house while they were gone. The boys were all away. I heard my parents turn the key in the lock, and went downstairs to greet them. We embraced happily. They looked great. Mom came into the living room and sank on to the sofa, while my father deposited their bags in their room. 'St John was stupendous,' she exclaimed happily. My father reappeared. 'Oh yeah,' he said. 'The best so far. Each cottage with its own pool. The food terrific. Really great. Just beautiful.'

They seemed, this time, to have licked the problem, and were still relaxed, still happy. I began to relax myself. After a bit my mother got up and went into her room. She was gone a while, and I heard her checking out the rest of the downstairs. I heard her turning off lights. Uh-oh, a mistake: I'd left them burning. But no: her footsteps remained light.

She reappeared in the living room. 'What about dinner?' she asked. 'Have you had any?' As a matter of fact I hadn't. I'd thought we'd have a pizza, or Chinese food – something we could have delivered, as I didn't know whether or not they'd have eaten. But she didn't want pizza or Chinese food. 'There must be something in the refrigerator,' she said, on her way into the kitchen. I followed her. I'd cleaned it the day before, made it sparkle. I waited for her squeal of pleasure. But she was opening the fridge when I reached her, and her shoulders were drooping. Uh-oh, I thought, what's that smell? I hadn't really noticed it before.

She whipped round. 'I mean,' she began in a slow burn which quickly turned to operatic fury, 'could you not tell that fish does not last a whole week? How could you not smell that? How could you have been so stupid to leave a fish – a fish! – for a week in my refrigerator? I don't know. I think finally you're OK, you've grown up, you're responsible, and then I find out you're just absolutely not. I mean, really! The stench!' She was almost enjoying the frenzy, as if she were stoking it. It made things conveniently black and white: in an instant I became the wholly unreliable failure of a daughter, and she ignored the fact that I'd tidied the house, kept it secure for a week, scoured and dusted the kitchen. Part of me knew she meant it with only a part of herself, that part taken over by misery far beyond this particular failure, but it still hurt. In her slitted eyes there was mockery.

In the silence punctuating my mother's rant, I faced a choice. I could capitulate: be contrite, repentant, protect her. This was what she ostensibly wanted, though I think the tiny part of her left observing was uncertain that this would do either of us any good. Or I could retaliate. I could – and should – have been measured, mature, but I let myself go. I was sick of her irrationality, sick of failing tests, sick of her being sick when she didn't have to be any more. So I turned primitive. Disgust and pent-up hatred spewed out; I screamed abuse and scorn, and my mother stood stunned, fridge door ajar, then all at once collapsed on to the floor. She uttered words which shocked us both – I'm sure she did not know she was going to say them. 'Kill me, then. Go ahead.'

I was so shaken that at first I almost wanted to laugh: 'What do you mean, kill you? I left fish in the fridge, for Chrissake!' I did not know then that her thoughts had so often turned to death, which was why the words had risen to her lips. I stood rigid over her, each of us stilled, while we caught our breath. Then I bent and scooped her up. She slumped into my arms. Momentarily it was confusing. Then the mood shifted. She held me tenderly. I was her baby, back in her arms again. 'I'm sorry, I'll never do it again,' we chanted.

Something was mended that night, for us as well as for her. It helped her shake off the depression. Perhaps she could even be well.

She had much more verve: her poems were successful, and her work, as a programme director and researcher for volunteer organisations in the city, was rewarding. She took on a further commitment: running what her neighbours referred to as her 'old people's home'. My father's Uncle Harry, childless and now widowed, took over my bedroom. We'd always thought he was gentle and unprepossessing, overshadowed by his buoyant wife, Aunt Rose. When he moved in, we realised he was vain and demanding.

Soon afterwards my grandfather was diagnosed with colon cancer. My mother's solution to the Uncle Harry problem was to bring her father to Great Neck, get him superior medical care, and force the two old men into a friendship. It flopped. My grandfather criticised Great Neck and disliked being stuck with Harry. 'He has nutting to say,' he confided to me. 'All day he can go vitout saying a ting.' He missed his Workmen's Circle friends in Paterson, and resisted and ignored Mom's efforts to care for him. After a few months he left. He chose his friends, again, over her, entering a Workmen's Circle nursing home back in New Jersey to be with them, and dying a fairly contented death, in the bosom of his Old Country friends and memories, about eighteen months later, in September 1973. Shortly after my grandfather left, Uncle Harry, who had been moved to a terminal care facility as a series of strokes incapacitated him, also died.

Although the 'old people's home' did not last long, it regenerated Mom, deflecting her concerns from her own death to these old men's lives. She read with renewed enthusiasm, booked theatre and concert tickets, had dinner parties, played more tennis. Gene became engaged to Cathy and they married, just out of college, in January 1972. I, like most of my friends, finally took my built-up pain into therapy. It worked: I found out what I wanted to do. I applied for PhD programmes in psychology and decided to go to the University of Chicago. (I was unaware, until I got my acceptance letter, that it was this university that my mother had planned to attend.) I needed to leave New York if I were ever going to end my on-again, off-again, going-nowhere relationship with Marc. We were rolling again as a family. Perhaps my mother could trust in life, after all.

Then, in February 1972, eight years after her mastectomy, as she entered menopause she began to bleed heavily, and not just during her periods. Scary clots appeared. She phoned the gynaecologist her anaesthesiologist friend Leona recommended.

'We should take a further look around,' said the gynaecologist, matter-of-factly, after he'd already had a look around on his examining table. The death knell began to sound in the distance again. My mother entered Long Island Jewish Hospital. Leona would be her attending anaesthesiologist.

My mother behaved as if she believed her new symptoms were unconnected to her cancer, and we, relieved, followed her lead: her sisters' disease hadn't progressed to either their wombs or ovaries, after all. She and her friends had bared their menopausal symptoms to each other, and hers were not in themselves alarming. Most of these women had been told to 'whip them out' if their womb or ovaries caused problems. Having a hysterectomy wasn't unusual; it was her history that made her different. When she entered hospital she mostly believed she was preventing illness rather than discovering it.

Each step my mother took in her battle against disease revealed both her luck and her sisters' misfortune. After her hyster-ovariectomy the doctors said she'd in effect had preventatively what her sisters had had as a necessary treatment. They'd found 'irregularities in cells', 'hyperplasia'. By removing the whole uterus they'd removed the path the 'irregular cell growth' would eventually have taken if they'd become cancerous. Her doctor reported a 'precancerous' condition.

'Your mother's fine,' my father phoned to report from the hospital, post-surgery. 'She doesn't have cancer.' He said, 'It's *pre*-cancerous,' enunciating very clearly, lingering over the 'pre'. When she came home we celebrated again, going out to dinner and a film as soon as she felt well enough.

Remarkably, without her ovaries my mother did not shrink or become brittle and wizened. Her skin remained almost unlined and she simply rinsed her greying hair with a caramel colour, which suited her pinky complexion, now sallowing through age. The lighter rinse, according to her friends, increased her resemblance to Joan Fontaine. Her hot flushes were not disabling – at least she never complained – and no ugly widow's hump formed on her back. Still, over the next few months I watched warily for signs of the return of depression. It did not come.

One day during my first year at the University of Chicago, on a break from scrolling through computer print-outs of a study on alienation, I wandered into the departmental office to check my tiny pigeonhole. The receptionist was chomping on an apple and reading a book called *Going Crazy*, by Otto Friedrich. It rang a distant bell. On a visit home five or six years before, I had taken a message from him for my mother. I'd wondered who he was. 'Oh, he's a journalist friend of Muriel's – he wants to interview me about work,' my mother had answered airily; then she changed the subject. He hadn't crossed my mind again till that moment in the department office, when suddenly the penny dropped.

Politely, squelching the impulse to snatch the book, I asked the girl if I could have a look at it. She must have seen the anxiety in my eyes, because she handed it over without comment. I tried to seem cool as I left, trembling, for my office. I locked the door. I scanned the chapter headings and chose the one entitled something like 'Facing Death', which was full of interviews with people driven crazy by an overhanging threat of death. There she was, as I knew she'd be, thinly disguised with a similar name and one child fewer than in reality: '"Jean," an attractive middle-aged professional, with three children, a husband and a house in the suburbs.' It went on to describe me – and my unsuitable boyfriends – my brothers, her feelings about my father, and, most of all, her private struggle with the fear of dying as her sisters had. She was reported as saying something like 'I used to flirt with death. I would stay away from home, thinking about how I could just not return . . . One morning

I was walking down the street on which I worked, and I stepped in front of a truck. The young driver pulled to a screeching halt and started cursing me furiously. I saw the terror and anger in his eyes, and realised how ruthless I had been to try to ensnare him in my continuing drama.'

I put the book down. If only I could have relived the angry scenes from the years since January 1964, I would have choked back my curses and replaced them with kindness. Behind that closed door, clutching that book as if it were something illicit, I at last understood both how she had felt and also her struggle to protect us, like a mother bear. But her struggle had been twisted out of recognition, too private, too underground. Still, I should have spotted it. Still I'm ashamed.

9

Regina's Story: Fighting Back

Chicago, March 1975

My mother had never taken a plane by herself. She was fifty-five and had travelled worldwide, but always with her children, her husband, or both. She was quite nervous as she boarded a United flight from New York to Chicago. But she was glad to be doing it, and on the plane she ordered herself a Bloody Mary, pushed her seat all the way back, sampled her roasted cashews, and took out her novel. She allowed herself a shiver of anticipation. It was as if she herself was flying; she felt curiously light: where were her children, the extra bags? Where had my father gone?

The big shadow, her belief she would die, had gradually dispersed. Perhaps her operation in 1972 had brought on a feeling of triumph. At all events, she permitted herself a sublime indulgence: pleasure in us. In consequence, like magic we'd come to return sweetness to her. It had been a relief for all of us to live by simple equations again: give, then receive; love, be loved back. We'd witnessed this elegant physics of emotion over Christmas when we'd all arrived, from Chicago (me), Buffalo (Gene and Cathy), and western Massachusetts (Rick), to join our parents and Mark (then in his last year of high school), in Great Neck. We'd played games, joked; friends home for their holidays stopped by. Mom and Dad were relaxed and she chuckled again at his silly punning. There were no arguments. We followed her lead – as she relaxed, so did we. She believed that, though she walked around with one breast, the other's absence did not signal death. Lee across the street had walked around single-breasted for almost twenty years. It looked as if she was the sister who'd win.

She was coming to visit me in Chicago, celebrating her prestigious and demanding new job. She'd been appointed the first executive director of the newly established New York City Commission on the Status of Women. She was the salaried director, though there was also a volunteer board, appointed by Mayor Abe Beame, who oversaw the Commission's work. Her mandate, amorphous and wide, was to create policies and programmes to strengthen the voice and position of women in the city, her first task to define the concept 'status of women in the city'. Such a job needed a life force behind it and my mother had once again found it in herself. We were proud: not so very long after leaving full-time motherhood and voluntary work, and only a decade after her mastectomy, she had a place, with secretary, nameplate on door, suite of offices, at City Hall.

At O'Hare airport she spotted me in the distance, jogging briskly into view, typically late, and hoping she'd overlook it. As soon as I greeted her I could see she approved. She checked off the list: I wasn't as thin as I'd been on my last visit home, not pinched with anxiety since I'd broken up with the last boyfriend she'd met, who'd scared her with his unsuitability; my hair was longer, straighter and pulled off my face, a style she'd always preferred; I was wearing muted colours and tailored clothes. I'd passed – but by now these maternal check-lists had receded to the environs of a normal generation gap. My style and my life were different from hers; there would always be some mismatch between my reality and her imagined ideal of it. But now in seconds the gap was bridged with affection. I flung my arms around her and she hugged me to her with joy. 'You're here!' I cried jubilantly.

My mother had never been to Chicago before. There was poignancy in her seeing it now through my eyes. I took her bag. 'What are you doing? I'm not an old woman,' she protested, but I didn't let go. Though she winced as she tried to grab it back, I barely noticed – the missing muscles had been so long integrated into her life that none of us registered it any more. She played tennis at least weekly, with tenacity and skill if not grace. That was something she would never regain; lymphodoema limited fluid arm movement. But my mother did not look in any way 'old' and, instead of feeling she was near the end of life, she felt the opposite: a new one had started. Having her there in Chicago felt as if I was introducing my best friend to my transplanted life; she had recaptured the enthusiastic responsiveness of the mom I'd had as a small child.

We drove in my roommate's dented blue Toyota the long way down to Hyde Park where the university was located. Hyde Park was a small, attractive and surprisingly green community studded with turn-of-the-century townhouses, imposing early twentieth-century and inter-war mansions, apartment blocks and six-flats, and a smattering of 1960s apartments and townhouses built round common green spaces. It was bounded on the east by the stunning sweep of Lake Michigan, which resembles a sea more than a lake, with its ribbon border of parks and beaches, and by filthy, dilapidated ghettos on its west, north and south. Tales of crime abounded then in Hyde Park, surrounded as it was by destitution. But we lived by making adjustments. No young woman went out alone at night; the university had installed security buses to take its students around after dark; the streets were eerily silent once twilight fell. 'Operation Whistlestop' signs were dotted around the streets, and we carried whistles on our keyrings in case we were attacked or saw anything amiss. If so, the community went on red alert: a whistle blown fired a cacophony of following whistles, which, like smoke signals, stirred the police till their car sirens took over from the whistles and, finally, police cars whined to the scene.

My mother was pleasantly surprised at the attractiveness of my airy, modernised 1930s apartment, shared with my friend Amy and our badly trained mongrel, Mamie, who was deeply irritating to all except Amy and me. She admired our polished light wood floors covered with rugs our families had donated, and noted Amy's mother's discarded once-smart office furniture in the living room. She did not fail to point out that we'd unwittingly left a 'Playboy' label stuck on a reclaimed filing cabinet – Amy's mother's law firm represented them. She commented delightedly on its unusual tidiness.

Her relationships with all of us children – in particular, Gene, married and in law school, and me, now doing a PhD, both of us now objectively respectable – were blossoming again. No longer did our phone conversations hover on the edge of disaster, both of us straining for decency and achieving transparent irritation. Now my mother could let things go. So could I.

We took an afternoon amble through the main quadrangles of the university. I showed her Beecher Hall where I had an office, which I knew would thrill her – my own desk, a nameplate on the door in these hallowed, if dirty, halls. In the March sun Chicago's winter snow had turned to grey slush and mud, and the floors of the buildings were stamped with drying bits of it. Outside, down the shared back steps of Kelly, Beecher and Green Halls, we entered a slushy green side quadrangle, and, as if sent by the gods, there was Saul Bellow, whose office was in the building perpendicular to mine. On our way out of the quad a white-haired, Einstein-lookalike, Professor Emeritus Sam Beck, the scholar of the Rorschach test, rounded the corner. I introduced my mother. '*Beauty in the daughter comes from beauty in the mother*,' he quoted to us in Latin, then translated. My mother had entered Academic Heaven and I was blessed for taking her there. She had got to the University of Chicago.

We had two days of meeting my friends, including a dinner party I gave at which both people and food were a success. She had fun. They liked her. People kept pulling me aside and telling me how nice, how interesting – and how beautiful – my mother was. We had walks along The Point, the park bordering Lake Michigan where I, like most University of Chicago people, spent a lot of time enjoying the lake. We had lunch in Reynolds Club, the august ivy-clad building with university restaurants and clubs, with my faculty adviser; and, finally, a dinner with Phil, a lawyer on Chicago's North Side, whom I'd been seeing for a few months. He was good-looking, prosperous and gregarious. We dined in a smart French restaurant on Halstead Avenue: linen napkins, filter coffee, cooking from Provence, and French-accented young waitresses in shiny black uniforms, dainty white aprons and black tights. She and Phil hit it off. 'She's so beautiful,' he, too, said. 'She's sure not like most mothers.' She'd dazzled him; she was her best social self, the gracious Great Neck lady of my past.

But at O'Hare we flirted with a moment of discord. I knew I

was taking a risk as I brought up the one disturbing moment of her stay.

'Mom,' I tentatively began. She stiffened and looked cautious. 'You know that dinner we had with Phil on Saturday?'

'Yes?' she replied, matching my hesitation with her own. Had she been too pushy? Had she taken over the conversation? Years earlier she'd confessed to me that she'd felt a twinge when boys showed up at the door asking for me. Were they really for me? Did that mean she herself was over the hill?

'Well, you know you're supposed to be in charge of women's issues for New York, the one who's supposed to be strengthening women in the eyes of the public, and all that?' I ventured somewhat more bravely, my voice stronger.

My mother was on her guard. This was her treasured job I could be driving horses through. 'Mmmm' was her deeply noncommital assent.

'Well, how come you let Phil pay for your meal, then?' I quickly finished. I hadn't believed my eyes when my sophisticated mother, now earning decently herself, sat back unresponsively – nothing to do with her – when the waitress brought the bill. Phil always paid for me – that was understood, as I was a poor graduate student and he a highly paid lawyer. But he wasn't my mother's date. When my parents and I went out, they always paid for me, for the same reason. I couldn't understand why she didn't offer to pay. I had apologised to him when we talked the next day, and he brushed it off. 'Oh, I wouldn't have let her pay,' he cried. But that wasn't the point.

The old defensiveness, the old 'What right have you to attack me when I'm already worn down?', the old, protective 'Don't even think of judging – you've got no idea' rose up; I could see it in her face. Then, quite deliberately, she let it go. She looked at me, the feminist. My friends and I, and other young women like us, were the standard-bearers to whom my mother and her friends would soon be passing the flame, and she thought, as I did, yes, we can have a dialogue. We can talk. I can learn. She can learn. In her new job she would have to. This was a step.

'That's interesting,' she remarked. She turned it over in her mind;

I could see her thinking about it, though she didn't immediately reply. Why did she automatically let him pay? He was the age of a son. She would pay for Gene or Rick or Mark, as she would pay for me. Had it been a knee-jerk traditionally female response? Was it cheapness – he earned a lot, let him pick up the tab? It was a fair point and she conceded it.

She nodded. 'I think it was to do with a lot of things,' she said, and enumerated the ones she'd just thought of. 'But I'll think about it.' We'd managed it.

New York, June 1975

I was home again; Memorial Day weekend had just passed, and I'd phoned, in great upset, to say I'd be bringing all my books and papers – and Mamie, the dog – home to study for my qualifying PhD exams in September. I wanted to stay, this summer, in New York. I'd just ended with the seemingly terrific, but actually mad, Phil. I needed my mom and dad. So here I was, thin and distressed. Within a few days, being home restored me. The weather agreed: we had meals out in the sunshine. My brothers and I went to the nearby beaches.

It looked, it seemed fine. No one but my parents knew it was not.

When my mother discovered a lump, larger than her first one, in her remaining breast, she felt overwhelmingly, intensely bitter. 'Again. Here you are again. You have marked me, you have marked my family.' As bitterness faded terror rose, this time deeper and more violent. For this time she felt cancer would – must – win.

But this time her defences were ready. She had projects to complete. She had poems to publish. She had to finish her task at the Commission. She had to see me through graduate school, Gene through law school. And she had to know that Rick and Mark would be all right: what each would become, how each would support himself. She had to know that we would find partners. And she and my father had by then made plans to spend years rediscovering their pleasure in each other; take more trips: to Israel, to the Bahamas, to Europe again, to the Greek islands. They'd barely started. She would fight, really fight, this time, for more time, even if she now knew she would indeed die from breast cancer.

She was treated at the new cancer centre at nearby North Shore Hospital, where Mark had been born. It had become a teaching hospital, an outpost of Cornell University Medical Center. Some regional hospitals were now hooking up with major teaching centres, to keep pace with the increased sophistication of their patients and compete in the medical marketplace. Cancer was a hot issue and lung cancer was the big bogeyman – it had even got John Wayne. The cigarette companies were on the defensive. Partly as a result, there were cancer centres springing up around New York. By the 1970s medicine in the US had become a consumer good. Women shopped around to find doctors who would give coherent explanations of what breast cancer was, what it did to their bodies, what was likely to happen next. Paternalistic doctors lost business to men – for there were still few women doctors, even though this was a women's disease – who talked to patients sensibly, sensitively and with dignity.

Breast cancer treatment was changing quickly. A small army of women, aided by a surging women's movement, were making their private medical questions public. What about access to quick diagnosis? What about teaching women how to look for signs of breast cancer to monitor themselves? What did medical research have up its sleeve to help those diagnosed? Doctors had had to cope with breast cancer in their own families. Their mothers, now living longer rather than dying of other things earlier, even their older sisters, in smaller but nevertheless increasing numbers, were being diagnosed with it. People talked about breast cancer.

The growth in the number of women affected, of women who were alerted, and of women who could articulate questions about breast cancer, was a sign of the times. Women were claiming attention and power, and the medical profession was having to take note. My mother's job title, Director of the Commission on the Status of Women, said it all. Women had arrived, and we all – New York City, the press, doctors treating them – had to listen.

Mammography was beginning to be offered as a diagnostic tool. There was resistance to it. X-rays had a bad name: wouldn't they produce more cancer than they were trying to cure? It was not offered routinely, not even to women past menopause, who, statistically, were more likely to develop breast cancer. But some doctors did use it, if only for high-risk women like my mother.

My mother's second bout with cancer was therefore an entirely different experience. Part of the reason for this was sobering. Her second cancer was a different and more aggressive one.

It was in an entirely new primary site in the second breast, not a spread from her first one. She had indeed been cured of her first cancer. We didn't know then that this was a likely indication that her cancer had a genetic basis. With a mutation in each breast tissue cell, which is what the genetic predisposition to breast cancer is, there is an increased chance that any breast cell will become cancerous. So the appearance in the same woman of more than one primary site of breast cancer does suggest the likelihood that all cells in her breast are predisposed to develop cancer.

However, we knew nothing about breast cancer genetics. All we knew was that this cancer was more aggressive than the first. Her lymph nodes were removed; it had spread to them. She again had radiation treatment, post-mastectomy. Her doctors, in the face of competition from other cancer centres, were developing research protocols.

And there were, they told her, developments. Scientists were working on whole-system attacks, against possible spread, or metastasis, especially against little micrometastases, or undetectable spreading cancer cells, which through the bloodstream could take off to distant sites that would not show up in the crude diagnostic procedures of the time. These included surgical sampling – taking out lymph nodes and checking to see if there was evidence of spread there – and mammography in any breast tissue still remaining (none in my mother's case). The possible metastases needed a scattergun war against them, which is what chemotherapy is. So in the pipeline there was chemotherapy, and medicine ingested or injected which would act like bullets spread through the blood system. But these treatments also attacked healthy cells. There were unpleasant side effects. It was unclear when and if my mother would be a candidate for chemotherapy as it became available. She would be monitored closely and treated as aggressively as possible, she was assured. They were watching her and trying to come up with methods to help.

She took two months off work to recover. It was the summer, anyway, and work was less demanding. When she did return she worked shorter days and shortened weeks. It was not the same. In her absence the chief volunteer at the Commission, the bossy wife of a philanthropist, used to getting her own way, but with no experience of managing people apart from her domestic staff, had assumed command. A tussle over territory developed. My mother had neither the taste nor the stamina for fighting on this additional front. Inevitably, after her new diagnosis, her focus had sharpened. She had no time for petty arguments. The woman was in the way, so my mother stepped aside. She resigned.

1975–76

In late 1975 my mother was exhausted and stunned. We were, too – it wasn't fair; we didn't want to let go of her well-ness; how could it have been so short-lived? Perhaps our disbelief, and hers, was part of why she reacted differently this time. She bypassed self-pity, so we tried to as well. This time it was much more matter-of-fact.

In the weeks following her surgery I had met Stephen, an Englishman finishing a post-doctoral fellowship in the US. Both parents – even my mother! – approved of this sweet man with his powerful intellect and quirky, unsentimental wit. In September, I returned to Chicago to take my PhD qualifying exams. I passed, came home for Thanksgiving, flew to England for Christmas, and then returned to Chicago. I talked to my mother at least weekly, from wherever I was. She sounded hopeful, increasingly energetic. Though devastated by this new cancer, we were all – my father included – curiously more optimistic this time. After our phone conversations, or after a visit home, I was newly persuaded this would be different, even if this cancer had been more advanced.

Between treatments she wrote more and more. She gave dinner parties. The triplets, Nina and other relatives came over on Sundays. Because it seemed she would be going on and on, I made plans to take my PhD research to Oxford, where Stephen had just started a job. Mark left for university in Maine, Rick took a job in Manhattan, Gene finished law school in upstate New York. We all carried on.

We fixed our sights on the short-term, eyes peeled for news of medical developments. Her doctors were responsive – they were happy to answer questions, and took my phone calls. That autumn my mother was offered another job within the City, as director of mental health education in the Department of Health. She was no longer top dog; her boss was the head of mental health, another woman, a psychiatrist, and we were all a little disappointed that the glory had passed from Mom to another. But maybe that was better, we sighed – part-time work would be easier on her. She and my father had planned to move into Manhattan when the last of us finished school, as the notable Great Neck school system would have done its job and the house become redundant for a couple essentially tuned to Manhattan. But now they realised how comforting the friends, the tennis, the pools, the garden, the greenery could be. My mother symbolically made a stand for her future: she began to plant flowers and vegetables.

She lunched regularly with her Great Neck friends – they jokingly titled themselves 'Les Belles Amies'. They were too elegantly dressed, too old, and the food too delicately prepared, to qualify as a consciousness-raising group, a phenomenon which I was then studying in Chicago, but in effect this group was a support group. I was touched to see the grass-roots sisterhood in action. My mother and her friends might not identify with my groups – politics was not the ostensible reason for their lunches, though politics were often discussed – but the confidences exchanged, the bolstering of spirits through discovering commonalities, the sympathy they readily gave, matched what I'd discovered in the younger women's groups I was examining. The sisterhood my mother had thrived on in her early years was powerful in a different way now.

1976–79

I moved to England the summer following her surgery: perversely, I landed on English soil on the day of the American Bicentennial. I went home for Christmas, and my mother and I planned my wedding the coming June. She looked fine. She'd had no recurrence and only went for frequent check-ups. We checked out possible venues – one being the Swan Club of that fateful New Year's Eve of 1963. It was fun planning together. Perhaps it made up for my not making her more central in my university applications. We chose the English-Speaking Union on Manhattan's Upper East Side.

She looked glorious at my wedding, on a hot sticky day in late June 1977. After a honeymoon on Cape Cod, Stephen and I moved into a summer rental in New Jersey, where he was doing collaborative research at Bell Laboratories while I worked on my PhD. Gene, now an assistant district attorney in Brooklyn, and Cathy had moved back to New York. Rick had started law school there; Mark, an undergraduate, was home for the summer break. My mother's life focused again on her children. In September Stephen and I would be moving to Oxford till September 1978. We children faced different rules this time about whether and how to talk about Mom's condition. We could talk about the facts of it, but never give it a name: 'cancer' was still the forbidden word. Enquiring about treatments or check-ups in the most matter-of-fact way was permitted. Asking about feelings was not. Similarly, we could talk about short-term plans but she wouldn't commit to a date for visiting us in Oxford.

In September we went back to Oxford, where I had a research job in the Department of Psychiatry and Stephen had a year to go on his job in the Experimental Psychology Department. He'd got an assistant professorship at the University of Chicago, which would make it possible for me to finish my research. Chicago wasn't New

York, but, especially then, it was much easier to fly home to Mom, to talk to her doctors, to be in the communication loop, from Chicago or New York than it was from Oxford.

As it happened the months we were in Oxford were dramatic. I still feel sad I was so far away. I've put things together from letters, phone conversations and the visits scattered over that year from Gene and Cathy, Mom, and my parents together.

During 1978 my father became distinctly unwell, which disturbed my mother's attempts to contain her own anxiety. His complaints multiplied. He stooped. His breath grew shorter. His complexion became continually florid, as if he were an advanced alcoholic; ironically, he couldn't touch alcohol because he was allergic to it – for the past ten years he'd been turning purple at a sip of red wine. I heard from everyone – except my mother – that she was becoming impatient with him. After all, she was the one with no breasts, she was the one with the death sentence, and she tried not to complain. His complaining upset her fragile coping. It made her think about illness when the trick, she'd discovered, was precisely to avoid that.

The desolation that had once engulfed her hovered in the air. Sinking into it was out of the question, so she tried to stay remote. She became uncharacteristically detached, not asking the penetrating questions we expected from her, taking no part in dissections of friends and acquaintances and passionate arguments about books and films. Her attempt to disengage was only partly successful. She still picked fights with my father, and still felt ashamed of her intolerance of his complaints, she still grew impatient with my brothers. She wondered how some of her friends could let their children drift, experiment with drugs and endure marital break-downs. How did they manage to seem so unrattled? Now and again, despite herself, she plunged into the old, familiar despair.

Unbeknown to me, on December 6, 1978, my mother had to return to North Shore Hospital. The following day was my birthday. She'd never missed speaking to me on my birthday, and was worried about doing so. Couldn't she be operated on a different day so she could phone me on the seventh? She couldn't. She decided not to tell me anything until she had the full story. No point in making me miserable, impotent on the other side of the ocean.

On December 7 a lump on her back was removed.

On December 8 she phoned me. I had gone to sleep the night before very unhappy – no call from home. But as soon as I heard my mother's voice I forgave her. She sounded terrible and her story of bad flu was entirely convincing.

This time I'd been the one left in ignorance. I found out when a long, handwritten letter dropped on the doormat (for months afterwards I was scared of the sound of the post dropping on the mat). Reading it, I felt ashamed for having been upset she hadn't phoned. I felt betrayed for being left out of the loop. I was angry that I'd been lied to, and the distance made me feel impotent and guilty. But my dominant feeling was fear. After all, how many reprieves were likely? This lump was a sign of the cancer's spread. Reading on, I tried to accept my mother's explanation of why she hadn't told me. She'd wanted to wait till she'd got the full story from her doctors. Maybe there'd be hope. Indeed, she was being given chemotherapy. There would be side effects: some hair loss, nausea, exhaustion. They would monitor her closely, take blood samples to make sure her white-cell counts were all right. If they were not, she would need to be taken off the regime, at least temporarily. She'd had her first treatment and was tolerating it well enough. She thought she'd be in good enough shape to visit me in late March. No need, she stressed, for me to fly home. I alternated between desolation and this new, medically based hope.

But she could not work regularly any more. She would resign, and become a consultant. That way she could work later, when she felt well enough, and have more time for poetry and travelling. She was upbeat.

She had chemotherapy for the next few months. It gave her diarrhoea and made her vomit. Eating was a struggle: even the taste of water was repulsive. But she was determined that it would work. She would take anything – you will not beat me, she vowed as she crawled back to her bed from what might have been the millionth visit to the toilet. She hated taking to her bed, as if it were admitting defeat, that she was weak and an invalid, literally in-*valid*.

She didn't want anyone to see her bedridden, so she slept during the day after treatments, hiding out. She got up to cook supper, and would dress, put on lipstick, comb her hair, which thinned but did not completely fall out. When my father, who was still working, came home she pretended she'd also been working. On her weeks off the medication she felt well, no charade necessary. She wrote poetry and embarked on a report for the Department of Mental Health. She even played tennis at Great Neck's new indoor courts.

She came to Oxford at the end of March 1978, on two of her weeks off chemotherapy. No one had warned me what she looked like: perhaps they'd got used to it. I met her at Heathrow. I did not recognise her. A short, squat woman with a fat face and severe, shorn, steely grey hair came through the barriers – only when she smiled and met my eyes did I realise I was looking at my own mother. And in that split second she registered my non-recognition. I had confirmed to her, despite myself – oh, how I wished that I could have stifled my look of horror – that she looked awful.

She was taking steroids to counteract the chemotherapy, and they had puffed her up and inflated her face; her eyes had gone slitty within plump cheeks; her upper arms had filled with water. She resembled the chilling photos of the old, fat Simone Signoret in her terminal decline. Her friends had tried to reassure her. 'This new look is chic,' they said cheerfully, trying to convince themselves as well. My greeting scuppered their attempts. She had been given sleeping pills but refused to take them, associating them with defeat. She was bone tired. She was hunched as Fannie had been, hollowed out completely.

It was difficult being with her in Oxford. Her detachment was unsettling. She was not terribly interested in meeting my friends. Her refusal to talk about cancer reasserted itself, so I was unable to apologise properly for my initial blunder and soothe her wounded feelings. Our conversations felt unnatural and distant. She and Stephen were stiff and formal with each other. He didn't know how to read her remoteness, the new coldness that surrounded her.

He didn't know what to say, and is anyway reserved, even shy, so they ended up saying little to each other. She grew impatient with his silence. I felt caught between them. Their relationship never quite recovered: Stephen felt hurt as I used to, felt that she'd unfairly judged him, thought him uncaring. He'd been frightened of getting things wrong with her, of disappointing her, of incurring her prickliness – that had already happened once the previous summer in Great Neck, and he'd seen her behaviour with me. So his reserve grew. She, I think, was ashamed. But still, she wished and expected he'd make a first move. Instead he backed off. Distance between them increased.

At the end of her stay the two of us spent two days in Paris, where we recaptured the quality of the relationship we'd so slowly rebuilt over the past few years. I think she might have been showing me she could pay her own way now – she hadn't forgotten our O'Hare conversation. She was intent on taking me over to Paris, going to museums with me, and having a great meal there, which we did near the recently opened Pompidou Centre. Except for the fact that she snored and kept me awake in our shared hotel room, Paris was sunny, fun and wonderful.

And that is how she remembered her stay with us. With this cancer, as opposed to her first one, she forcefully looked on the bright side. 'How was England, Regina?' her friends asked on her return. 'Terrific,' she replied. And believed it.

By this time breast cancer was losing its cloak of impropriety. Betty Ford, the ex-president's wife, had 'come out'. Betty Rollins, an NBC broadcaster, had written a book about her breast cancer, *First You Cry*, which had been a best-seller, and they were making a Mary Tyler Moore TV film from it. Neither had died. Neither had literally bared her breast, or lack of it, but each had done so figuratively, by coming out as a one-breasted woman. I wonder whether people ever pictured their nipple-less flatness. I never did, because there had been such shame attached to it, my mother being careful none of us ever caught even a glimpse of her scars.

At the hospital, nurses now talked to her, rather than just taking her blood – they had become a more active part of treatment, sitting in on consultations – and got to know their patients. My mother's nurses knew I was in England, that Gene was an assistant district attorney, that Rick was in law school and Mark was still deciding what he wanted to be. The hospital had become a focus of my mother's life, and the nurses tried to make it as pleasant as possible, mixing warmth into the clinical drug trials in which she and other patients were participating. Nurses – mostly women, of course – had taken breast cancer out of the total control of doctors – still mostly men. On the front line, tending women sick with pain, they'd seen the devastation in their patients' eyes when the dressings were removed. Largely through the nurses, 'quality of life' issues had entered breast cancer treatment.

Another change: my mother told me later that summer when she and my father visited us that the nurses had offered her contact numbers and addresses of breast cancer support groups. I was impressed: she told me because she knew I was studying the effects of different kinds of therapy and self-help groups, and that I believed such groups could help people through difficult times. But I also knew she was telling me she was *not* like the people I studied. It was OK for them, but not for her. In fact, she was dismayed by the offer: she would *not* be defined by her illness. She had plenty of friends, she told me, she knew where to get information, and she had all the support she needed. To give her credit, she was generous enough to realise she was privileged, and said that on the whole the groups were a good thing. They were part of the vast change since Fannie had suffered in shame and isolation.

During my parents' visit, I met them one day at their hotel in London. At their door I overheard the sour sounds of an argument. 'I disgust you, don't I?' she was accusing him. The old gloom flooded back – here we were again. And then I remembered her words after her first surgery, when we were sifting through the rejects of her wardrobe: 'You feel like you're not a woman.' Freud was right: projection is distortion, a disfigurement of a relationship. Maybe she did disgust my father. I never knew. But perhaps not. Being without breasts is ugly. It's hard to love your body when they're gone. And it's hard for anyone else to love it, also – if you hate it yourself.

In 1979 Stephen and I moved to Chicago. We visited New York at Christmas. It was not my mother but my father who alarmed us. His symptoms had multiplied: he was constantly forgetting things, he'd fallen down, unconscious, in midtown Manhattan twice. He waved our concerns away. 'I'm on medication. Don't worry. Dr Blum's investigating.' Of course we worried. I never considered my father might be the vulnerable one. None of us took his symptoms seriously; in fact his 'hypochondria' had become a family joke. Two parents ill? Not possible. He just wanted some attention.

By Easter when we visited again he had lost thirty pounds. He had tried stuffing himself with calories. No matter how many chocolate éclairs, tubs of chocolate ice cream, or chocolate cream pies he ate, the weight dropped off. His face was now almost constantly reddish, with purpled veins, and his arythmia was worse. But he didn't want to go to any more doctors. He and we were very frightened. I'd grown used to the idea of losing my mother early, but not my father. He was a rock. He was the one who'd saved me from my mother when I needed saving; and her from me. He was happy just that I was alive – 'Look! She walks! She talks!' – not because of anything I'd achieved. He had to be around. Always.

But eventually he did go to a specialist: his symptoms, it seemed, were very unusual, but they did fit a pattern.

We got the diagnosis in June: carcinoids. Cancer again. A rare, unusual form, not inherited. Unlike breast cancer, easily curable if caught early. It almost never was.

Great Neck, June 1979

My mother and I sat on the sofa in the den. I had flown in from Chicago. She had been in constant touch with my father's doctors at North Shore Hospital where he had been for a week of tests. Some of his doctors were her own. They'd become a double act, the only husband-and-wife team on the oncology ward, though my father had his own specialist for his disease. The cancer was in his colon and liver, where it had settled, and it was incurable. My mother stopped listening when the doctors used those words. My father did not probe further. They both asked to be given whatever treatment was available. Where? How soon? They would be pleased to be guinea pigs. They wanted to live.

We children had our own tele-conferences with our parents' doctors. Though my mother was touched by this, it made her uncomfortable. She knew I would have asked the doctors for a prognosis.

And so, I asked, 'Mom, what have the doctors told you? About what to expect?' I held her hand.

She shrugged. Dangerous territory. Watch out for pitfalls, she must have been thinking. 'Just that he isn't going to get any better. That they'll give him whatever they've got in their arsenal. And that they think it won't be possible for him to keep working much longer. He wants to, you know . . .' She stared ahead, at the door to the cupboard where my father's suits, pushed out of a joint one in their room by her burgeoning clothing collection, now hung. To its right was a portrait of his grandfather, sweet-faced Abraham Gam, with his white hair and handlebar moustache, painted in gratitude by an immigrant, a beneficiary of my great-grandfather's generosity. She dared not look at me – she knew I would start crying and then she would.

'But, Mom . . . The doctors, they told me he only has six months . . .' I began. It was as if I'd smacked her in the stomach. She leaped up from the sofa. 'You will never say that again. I never heard that. Never,' she hissed, not looking at me, and she darted from the room.

10

Shadows

Great Neck: 1979–80

My father, even with his more gentle disposition, proved almost as tenacious as my mother. He finally sold his company, all in a rush, when even he had to admit he could no longer manage the commute nor keep track of business. But that took about six months. When he stopped commuting it was an admission of defeat. My mother campaigned: the pattern established years earlier when he'd begun to complain prevailed. She'd push, he'd resist, she wouldn't listen, and in the end he'd capitulate. She made him get dressed, take walks, go to the cinema, see friends, even bat tennis balls around, and she still entertained frequently.

He got more ill. His resistance to my mother's tactics grew and about a year after his diagnosis, he became mostly bedridden. The rhythm changed. The social flow increased inwards, towards the house; women visited during the week, men at weekends. That was interesting in itself: my mother had been the cultivator of social life, so it was revealing that their friends were so attached to my father. I glimpsed one of his friends – a captain of industry, normally stern and restrained – leave my father's bedroom sobbing. Friends had warmed to his soft shine as much as to my mother's bright one.

At the North Shore Hospital clinics, my parents sat next to each other in the waiting rooms, reading their respective novels. They were now a Cancer Couple, sharing drugs, surgery and the spectre of death, in addition to their joint history and family. My father took new, increasingly debilitating drugs, and had a long and dangerous operation to tie off the cancerous part of his liver. He looked more and more frail, his voice grew thin and hoarse, and his hair fell out, then grew back white, but he did not die in the six months his doctors had given him.

Chicago, 1979–80

While my parents were in decline I became a patient, too. With the end of my PhD in sight, Stephen and I had begun to try to conceive a child. For more than a year nothing happened. Not to have children was unimaginable, and each month we sank deeper into despondency. After the obligatory year's wait, we began infertility investigations in 1979, just about the time my father was diagnosed.

In March 1980 I was rushed in for emergency surgery, having suffered searing abdominal pain – ectopic pregnancy everyone thought (I've conceived! I was momentarily jubilant). An ultrasound showed a large mass on my ovary. Briefly I found myself in the abysmal limbo my mother and aunts had shared between examination and firm diagnosis. Until the doctors operated it wouldn't be clear what that darkness on my ovary was. My mother came out to Chicago to help nurse me. When I phoned to tell her I was going into hospital I did not mention the 'mass', but said it was probably just a fibroid cyst.

It wasn't a fibroid cyst, but more importantly it wasn't cancer. I had an advanced case of endometriosis, and the mass was an endometrial cyst. Endometriosis is an abnormal but quite common proliferation of the uterus's endometrial lining which during menstruation – when the lining is sloughed off – deposits itself in various parts of the abdominal cavity (and sometimes beyond). This abnormal growth and renegade colonising suggested to my non-medical ears the abnormal proliferation and colonisation of malformed cells which defined cancer. But medics who understood the workings of both assured me these were entirely different processes. Endometriosis often causes infertility, so we were ushered along the assembly line of infertility investigation and treatment. Nothing was going to prevent me from having babies; I would try everything.

The infertility work-up was relentless – we were submitted to undreamed-of and humiliating procedures while scientifically trained strangers scrutinised and evaluated our sexual and reproductive functions. Another year passed and I was still not pregnant. With my father now in a terminal state, and my mother – remarkably – in apparent temporary remission, the pressure to produce a grandchild for them was intense; not from them but from me. I had discarded dreams of my father crooning Bing Crosby standards to my child, taking him or her to the cinema as he had me, or tossing footballs in the back garden with him or her. I just wanted him to see my child.

I was getting older, my parents were getting more ill, and my body was not cooperating. I had been on hormones, I had stood on my head, I had taken my temperature every morning, had calculated my ovulation; Stephen and I had been good little scientific specimens, applying ourselves and our bodies studiously to the protocols, and still we had not conceived a child.

March 1980

I sat in the Department of Obstetrics and Gynecology, University of Chicago Hospital, waiting for the results of an endometrial biopsy, part of the infertility work-up protocol. Ten days earlier a needle the size of a small drill attached to something resembling a turkey baster had been inserted into me, and, though I had quickly looked away and willed myself into a parallel world, in some dim corner of my consciousness I had been aware that this monstrous instrument was invading my insides, pushed in there by a team of cool and impassive men ('As you know, we are a teaching hospital. Would you mind if students observed?'). I could not escape the involuntary spasmodic cramping of my pelvis, as if it was being attacked and was fighting back by crowding all its parts in on itself and silently screaming.

Endometrial biopsies were tests I wished to avoid for the rest of my life, if I possibly could, but I would do anything if there would be a child at the end.

The biopsy, I was told, was not informative. Nothing there was responsible for my failure to conceive. The doctors and their students greeted me in the consulting room with serious, long faces, took deep, meaningful breaths, and turned their hands upwards as if to say 'Don't know what next' – there is always a 'next' in American medicine. I waited patiently for their suggestions.

The chief consultant, with his deputy next to him, was new, not my normal infertility doctor. Every time I saw a new doctor I had to go through a tedious family medical history ('No, no diabetes. No strokes. No high blood pressure. Yes, heart disease – all old people, though'). When we got to the cancer section it was both uncomfortable and grimly amusing to watch the new doctor's reaction to the litany ('How old did you say your aunt was? And your mother? And your other aunt? And not – you're sure? – not your grandmother?'). Sometimes I thought they thought I was embroidering for effect ('Oh, how terrible. What a tragic history that is'). Why couldn't they read the other doctors' notes? Working in clinics later, I came to understand how little time they had to read, or retain, notes. But, still, you'd have thought something like that history would have jumped out at them and stuck to their brains. So there I was, having to recite it all over again, as dispassionately and politely as possible. But it did show that thinking had changed about breast cancer: data were being compiled on diseases that ran in families – diabetes, heart disease and now cancer, including breast cancer, were part of the medical histories taken as a matter of routine. The genetics and breast cancer link had been made. My female cousins and I had to be considered at risk. The fuschia curse was real.

The consultant's eyebrows rose above his horn-rims. 'And have you ever noticed any changes in your own breasts? Any discharge?'

That brought me up short. Even with my family history, I didn't know properly what to look for. Lumps, that was all, and I couldn't tell the normal from the abnormal. Only when I went to the gynaecologist did I have my breasts checked, as part of the general exam. They were usually lumpy, particularly around the time of my period, and painful. Discharge? Recently I'd seen something like a crust, but I hadn't paid much attention. The consultant locked gazes with his deputy. They missed a beat, and that sliver of silence made me feel sick.

The consultant returned to my notes. 'I see you've never had a mammogram. Is that correct?' I nodded. Oh no, this was not happening, I thought. I was there to have a baby. Indeed, I was scheduled to have a laparoscopy – an investigative operation – in one month, for another look-around. Please could we return to the subject: babies.

'I see here you're scheduled for surgery in a month,' he continued, thumbing his notes. 'I think we ought to try to get a mammogram in before you go in, before you may be put on more medication. I think it's just as well to have a look, get a baseline on the state of your breasts. You're really old enough now, with your family history, to be having regular mammography – yearly, I'd say.' Another change, even from five years earlier, when my mother had had her second cancer.

The mammogram took place the following day. It was to be the first of many. I was astonished at how pliable breasts were, and how dispassionate one could be about them when they were treated objectively by others. The cheerful, matronly technician took each in sequence. She lifted the first, like a pound of disembodied flesh, pushed and pulled it, flattening it against a portable table with a photographic plate till absolutely all of it was stretched, to position it so that all of it could be X-rayed, pushing the flesh down and securing it under and next to the plate. (She wore a protective leaded apron, I noted bleakly, a courtesy not extended to me: I still was afraid of radiation.) Then she left the darkened room in which I stood, naked to the waist. She X-rayed the breast from one angle, then repositioned it for another shot. The procedure was repeated for my other breast. It wasn't particularly painful, just disorienting, but the room was dark and silent and, in its own way, quite peaceful.

A few days later I again saw the chief consultant and his deputy. This time he was far less clinical. He had become avuncular. I should have gone with Stephen. I was alone when the doctor said things which, without my realising it, I had been waiting for about fifteen years to hear. When I did hear them, I knew. They were the same words my father had used when he told me about my mother's womb. I had been reassured then, but I'd known he was saying she'd been on the road to developing cancer.

'You have what we call "hyperplasia",' the doctor said. 'Your breasts already show that the cells have abnormalities. There are lots of reasons women's breasts show these: for instance, you have noticed your breasts are lumpy, and many women have what you probably will turn out to have, from your description – it's called fibrocystic breast disease [now called fibrocystic breast *condition*]. Women with that very common condition do not necessarily go on to develop breast cancer, but with your family history I'd recommend you be watched very carefully. I want to send you to a breast specialist now and get a firm opinion from her about what she would recommend, but I suspect, given your age and that you are trying to conceive, she'll recommend what I'm suggesting: just watching you for the moment.'

I returned to my office, stunned. I called Stephen. We met for lunch so I could tell him face-to-face, and so, I hoped, he could calm me. Of course, what I might be telling him was that perhaps he shouldn't be trying to have a child with me, so why was I expecting him to comfort me? It looked as if I, too, were damaged goods. What if we did manage to have this child, and then I did turn out to be like my mother? Aunt Fannie had been even younger than I was when she was diagnosed, so it was not unthinkable. What were we doing here, with this baby-making business, when my breasts might be telling us we should be making quite different plans?

The infertility conversation took us over. It resumed each day in a new way. Often we went down a logical road that ended in 'Don't go ahead now'. Stephen's first line of defence with hot subjects is logic, which in this case was like bringing water to a parched throat. But it was never enough. We always returned –

and we didn't know if it was logical or illogical – to the desire to have a child.

I went to the breast specialist, unusually, a woman. Another change. I found it useful: she'd more readily grasp the emotional point, I thought. She shocked me. Gently but clinically she described a revolutionary new procedure. I would be a candidate for it, as it was designed for women like me, with my family history. She told me about prophylactic bilateral mastectomies, the removal of apparently healthy breasts protectively. The procedure pre-empted cancer. But it still left women without breasts.

I was at that point a research associate in the University of Chicago Hospitals. I talked to medically trained friends, and they gave me abstracts of whatever research existed, which was very little. In theory, the procedure made sense, but only a handful of women in the world – most, if not all, in the US – had undergone it and no statistics yet existed to determine its success.

The specialist had drawn a family tree, or geneogram, for me. Lots of big Cs were written across circles representing my aunts and mother on my mother's side of the cancer geneogram. Over on the other side of the geneogram, my father's, were my grandfather and father. I was assured these were entirely irrelevant to the possibility of my developing breast cancer, though emotionally they added to the conviction that cancer would get me.

Years later, in a consultation with a geneticist in the 1990s, I discovered that the colon cancer on my maternal grandfather's side was not irrelevant. There are indications that colon cancer in men in families with breast and ovarian cancer may be part of the same genetic configuration. I didn't ask the breast specialist where this condition, which so far afflicted only one generation, might have come from – my grandmother, her sisters, their daughters and granddaughters were unaffected. (In my later consultations I discovered that men could be carriers of the gene, even if they didn't themselves normally develop breast cancer.) This early consultation confirmed that I had a higher probability of contracting breast cancer simply because I had one first-degree relative (a mother or a sister) and two second-degree (two aunts) who had done so. This meant

I should be thinking about ways of preventing it, and one way was to chop off my breasts.

I certainly was not going to have a prophylactic mastectomy at that point. I had to have babies first. I was not going to think about not having breasts when I was still young and not yet pregnant. So I asked the specialist about getting pregnant. She was sympathetic. She assured me that I had time to think about it. There was no rush: if I was unfortunate enough to develop breast cancer it wouldn't be likely to happen for years – the chance of its developing increases with age. At that time, though there had been an increase in sufferers in their fifties, breast cancer was (and still is) a disease primarily of older women. I was then in my early thirties. I could put off my decision. By all means, she urged, I should try to have babies. But afterwards she'd recommend I seriously consider prophylactic mastectomy.

'This operation has been designed for women like you.' Her words stuck with me. But then, most women with fibrocystic breast condition, while showing breast cell dysplasia, do not go on to develop breast cancer, the other doctor had said. There was no definite reason to believe I had anything more than that. We were only talking probabilities, only making guesses.

Well, that was one route to pregnancy. The day before my laparoscopy I had a pregnancy test, and got marvellous results: the paper turned whatever colour it was supposed to turn and confirmed my pregnancy. The only explanation I can give is that I had stopped focusing on getting pregnant, and my breasts had become the target of our anxiety. I had wavered about the wisdom of pregnancy, and, in the supreme perversity of things and of my body, conception had occurred. I must have conceived in the week of my mammogram. (The perverse notion that shifting the focus of anxiety from pregnancy to something else might reverse infertility was supported when our second son was conceived, in 1985, after another three years of infertility, with more testing, hormones and finally radical surgery to reconstruct tubes, with a warning not to expect conception. Then, one month after my mother died, a month in which mourning took the focus off reproducing, I was pregnant again.)

Though shocked by the notion of a preventative bilateral mastectomy, its logic was somehow persuasive. I tucked it away, aware already of how repelled people would be if I ever chose to have one. The medical friends I'd taken into my confidence were split over it. One wrote angrily about the male medical fraternity's conspiracy to use women like me as guinea pigs in mad experiments based on their contempt for women: chopping off their breasts, indeed! Others urged me to think about it seriously. One (male) joked that when I was fifty I'd have the fittest breasts on the beach. He obviously didn't know much about plastic surgery, though at the time – in my case, he would turn out to be wrong, unfortunately – his joke was reassuring.

I did not tell my mother. The moment the doctor told me that I had hyperplasia, I vowed never to let her know. I had only to tell my brothers, Stephen and my cousins for them to know immediately she shouldn't be told. It would have opened the door to misery all over again. She and my father were getting by by never thinking long-term. I'd disrupt that. She'd have to worry about my life and her terrible gift to me. Our relationship was so much better now that I was trying to respect her boundaries. I was trying hard not to repeat my blunder about my father's prognosis.

My mother had made only two allusions to my own vulnerability. The first was after her second mastectomy, when I was already married, and she asked me, carefully avoiding the word 'breasts', if I examined myself. I assured her that I did, that I knew how to. It wasn't true – as I've said, women with lumpy breasts have difficulty examining themselves, because it is hard to distinguish a normal lump from a suspicious one. In fact, it is so hard that many, if not most, general medical practitioners cannot tell the difference, either. For that reason breast specialists are the people to go to whenever you find a lump. The second allusion occurred a few years later when she pointedly advised me that wherever I was in the world, if 'anything should ever happen' to me, I must ensure that I got the 'very top treatment'. 'The Strang Clinic [in

Manhattan, where she was then being monitored], that's where you want to go, or someplace that you're sure is its equivalent. You make sure of that, OK?' And she went on to something else. She had tried to be offhand. Her words sounded rehearsed; my heart, and probably hers, was pounding.

I told my cousins. They hadn't yet heard about prophylactic mastectomy, but within the next few months they were discussing it with their own doctors. To bring it up was awkward. We'd never talked about our own risks before. I didn't want to alarm anyone. We were all equally at risk.

After that, though we didn't speak frequently and never had, whenever we did, we'd ask, 'Have you been for your check-up with the breast specialist? When's your next mammogram? What did the doctor say this time?' At regular but less frequent intervals, I'd also ask, 'Any discussion of the operation?' None of us could name it. None of us got any closer to thinking about the horrid surgery.

11

Regina: Ending: I

December 1981

On Christmas Eve Adam was born. The most perfectly formed child – of course – in creation, or so Stephen and I believed. When the baby's eyebrows became clear, on his second day of life, and they exactly mimicked the distinctive V shape of his father's, I thought I'd literally burst with the love of them both. My father, by now faded into almost nothingness, heard his gurgles on the phone. He heard me say a million times, 'He's beautiful, Daddy. He's perfect.' 'Of course, PuPu,' he laughed, calling me by his baby name for me.

At our last visit, two months earlier, which had been the latest date on which I could fly, he'd promised me he'd stick around till December 24, my due date. 'This is no life,' he'd said, shaking his thin, almost hairless head, as I sat at his bedside. 'I'm just waiting till December 24.' 'But then you'll have to see the baby,' I'd stubbornly urged. He'd smiled wanly, shook his head ruefully, and patted my hand. He could do nothing – everything hurt or itched or took huge effort. I dreaded life without him. He had to fight, like Mom – look how many years she'd gained.

He'd kept his word: he had waited. More, he hadn't deteriorated; with care arrangements in place my mother could come to Chicago, which she did the following week. He might have been skeletal but he would not die without her; it was an unspoken deal. All this staring death in the face had made us believe people can control exactly when it will come. When my mother left for Chicago on January 2 my brothers were on nursing duty, shared out between them at night and friends and neighbours during the day.

On the night she returned my father developed a fever. Delirium followed, and an ambulance took him away; my mother admonished herself afterwards for allowing him to be taken from her. Two days later he was dead; his new grandson was only two miles from my father's bed but was not allowed into the hospital. Stephen and I had made the last plane leaving Midway Airport before it was closed down yet again by a snowstorm.

Among my father's last words were 'Janet!' I'd raced to the hospital from the airport. 'He's in a coma,' I was told, and then I was led into his room. He lay there, ghostly. I took his hand and called to him: 'Dad?' All of a sudden he started, eyes wide open, and breathed an astonished 'Janet!' I swear he grinned. Then his eyes closed and he sank again into unconsciousness. The doctors didn't believe me. My family did.

So my mother became a widow, something she'd never expected to be. A widow whose cancer had stopped growing as if to let her nurse my father to his end.

Chicago, March 1982

My mother was back in Chicago.

She was comforted by knowing my father's last documented actions were to see me, utter my name and smile. Apart from that there was nothing comforting about his death. She learned one thing from it: she wanted to die at home. She made it clear that she would not deny us what she felt she'd denied my father and what his death in hospital had, in turn, denied her. She lived with sadness that she hadn't been there as he met death, holding his hand. She treasured the fact that she had been there before, even if carping – cleaning up after him, sharing his bed, feeding him, responding to his moans. And then the hospital had replaced her. (Months after he died the oncology unit set up a home-care hospice team.)

So there she was. She sat on my brown corduroy sofabed, a fire crackling in the fireplace, and watched me glide in circles in front of her. I clutched my baby son, my dancing partner, his tiny hand in mine, our arms outstretched . . . I'd taken a chance and put on 'If I Were a Rich Man' from *Fiddler on the Roof*, with Zero Mostel. We both imagined him – he was dead, too – rolling around the Broadway stage, where we'd seen him with my grandparents to celebrate my high-school graduation, propping up his enormous belly like a balloon, dancing lightly and gracefully, as some obese men can do. Both of us had tears in our eyes, though we pretended not to notice. This dance was a tribute to my father. I wished he could be watching his grandson being inducted into the Zero Mostel fan club. In the air of our Chicago flat, which he had never visited, there was almost a faint echo of his high-pitched laugh. For if he had been listening to 'If I Were a Rich Man' he would have been shuffling to the music, pretending to be Tevye, or, rather, Zero Mostel, the funniest man in the world, the man whose startled eyebrows alone could summon my father's laughter.

My mother tried to believe in life again but failed, though she gamely did her best to conceal it from me. I had come to respect such defences. I let her be. We treated each other with delicacy and as a result we were restored to harmony. Adam delighted her. But I noted moments of distraction in which she seemed not to hear people or when she gazed into the far distance. She seemed disconnected by grief. It must have felt as if she'd broken both legs and her crutches had gone, too. She could still get around, but it was painful, awkward, and took a huge effort of will.

Her grandsons kept her going. She had the A to Z of grandsons, she crowed to her friends: Zack, at home with Gene and Cathy – she was comforted by the fact that my father at least got to know him – and this one, Adam, here, in Chicago. She also took comfort from the fact that Dad had seen him in photos before his fever began. And her children. Rick – he'd not yet met the right woman; Mark – he'd not yet got the right career. There was more to stick around for. She had written a poem about her fierce love for us in the face of my father's death and her dying.

The One Condition

My mother climbed into her box
alongside sisters and my father,
still unwrinkled, dapper
in a black serge suit reserved
for somber occasions.

I served coffee, homemade bread
to relatives from Albany.
They swallowed loudly and admired
the silver teaspoons and
my fortitude.

I'd settle for a cup of air:
my pride is small;
and crawl until they made me stop.
I'd praise the sun and fondle
worms, entranced with silkiness.

Unless they take the children.

Yes, she was broken. Curiously, though, she found she still wanted to be around.

I arranged a brunch for her. I was trying to bring her back to the land of the living. In our bright living room, with its huge bow windows and blond wood floors, on a nippy, clear Sunday morning, she rocked slowly in the bentwood rocker my brothers had given us as a wedding present. I watched her quietly survey our friends. I'd hoped a party would summon her vivacity, but she was detached, assessing my guests: they were interesting, nice people, people concerned to make her feel comfortable, making a kind effort for the recent widow. She went through the motions, but she was watching herself, not really there with them.

She was numb, thinking how was it that she found herself there, sixty-two years old, at the end of a life? How was it that she could have put the one and only man she ever loved into the ground? How was it that that woman over there – me – was her child, that this tall, elegant man with an English accent was part of her family, that she held a tiny, perfect new baby in her arms once again, only this time, disconcertingly, he was not hers but that Englishman's and that daughter's?

She nodded to people and smiled politely. Sometimes she shook her head to bring herself back to the present. She smiled and nodded at the intense woman next to her, wife of a colleague of Stephen's, who I knew would not notice my mother's reluctance to engage but would keep prattling on. She was a pale, wide-hipped woman with an unflattering haircut and eyes too close together, who indeed had not noticed Mom had been a million miles and many years away; the woman seemed to be talking about research she was conducting into emotions.

I observed this interaction with caution. My mother's smile began to falter – it looked as if she was becoming alarmed. I prepared to intervene. I knew my guest. She was trying to capture my mother, make her a research subject. Then, as I looked at my mother, I saw in her face not alarm but self-consciousness. She was wondering if she looked dopey, suspecting her social smile might be inappropriate. She leaned forward. If she looked intensely attuned, maybe she would become intensely attuned. I edged my chair closer to hear what was going on: something about 'trauma' and 'processing the turmoil of emotions'. My mother sat back: 'Serious', she registered. Oh dear. Smiling as she had been probably looked crazy. She tried to stop drifting away. She nodded fiercely. My guest went on. My mother's brows knitted tightly.

I shifted closer. My guest said that she wanted people who had experienced trauma to keep diaries. She was interested in the process of getting through life-changing events. I knew my mother was not sure she actually was getting through life-changing events. But the fact that someone believed there was a process worth tracking, and that the mechanism for doing so would be through writing, might engage her. I was on high alert. My mother was being exploited.

'So would you be interested in participating?' my guest asked. My mother looked over at me. I was darting poisonous glances at the woman but she was completely unfazed. Then my mother did just what I'd done to her so often as a teenager: exactly the opposite of what I wanted. Of course she could write a journal. It would be interesting and helpful. She would be contributing to science, and here at the University of Chicago! Suddenly she was animated, best pals with my obnoxious guest.

And with that, my mother had a new project. Something to believe in, something to recharge her, something to organise her day. She would be writing a journal. For this I have to reluctantly thank that woman. Mom left Chicago happier than when she'd arrived.

My mother began her journal in March 1982. At first she wrote mainly about reconstructing life after my father's death. She reflected on what made it possible to rebuild when you yourself faced a shortened life. The journal helped my mother realise she wanted to live. Between 1982 and 1984 she published a number of poems and was invited to give poetry readings in Manhattan. We children – who had been raised, studiously, without religion, on the one side from a irreligious socialist position, and on the other an a-religious, assimilationist one – found it funny that she was becoming identified as a New York Jewish poet. She drafted a novel she'd plotted, about a marriage between two unlikely people; it was inspired by her bemusement that such temperamentally different people as she and my father came to love each other.

Her days, when she felt well – no chemotherapy, radiation or pain – became structured around the journal, writing poetry, playing tennis and seeing friends. Then, in the summer of 1982 she began a completely different project, which she continued until she died. It filled evenings, when she was aware of her loneliness but too tired to write. As she listened to music or the radio she stitched together pieces of patchwork into baby-sized quilts. At first they were for particular babies – her friends' grandchildren, or Zack or Adam – then she just kept making more, for no specific child, for grandchildren yet unborn, even unimagined. Perhaps as she sewed she felt connected to her own childhood in Paterson, with the sound of the sewing machine in the background. When she went shopping, instead of looking for clothes, as she had for so many years, she looked for pottery and china. She bought seconds and end-of-line dinnerware. She bought so much that the cupboards bulged. Other pieces she stored in the musty, crowded basement. She hunted for replacements for pieces she'd broken years before, to complete sets. I think she was arranging heirlooms, just as my father's mother had done for her. None of us particularly cared about pottery or china, and to a degree each of us had inherited my father's proneness to break things, but that didn't stop her. She kept collecting. She arranged for repairs to the leaking roof, for broken furniture to be mended, and had parts of the house painted. Projects kept her going.

As she tended the house, her relationships and her writing, she was refusing to die. Within six months of my father's death we had mounting evidence of her continuing will and talent for survival. My brothers and I came, perhaps foolishly, to believe her indestructible. She might go on and on. She'd lived so long with cancer. Now she was adding another chapter to her life, one without my father. We used to worry about how Dad would survive after she died – unless he met another woman. Even to think that was disloyal. They were like the song: 'love and marriage', 'horse and carriage', 'Lou and Regina'. No one could be put in her place. We were spared the need to think about my mother's meeting someone else. That was where we came up against her mortality: we knew her cancer was advancing. There would be no time, belief or energy for a new relationship. Besides, I knew she would never contemplate standing naked in front of another man.

She had plans to see more of the world. She wasn't bored with travelling yet. In November 1983 she went to Egypt, sailing down the Nile with a friend. Over the next two years she travelled back to Paris, a few more times to Chicago, to Boston a number of times to see Phyllis and Irvin, to Philadelphia, and to her friends' summer homes dotting the eastern seaboard. She kept her journal, off and on, from March 1982 until the early summer of 1984. She called it *Endings*.

Endings was divided into sections, titles given when a writer friend had encouraged her to think of publishing it. Part one she called

'Widowed'. She started with a poem which she wrote the night my father died; her cousin read it at the funeral.

No Fitting Eulogies

The poets of my childhood fail me:
words in Greek or rhymes too stiff,
reminding me of schoolrooms
where I sat with folded hands.

The poets of my time,
well-trained in whining or restraint,
disguise their pain with irony.
Their words are not for me.

Despite embarrassment at sentiment,
despite a style informed by shyness
and a fear of scorn of cynics,
I must compose my own encomiums,
a patched together hymn
of praise, excuses and confession,

Reaching back,
recalling all,
the broken promises,
the jokes, the foolishness.

You understood when I was silent,
slowed your pace to match my stride,
forgave my ridicule and spite.
And charged with rage at anyone
who dared find fault with me.

We played at children's games,
at fantasies,
until we had no need of them.
The children gave us different
dreams to fabricate.

Our hopes were modest,
realistic as befit our station.
Never did you think me less
when I was less.
Nor did I ever crave for more.
I wish I could be sure
you knew that.

The other sections she called 'Shock', 'Disorientation', 'Alone', 'Embarrassment', 'Rebellion', 'Detachment', 'Endurance', 'Regeneration' and 'Adjustment': they spoke of how she got through that first year without my father, to show other widows the line of progress. In that year her cancer remained steady, showing no growth, as if giving her a chance, slowly, both to lose my father and to retain him in her heart with some measure of peace. It fuelled our belief that she could carry on indefinitely.

That summer, the first summer without him, my mother tentatively began to resume a social life amid couples. She thought of herself as half of an unseen pair. Returning, for instance, to Leona's summer house in New York's Adirondack mountains without him was a first step. While carrying my father inside her, she managed to seem whole. She saw herself more clearly etched than she ever had been: no sisters, no husband, no children defined her. It was a babystep to go to Leona's, where she felt at ease. But while there she made a profound discovery:

August 23:
Yesterday, Leona (who was the anaesthesiologist attending my hysterectomy) told me that operations for uterine cancer, such as mine, are almost always successful because they are generally enclosed in their containers and can be readily excised before the malignancy spreads. 'I thought I had a "precancerous" condition, not cancer of the uterus,' I said. It turns out that Lou had asked the surgeon to tell me that. He evidently had told some of his friends the truth (I don't know how many knew at the time and have kept the secret all these years). I remember a few years

ago, my friend, Horty, mentioned I had had uterine cancer, and I corrected her: no, I said, I had hyperplasia, I said, a precancerous condition.

I was very contrite: she [Leona] thought she had blundered. But I felt triumphant. First of all, I was not upset by the disclosure; the operation was ten years ago and obviously it had worked.

Curiously I felt like the winner of a match: I had outwitted Lou; the deception was exposed. I always used to say Lou was absolutely unable to keep a secret from me. And he would agree (but of course who knows if that is true, and wouldn't it have been clever to let me believe that I knew it all). It appeared that he couldn't keep anything to himself for any length of time. He would always share confidences, which he had sworn never to reveal. The secrets he held were too large and lively to be contained, and they would come bubbling out like milk running over the side of a saucepan. Usually, his own secrets, like a surprise present, were so ill concealed anyway that I had no trouble guessing what he wanted to hide. He didn't really have to break down and confess.

Perhaps it is my typical response to crises – which is to avoid questions which might lead to answers I don't want to hear – that made it easy for him to keep the secret. I may have refused to acknowledge the clues. Certainly, I know that I never pursued a doubt about the nature of my operation.

It may seem ridiculous that I should feel such elation on discovering that I had had uterine cancer. That is something to crow about? But the point is that it is something long in the past. It is an obstacle surmounted without any pain or effort on my part. And it is a puzzle cleared up. I can feel smug about it: see, smartie, you can't hide things from me. I'll find out sooner or later.

So she hadn't been cancer-free all those years, after all. Because I did not read my mother's journal till after she died, I hadn't known this, and nor had my brothers. By the time I read about it, Leona herself had told me, and I'd told my shocked brothers. Poor Leona, again assuming that of course I knew, visited me in Cambridge shortly after my mother had died, and mentioned it to me. I, too, was utterly shocked. But I, too, smiled wryly at my father's canniness. So did my brothers. Dad won, actually, I concluded. He was right to have tricked her. His had been the same impulse I'd had when I hadn't told her about my dysplasia. We'd lived with the Regina of then.

The journal was a place to reflect. She had never fully realised till then the pain of the years following her first mastectomy. At this distance, within the quiet house, she could recall on her typewriter the turmoil we had lived through and lay it to rest. Ironically, even though she was much nearer death than she was then, the turmoil was gone. She could never have responded so equably to Leona's revelation then. She was changed from only the previous year, when she'd visited Chicago in a state of shock and bewilderment. She had moved out of numbness punctuated first by sharp grief, then detachment, and into a stage she labelled 'Regeneration'.

Regeneration (March 1983):
I am back, more than less, in the world. All things remaining equal, I don't mind sticking around for as long as is comfortable. Interest in my surroundings is often piqued; how will events turn out? Who will run in the elections? Who will win? Will Sandy become pregnant? How much did Mrs Davis get for the house across the street? None of this adds up to a major purpose in life. Or great drive and verve. But it's an improvement over massive indifference. It's sufficient.

With customary irony, my reawakened interest in life coincides with new symptoms of disease. There seems to be a malicious symmetry in the plan. If I spurn life, if I am sickened by the sight of food, I can have a limitless amount. But if I savor a sweet and show the slightest appetite, the feast will be removed. No seconds, no refills; that's it.

I have had cancer, or more precisely, cancers, for almost twenty years. My first cancer operation was entirely successful and there was no metastasis. I was not convinced by medical assurances, however, and for the next ten years I assumed I was on the verge of death, suspicious of the least symptom, waiting for the pronouncement, terminal. I adjusted to my fate by excising hope, by suppressing any dreams or plans for the future, denigrating the richness of life, emphasizing the fears and perils, so it would be easier to leave (why would anyone want to stay? Nothing good was likely to happen; nothing could tempt me). Thus I could move calmly toward death: my refuge, my escape. I relied on death as an excuse. I had not accomplished what I had earlier hoped I would, not because of lack of talent or capability, I could rationalize, but because death had robbed me of the chance. It was a convenient and appealing explanation. Death could make my apologies.

Long before I became ill I had promised myself to take my life when I became helpless. My sisters had both died of cancer. They had lingered and suffered. One clung to life despite her misery, grasped it on any terms, held on by her fingernails, unaware, unconcerned with indignities. The other sister faced her death squarely and bravely, ashamed of being a burden, regretting her months of dependency. I resolved not to permit futile life-prolonging efforts. My greatest worry (still is) was that cancer would affect my brain and leave me incompetent, a witless burden against my will.

I was determined to maintain the initiative, to end my life before terminal illness made me helpless and disgusting. Illness is not a disgrace or a sign of innate weakness, but in my mind reducing people to extremes such as starvation, thirst, imprisonment and narrow confinement or subjecting them to overwhelming pain removes the veneer of civilization, the refinements of socialization and exposes them as quivering, sometimes hideous animals. Lingering illnesses are often ugly and shameful. I hold dear the ideals of courage and dignity. Some people I know have been able to exhibit admirable gallantry throughout their ordeals. I don't know if I can. I'd rather not test myself. Particularly when it is known that the end is inevitable, the additional few months to be gained are a poor exchange for the trial.

My fear of the degradation of the flesh and the spirit through terminal illness was just one of the reasons for my sinister infatuation with death. Death attracted me in other ways. I enjoyed things less and less, hoped for fewer things, eventually nothing except surcease from continual effort and failure. Death would release me from the struggle. And I lived with the thought constantly. It comforted me. I became death's comrade, enjoying the casual, easy relationship, proud of the apparent indifference, clearly able to trivialize the awful prospect. My friendship with death became not only an escape valve but a game and a pick-me-up: this may be the last time I have to clean this closet, buy a new winter coat or a new package of sewing machine needles or a spool of pink thread or a box of sesame seeds. It was soothing to believe I wouldn't have to keep on doing these boring or irritating chores. I was on my mark, ready to split any day.

Death held no terrors for me. It was my friend. But the preoccupation was depressing, and I tried to hide it. Occasionally I blurted out my attachment and Lou would argue with me: I don't mean it. I have so much to live for. I don't appreciate what I have. Anyway, he didn't really believe me, attributing my outbursts to illness or hormones or to my explosive temper which confounded him completely. It was not something he could readily recognize or identify with. He rarely lost his temper, and when he did he was able to forget the incident quickly and completely, a very accommodating and protective amnesia.

I no longer cultivate the notion of death. I don't speculate on which kind of exit appeals most to me. I am older and sicker than I was when I mused endlessly and fancifully on my means to an end. I have more humility now. Perhaps, after all, I will be only too willing to accept restricted mobility, to spend the hours gladly doing very little.

I have spent many days in bed and they haven't been wretched. Some of the bed-ridden days, when my stomach and head were quiet, I've enjoyed listening to music, reading, talking with friends, eating. It would not be so demeaning, I now believe, to accept help and favors. I am not necessarily abject or disgusting if I am able to do less for myself than I was, if I am more slow-witted or slow-moving.

In the meantime, I am making small-scale plans, appropriate to my status, suitable to my tastes. I negotiate a narrower territory with lateral, crablike mobility. I may get worse sooner than I expect; I won't think of that. In the interim, I am broadening my vistas and moving energetically within a circumscribed but new and agreeable arena.

Great Neck, 1983–January 1985

My mother, the widow, was entering unmapped territory. She made up her route as she went along, keeping her sights on one lane – that of living. Unlike her sisters, she was aware of others on similar territory. Though, it's true, her breast cancer colleagues hadn't suffered the double whammy she had: being ill while nursing a dying husband.

Breast cancer had exploded on to the national consciousness. Even young actresses admitted having it. She had a choice of three hospitals to get her radiation treatments from! A subculture of breast cancer patients was developing. Even though at this point all she was doing was getting her blood drawn every few weeks, she couldn't leave the little club they formed. They saw each other at Waldbaum's Supermarket and Food Emporium's delicatessen counter, shopping for their families, or on the train to Manhattan; they greeted each other with detached but nevertheless intimate recognition. In the clinic waiting areas my mother heard other women discussing their prostheses. That was more intimate than she wanted to get.

Meanwhile, in Chicago, friends of mine had mothers who were facing breast removals. As early as January 1980 I had returned to my university office after the Christmas break to see a graduate student – a few years younger than I – wearing a headscarf, her skin a telltale yellow. She'd just had a mastectomy. She was finishing a course of chemotherapy. She was optimistic she'd beat it. She wasn't a friend, but I monitored her at a distance, through the university grapevine. Now, three years later she was thriving. She'd moved away, taken an academic position, and was planning to become pregnant. I knew my mother was in an advanced stage of the illness, but I also knew that her treatment team had a fighting mentality and a seemingly endless supply of new medical interventions. And she hadn't had a single recurrence since long before my father died. Besides, my mother was unusual. She'd been a pioneer among her peers: first to get a postgraduate degree, first to go back to work and finally, first director of the Commission on the Status of Women. Maybe she'd be the first to outwit advanced breast cancer. Besides, she was a wonderful grandmother, with passion, energy and time for Adam and his cousin Zack, and I thought she'd probably be around for them for quite a while. I couldn't think otherwise; I was raw with missing my father.

12

Regina: Ending: II

My mother began a second year of her journal. She called its first section 'Continuity'. She was seeking threads, continuing themes. 'Continuity' for her meant simply to live, miraculously, now packing away the pain of her loss of my father – with the grief it aroused over her sisters and parents – as if in an ever-ready, ever-present, bulging suitcase. Indeed, at the beginning of the year she was able to work again. She took on consulting projects for City Hall.

But on February 21, 1983, the inevitable struck, shattering our illusions: the loitering cancer, perhaps tired of waiting while she marshalled her strength to care first for my father and then for her grief, had pounced. Once again, she became a fully paid-up member of the breast cancer club; once again, she had to attend the clinic for treatment as well as check-ups:

> I have just learned that I must have a new series of radiation treatments for cancer in the bone of my left leg. I was not surprised, mainly annoyed that I must curtail my activities. Clearly, it was foolhardy of me to have gone ice skating last week. I did not feel at ease at the time, fearful of falling. But I did not realize how dangerous it really was. A fall could have meant a fracture, immobility, no one to care for me, and dependence on the generosity of others at their convenience. The X-ray of my leg was ominous; a sharp blow could easily have cracked the bone.
>
> I suspect that my disappointment [about having to cancel a

trip to Nassau with friends] is another example of evasion, of suppressing fears or refusing to look obtrusive facts in the face. It doesn't matter to me how it is characterized. If it's pretence or escapism or folly. It's better than palpitations and nightmares or paralysis . . . I'm assuming things will not be very different for the next few months, and that's as far ahead as I can think.

The explosion of cancer therapies and treatment centres actually aided and abetted my mother's – and our – 'evasion': hope was offered at every turn; there were always new treatments available. Right up to the end my father had been getting new chemotherapy regimens. My mother's task was to negotiate her way through the setbacks her body meted out to her, to find a kind of map for understanding who she still was, in the midst of advancing cancer and still-present grief, and not to face death. She turned corners in her mourning and accepted the return of the cancer that had become so familiar. She was 'savouring time' – which, she thought, was a neat title to lend to her next series of entries.

March 1983:
I am . . . like the traveller [who feels she must absorb everything about the place she visits, who must not waste the opportunity]. I suppose unconsciously I feel it is wasteful to walk around blind, numb and unknowing, or to postpone important summations. A report is due. I have to look deeply and seriously; I have to understand, and I have to try, at least, to evaluate the worth of things. It turns out I'm not a harsh critic. Most of what I see and hear is interesting. Not only do I enjoy music, a really good book, and looking at the sky and bare trees, and the earliest spring flower. But I know I'm enjoying it and I'm not wistful or rueful. It doesn't matter if it's for a long or short time. It really doesn't matter. I think this may be my last spring. I am unmoved, neutral. It's a possibility. Meanwhile, it's just good to be alive and to respond to so many good things.

She could go for weeks now without seeing doctors; now not only were there new treatments, there were also new ways of administering them:

> I had not been there for a month since I am not getting injections but only taking medication daily on my own. The doctor decided to add some new medicines because I have new lumps in the soft tissue and some of the old ones are noticeably larger and harder. The lumps don't hurt. At least I don't know whether my stop and go pains or the insidious constant ones, like an unreliable back or tennis elbow or a stiff neck, are due to disease in the bones or the soft tissue. And, according to the doctors, they are not life-threatening (another useful term that has come into fashion recently; in the old days they would just say it's not serious).
>
> At any rate, a new kind of chemotherapy has been prescribed, and I started the programme today. No adverse side effects as yet. But the cost is very high. The last few regimens ordered for me were special studies, financed by the National Institutes of Health, so I didn't have to pay for the medication. This will cost several hundred dollars a month. I've grown accustomed to moderate medical costs in the past year. Unfortunately, I'll have to readjust.
>
> I am more tired than before, but I still can do a lot. I play tennis and I do all the household chores . . .
>
> I wake up fairly refreshed and energetic but I wear down rapidly. In an hour or two my knees weaken and my breaths are short and strained. I go back to bed, usually fully clothed, to read and sleep. Though my eyes get tired, I rarely fall asleep, and if I do it's for a few good minutes. The bed is my best friend, my refuge and comfort. I don't even mind the nights when I am restless and awake . . .
>
> April 18, 1983:
> . . . I want to go on living like a normal person, healthy or at least unaware of an illness she may be harbouring. I don't want to be coddled; I don't want people hovering over me, and I don't want to defend what some people think is my compulsion to overdo,

as though I have to prove my mettle and superior quality. On the other hand, I am often tempted to exploit my position. I expect and want special attention and I want to be excused from onerous chores because of my poor health. It's a convenience, an unanswerable argument, a credit card that never has to be paid.

I also continue to plan and make arrangements as though there are no reasonable constraints. I agreed to join the tennis players next season. I have bought a subscription to the Y [the 92nd Street Y in Manhattan] Sunday concerts. I go blithely along with the rest of the crowd on any forthcoming plan – count me in, by all means. At the same time, I privately settle differences with my conscious appointments secretary; we'll see; it's easier to pretend I'm just like everyone else; it makes other people comfortable and they appreciate my tastefulness. The ultimate deception, however, is that I am playing a game that eases my discomfort. I'm the one who wants the deception.

I am constantly aware of a deadline. Something must be completed within a specified time or else it won't be done at all. Often the prospect relieves me, like not having to do next year's taxes. Without any apparent conflict – just another thought taking up equal space – I operate on an open-ended schedule. I can procrastinate. I have plenty of time for the modest projects I've laid out. What I don't do today, I can finish tomorrow, or within the short space of time needed. Is this another contradiction – deadlines and postponement? Not really, because the deferments are for short periods, and what is put off indefinitely is deliberately put aside because I don't want to deal with it and hope I never have to.

May 27:
If I'm dying I'm doing it in the most unobtrusive and inconclusive fashion. I'm different from what I was, but no one, including me, would ever notice the difference. I have less energy than before, and I accomplish far less than I set out to do each morning. The energy level is quite uneven and some days I'm very productive, proudly completing all the tasks listed.

My disappointment, however, that I cannot work and play as hard, as long, and as tirelessly as I used to is not unlike what all my contemporaries are discovering with a harsh and unpleasant jolt. For them – and, who knows, maybe for me too – it is a sign that they are aging, not ailing.

Despite the fact that hope was meted out to her each time she visited the clinic, one fact was inescapable: she had end-stage breast cancer. We all knew – and, really, had known with the cancer's return a few months earlier, though it had taken time to seep in – that her time was limited, though we were not sure to what. In this respect she, like her sisters, was still alone. There weren't groups for dying people, not that she would have gone if there had been. Her journal was her therapy, where she'd think things through. My mother wouldn't know whether her mourning and dying was like anyone else's, nor would she have needed to. But others might. Perhaps that was where cancer treatment would move to next: helping people learn how to die.

Belatedly perhaps, I understood her desire to protect me, to keep me her daughter. I neither probed her feelings nor showed my anxiety. My brothers seemed to have learned that lesson long before I did. They treated her with delicacy. Our reunions in Great Neck were full of affection, laughter. They'd been lively, actually, since my father's death. Even more since her recurrences. She was peaceful now. Turmoil and worry about us had evaporated. New pains and lumps continued and she knew there would be more.

May 1983: Ready and Willing:
Many old people and those who are chronically ill are disappointed that their eyes open to another pointless day. Not bitter, just weary and resigned, they say, enough already. I've had my share; I've overstayed my welcome. It's time to leave quietly and decorously.

I plan ahead activities for a week. I always have jobs to wind up but I wouldn't mind leaving loose ends . . . Nothing seriously engages my interest . . . I am past ambition and envy. Concern for the children rules my emotions, and when I'm not with them and diverted by their charm and solicitude, I worry about their lack of sophistication and aggressiveness . . .

I used to save the maraschino cherry on the grapefruit for the end. My mother, before clearing the table, would remind me it was hidden on the plate. But often in restaurants, I was gypped out of my prize by overly efficient waiters. Of course, now we have discovered that such cherries are carcinogenic, but what a pity my restraint and economy prevented me from enjoying in the prime of my ignorance and sensuality what was desirable and accessible. My advice – how heady it is to give advice; I have large stores of advice but no demand for it – is seize the opportunities for pleasure, indulge yourself, feast while the tastebuds are lively.

I miss Lou very much. He grows more perfect every day. I never think of the bad times together. I remember only the fun we had. Our separation has lasted long enough, I often think, as though I can call and apologise and he'll come back. Why not? I learned my lesson. I'll never be mean and shrewish again.

May 9, 1983:

. . . Despite my desire to crawl into a hole when I'm ill, I don't recommend do-it-yourself . . . surgery. Short of [that] . . . I expect to heal myself. The sickness will get tired and go away or I will. I don't expect doctors or nurses or friends or children to make me better. That is, so far. But as I've said earlier, I've grown more humble and less sure of what I'll do and how I'll act at the moment of truth, when I get worse, perhaps immobilised and more frightened. Maybe like Lou and like my sister I'll want all the attention I can gather; maybe the certainty of love will warm me, as it did Lou. As of now, it seems improbable. Actually, the sicker I get, the colder and more detached I become. As though preparing for rejection or a break-up, I become more convinced that love is evanescent, portable, and reusable in another context. It doesn't take away pains in the head that prevent one from sleeping.

That's not entirely true. Proof that people love me may often seem irrelevant, but I think no matter how sick I get, I'll always love the children and will always be willing to make bargains and deals to save them at whatever sacrifice. You can do this to me but deduct it from the children's debts; let me build a reserve they can draw from. I can't imagine that my love for the children could ever fade, unless I am reduced to a senseless shell before I die. I suppose that's everyone's greatest fear.

June 23:
I'm feeling a lot better than last week. I'll tell the doctor about the pains in my arms and various other places but I'm sure he won't suggest doing anything drastic. The pain seems to follow a regular pattern: it begins and becomes intensified usually a few days after my treatment [with chemotherapy]. The arm becomes discoloured and swollen and the pain shoots up from the point of injection, through my arm, to my neck and back. Sometimes both arms, not just the one injected, are affected. I get a stomach ache too, or some other apparently unrelated illness. The assault lasts about a week and then disappears. I think the symptoms are probably due to a churning up of dormant malignant cells and a battle between them and the medication. Since I feel better after a week or so and since I haven't observed new symptoms, perhaps the medication is winning . . .

I feel as though I'm serving as a passive but interested host to a bunch of unconcerned interlopers – they don't have any malicious intent; they're just going about their business – in a drama being enacted inside me. A lot of people at the clinic seem to have a similar attitude. I hear them discuss their cases with each other, displaying the same kind of detachment as though they'd read in a magazine a fascinating account of this curious condition.

I've had a good week. I played tennis one morning – not long; it was hot and I was out of breath very soon. I invited some women to lunch, had dinner with friends, and sewed an old dress to wear to a wedding this coming Sunday. I needed a dress (nothing fits me since I gained about ten pounds from the medication) and hated to buy a new one. I was delighted to find this dress in the closet. I had given it to Janet many years ago because I thought it revealed my under-arm surgery scars. I don't think Janet ever wore it after I gave it to her officially. She used to wear it when it was mine. I altered the dress and it fits fine – not the way it did when I was slim and flat-bellied, but good enough for someone with bumps, lumps and depressions in the wrong places.

June 29:
I stayed at Shoshonna's house [in Manhattan] and the next morning Rick and Stephanie picked me up and brought me home. Gene and Cathy came in the afternoon, and at night we celebrated Rick's birthday. Phyllis and Irvin [down from Boston] came and stayed over, and I invited Stephanie's parents to Rick's birthday party. It was a happy, merry party.

Phyllis and Irvin left Sunday afternoon, and at 5:30 I went to a wedding . . . It was a full weekend. I survived it . . . enjoyed it.

I had a treatment on Monday and spoke with the doctor about my complaints. Velban, the milder of the drugs injected, is the culprit, he believes, causing muscular pains and abdominal upsets. The doctor decided to lower the dosage and to dilute the medicine as it is administered. Maybe it will lessen the reaction during the cycle, but so far I have felt nauseated and weak and have spent most of the last three days in or close to my bed. I'm just mildly sick, queasy and drained of energy. I read and doze during the day and night. It's not bad . . .

August 10:
I've been in bed for the past three days because I have phlebitis, probably caused by the medication. About a week ago I noticed that my left foot and leg were swollen and that it was more difficult than usual to start walking when I got off the bed, that my legs were stiff and heavy and hard to push forward. I thought, however, that exercise was good for whatever odd condition I had, and that once my legs remembered their accustomed duties and motions, they would move easily. Exercise, I have since

found out, is the wrong prescription for phlebitis, but I did find that after the initial resistance I was able to walk almost normally. I played tennis, without running after balls, but I never do anyway. My kind and patient friends hit the ball straight to me so I hardly have to move my legs. I assumed that the heaviness in my legs was due to poor circulation, age, or a quirky reaction to chemotherapy, all conditions which could be conquered or put in their place by deliberate neglect.

By Monday, I had great difficulty walking . . . and the doctor diagnosed the condition as phlebitis. After sonar tests, it was agreed that it was only superficial phlebitis. I didn't have to be hospitalized, but I was ordered to bed . . . I do go off the bed from time to time and I do simple things around the house. Surely I'm allowed to do that. Nobody is expected to follow doctors' instructions without any deviation. My mother-in-law used to. When the doctor said no salt she never again used a grain of it. When he said lie quietly, she didn't turn or move an arm. But I've never met anyone else who believes so implicitly in doctors and follows their orders so religiously. Nor do doctors expect such unwavering fidelity. She must have been the best little girl in the world, and she never got any medals for it.

August 18:
I am undergoing radiation treatments because of recurrence of disease in the bone. The pain has largely subsided. I can't do everything I did three weeks ago when the pain started, but almost. I'm pleased that I'm not afraid or depressed. Life is very much the same and I'm planning a few little trips within the next month.

To others I may seem brave and courageous, but I really can't picture myself getting very much worse. Perhaps that is just as well. I don't need to conjure up scary scenes of the future. I don't think it serves any good purpose to indulge in self-induced nightmares of what it can be like. On my way to the radiologist's office (called Ground in North Shore Hospital, Basement in Deepdale Hospital, and Lower Level in other hospitals) I pass very sick people on stretchers. They look awful, many like corpses, and even the young and less emaciated look frightened out of this world. The old ones moan and shriek. The young ones are quiet, perhaps too bewildered to cry out. I cannot imagine that I will be one of them. I will not contemplate it. I don't think it reveals a lack of compassion if I refuse to face the fact that fairly soon I may be among them, and I should give a signal of sisterhood. I breeze past them with only a side-long glance . . .

September 8:
I am very much weaker and sicker than I was a few months ago . . . I would say 100% weaker, but that would mean I've hit bottom. It's far from that, I fear . . . I know it's not psychological because I do get up in the morning with every intention of behaving like a suburban housekeeper-accountant-flibbertigibbet. I get dressed and force myself to go on errands. I usually last three or four but after two, I'm not sure I'll last so I go home and retreat into my bed.

I've tried all kinds of surprises and dodges. I'll triumph over weariness, overtake my inertia while my unconscious is off guard. A small tennis game is what I need to perk me up; I'm always ready for that; I never refuse. I'll get caught up in the game, I figure. The necessity of returning an oncoming ball is urgent. My legs will move freely if my concern is not apparent. The body will automatically win the argument, refuting the brain's injunction against strenuous activity. Anyway, the way I play it's not strenuous.

I tried it and it was awful. I asked Miriam to play with me last week. After five minutes I was panting, and in ten minutes I had no breath in me. Rest, I called. Evidently I looked so ashen (I used to get red as fire) and was breathing with such difficulty, Miriam called a halt. 'It's too soon after your phlebitis. Maybe it's the medication.' She's very tactful.

A few days ago, determined to test myself again, to stop coddling myself and to return to a normal though modified life, I persuaded Mark to play with me. We played for ten minutes, rested for ten, played again at my insistence, and then quit at Mark's.

I have assorted pains almost everywhere but I have had worse. They're not bad enough to require pain-killers. It's the debility that's new . . . My chest is also filled with a heaviness and burning, like depression's freight. But I am not depressed. Just lethargic and weary . . .

October 4:
I am the boy who cried wolf. I'm feeling much better again. More pep than before; as well as I did in the spring. And the pain and stiffness in my leg are almost all gone . . .

Another false alarm. How much longer will anyone pay attention when it seems no more than a macabre game I'm playing?

October 17:
In a movie I saw recently, someone says, 'I never knew a happy person so I didn't understand what he meant.' . . . All of us know that hardship and sadness lie beneath the surface of the most fortunate and satisfied contenders for the model family happiness prize . . . But some nights I lie awake reviewing what I've done during the day and planning the next day's activities. Nobody's asked any questions; I'm not defending a position. But often I say to myself, 'It's been a good day. I'm happy.' And somehow my old cynical self does not intervene to warn it won't go on for long, tomorrow disaster will strike. And anyway what do you mean happy?

Did I have to get cancer, did I have to become a widow in order to shed my anxieties about the whims and instability of happiness? Does acknowledgement of a curtailed and limited life span induce greater enjoyment? Does it make people more humble, less demanding? Maybe we have to be half-starved before we realize a soft-cooked egg or a boiled potato is unbelievably delicious. It doesn't matter if the pleasure is fleeting. Who needs a promise of fidelity and permanence if I have no assurance I'll be around to test it? Surely it would be audacious and irrelevant to demand more than what the present can provide.

Live for the present is an old motto. I may have believed in it before but I certainly didn't live by it. Now, without deliberation, I seize the day. And appreciate it.

Or is this stability and tranquillity no more than chemically produced? That would be an ironic explanation of what I like to think is wisdom and maturity. I rarely lose my temper anymore. I do get depressed and morose at times, impatient often, but rarely furious. The hormones I am now taking inhibit the manufacture of cortisone and adrenalin. I have to take prednisone to bring my blood pressure up to a normal level, but nothing to replace adrenalin. I guess people can get along fine without adrenalin. So much for philosophy and psychiatry. A daily dose of hormones is the recipe for peace and happiness.

The happiness – I know when it's here but it's free to come and go – is very simple, an unselfish kind of happiness, unsullied by complaints about its fickleness and undiluted by fears of tomorrow. Perhaps a few lucky people have always taken and enjoyed life this way; I never did before. And I would recommend it, except the price is heavy. It's like my soft glowing complexion, also new and the result of my medication. Some of my friends who are beginning to wrinkle envy my youthful skin, but again, I don't recommend the cure. The disparity between appearance and reality reminds me of the Thomas Mann novel, *The Black Swan*, in which the main character becomes more lovely as the disease inside becomes more virulent . . .

Sometimes my sister Fannie, who died almost thirty years ago, appears not only in my dreams but next to me, to advise me on how to iron curtains, to raise children (she never got beyond sixteen-year-old children) and how to die unobtrusively. She tells me it's not hard – a relief for all. I also see her as a confident, resourceful, unsmiling child, more than fifty years ago. I realise now she couldn't have been very happy, torn between jealousy of a handsomer older sister and her responsibility to me, her younger sister. While I considered her all-powerful, more omnipotent than my mother, who was not as accessible, to tell off the kids on the block who were harassing me – Fannie would always defend me, very effectively, and then admonish me for being a scaredy cat: 'After this, you have to fight your own battles' – she was not as much fun or as interesting as my sister Mary who made up stories to amuse us and gave us fantasies to nurse and cherish.

On those days, I live in a seance, on and off, with the dead. I don't know why these days begin and end. Like dreams they determine their own course.

My mother's once painful striving had curiously been replaced by contented appreciation. She still collapsed into hilarity with Phyllis. She still loved to shop every weekend for her children's visits and she still cooked too much and made a huge Thanksgiving feast for over twenty people. We talked about Rick's wedding in May; whom she'd invite, what she would wear.

She managed her life within carefully wrought boundaries, withholding confidences she might once have wished to make (and, anyway, without my father around, there wasn't anyone she particularly wanted to confide in), circumscribing what she would allow her friends and children to elicit. She created clear parameters for her relationships, without rancour – indeed, with gentleness – but firmly: no, we will not discuss my symptoms, nor how I feel about Lou's absence. These boundaries helped her maintain her sweet if surprising contentment. The doctors and nurses at the clinic helped: they looked no further ahead than the next clinic appointment, and asked only about her current tolerance of the drugs.

My mother made her last few journal entries in a section she titled 'Waiting'. For she knew now that she was waiting. The number of days, weeks or months was the question, as was whether she would be lucky enough to avoid a painful death, inconveniencing others. 'Waiting' began just before Rick and Stephanie's glorious picture-book wedding, on a perfect, still May Sunday, in the garden of Stephanie's parents' house, only a few streets away from our house in Great Neck.

May 1984: 'Waiting':
I have many new symptoms, new lesions, some pain from the disease, mostly in my skull, where many lumps have appeared, and discomfort, fatigue, nausea ranging from mild to intense, and stomach upsets from the chemotherapy. On my good days, and they are in the majority, I function as well as my healthy friends. Since I have always had more than the usual measure of energy and stamina . . . I still can outperform most of my peers; that is, the over-sixty-year-olds I know.

'So far I am scarcely changed. Whatever differences have occurred in my routine and activities have been gradual. In the past five months, I have received a variety of chemotherapeutic programs, and I was intermittently knocked out of commission.

Only sporadically was I disabled, and each time I had an adverse reaction I was promptly given a new regimen. For the most part I went about my business as usual, just a bit more limited in my activity. The bed has been an irresistible magnet, drawing me in at any pause in the day's occupations. I haven't resented the weakness; I submit graciously to the bed's lures like a Victorian lady with vapors. Only when my head is heavy and hurts does the bed fail to comfort. I am a reluctant pill-user, but I am beginning to be more reasonable about it. Pain-killers, I am always astonished to learn, do work. Pain is neither ennobling nor necessary. I can do without it, so I no longer fight what I used to think was a siren song of pills. I even get up at night, out of my warm but hostile bed, to take a pill because I'm finally persuaded it will take away the pain and let me sleep.

Up until last month the doctors spoke in very reassuring tones. If this treatment doesn't work, we'll use another. The pool of possible remedies sounded enormous. The doctors seemed to have an infinite supply of arrows in their quivers. By this time I suspect I'm pretty much down to a last resort: hormones which sometimes retard spread in protracted metastatic breast cancer cases. This approach seems to be working and the side effects are minimal. So far, I've had little discomfort or pain and hardly measurable inroads in my daily functioning.

I don't ask a lot of direct questions, partly because I am not sure the doctors are entirely candid or omnipotent or certain of what they're doing. Some of them think patients are heartened by a posture of infallibility and self-confidence. I'm not one of those patients.

I don't ask because I don't know what to make of the answers, anyway. Are they painting a bleak picture so that my hopes will not be unrealistically lifted? If I should go into remission again and prosper, would I then not be enormously grateful for their efforts and impressed with their skill and expertise? Are they, on the other hand, being unduly optimistic to brighten my days? Isn't it the better part of valor and generosity to allow me as wide a ray of hope as can be contained in a curtailed future?

At any rate, I don't ask heart of the matter questions. And life goes on, quietly, uneventfully, and for the most part, pleasantly.

The difference between her late-stage breast cancer and her sisters' was enormous. There seemed to be a never-ending supply of treatments. Even when it looked as if she were at the end of the line, up popped a new, experimental one. This time it was hormones. Her sisters' hormone treatments had been harrowing; hers had few side effects. Indeed, this Tamoxifen, one day she confided to me, was terrific. She'd never had such an innocuous treatment. She watched the younger women enter the clinic, remembered herself at their age, knowing they'd be bombarded with helpers, information, helplines, and names and addresses of other cancer patients willing to talk to them. She no longer identified with them. Though she did with the women she met at radiation, waiting around at the hospital pharmacy, getting their blood drawn. They compared symptoms dispassionately but kindly. This was just a bit more than a decade after Mary's death.

But still the cancer grew, lumps appearing most worryingly on her head and neck, perilously near her brain and spine. This time

I was not restrained: I asked exactly what she wished I wouldn't. (In the meantime, my brothers, myself, the doctors and some of my mother's closest friends had been engaging in a buzz of phone consultations. What should we prepare for? How much can she manage by herself? How would she be nursed if she needed nursing at home?) I was in Chicago, and in October I'd be even further away, back in England – in Cambridge, where Stephen had been offered a job. Moreover, because I'd been infertile again, that July I was having surgery, a tubal reconstruction, requiring at least a month's convalescence. Rick and Stephanie would be moving in June to Boston, where he would be taking the requisite revision course for the Massachusetts Bar exam to sit that September. Mark was contracted to take a group of kids that summer on an Outward Bound-type expedition. Gene and Cathy were expecting their second baby at the end of June. There were going to be long periods when we'd be no use to her, and I wanted to figure out how to help. My mother refused to discuss it. 'I'll be fine, and I don't want you meddling,' she said, gently pushing me away.

Panicked, I appealed to her doctors. They said, 'Your mother is a remarkably tough woman. She's made it this far by believing she can manage anything. Let her believe that now. If she can't, put something quietly in place.' Which is what I did: I made nine copies of her house keys, drew up a rota for her friends to look in on her, distributed the keys, the rota and each other's phone numbers, and never told my mother.

April 20, 1984:
Today I had a radiation treatment. It is not painful. In some ways it's pleasant. For this series, I have to lie on my stomach on a hard table, my face sunk into a hole of a rubber pillow, so that my shoulder and nape (the focus of the bolts) are flat. It is not comfortable, but the sessions are short and what makes it bearable is that I can't see the machinery, which is menacing in its massiveness and technical prowess. As the technicians adjust the mechanism, bringing what looks like a James Bond pulverizer

ever closer, the patient, who has been positioned precisely and admonished not to move, is certain the machine is about to run amok. It is drunk with power, cannot be checked in its inexorable descent, determined not to irradiate but to crush the cancer.

Lying on my stomach I am spared this spectacle and apprehension. What is pleasant, for me anyway, is the knowledge that the treatments will stop the pain. The treatment itself, except for the relatively uncomfortable position required, is restful. The machine hums softly. It reminds me of summer background sounds or a warm kitchen with the low comforting buzz of peaceful activity. Odd that this huge machine, shaped like a monster, a masterpiece of cold modern technology, should speak in human tones of a solicitous mother or a harmless creature of nature.

In the past I've had treatments directed to areas where I've had considerable pain and the results of radiation have been swift and positive. The pain miraculously vanished. I look forward to similar relief this time.

I have many areas that could use radiation, but the main sources of pain are the head and neck. Since radiation treatments have to be rationed, only that area is being treated. The effect has not been instantaneous. Of course, I've just had one treatment, so I'll have to be patient . . .

Usually the pain comes during the night and awakens me. The complication in recent weeks has been an adverse reaction to pain-killers. That has been very disconcerting. Now I am less calm and confident about how I will be able to handle the future. I used to reassure myself that it will not be necessary to bear excessive pain. Modern medicine provides appropriate drugs and compassionate doctors prescribe them as needed. The main obstacle, I thought, was my own stubbornness, an obsolete bravery and misplaced stoicism. If I am no longer a good reactor, if my body is rebelling and betraying me and is no longer willing to cooperate with me and modern science, then where will I be? A helpless victim of pain, no longer convinced that stoicism is admirable and that pain is the price paid for pleasure, like having a baby as a reward for struggle.

These past few weeks I've become totally preoccupied with my body: what it is doing now, its quirks, malfunctions, breakdowns. I am constantly on the alert, awaiting a signal or another siege. My friend scoffs at her husband for being oblivious of his body. It's attached to him, he admits, but it's really a separate entity, and as far as he's concerned it has to watch out for itself. He's right. The encroachments and demands the body makes are cruel and demeaning. Such overweening attention robs us of our personality. It makes people very dull. All I talk about, to the children and my friends, are my pains, my symptoms and what the body did to me today . . .

May 8:
I've been in the hospital for the past four days, for tests and procedures, but little has been done. Scans have been scheduled and then canceled. Physically, I am feeling better, probably as a result of enforced rest. At home I exert myself, but here I lie in bed most of the time and my back naturally feels much better. That may not be a permanent cure but as long as I lie in bed it gives me no discomfort. Some of the unpleasant effects of radiation are beginning to wear off. I'm having less trouble swallowing and I think my tastebuds are returning, which is probably a mixed blessing with regard to hospital food. Today I tasted a black olive. The other taste that I am beginning to recognize is the chemical taste of mashed potatoes made from ersatz powders. No matter how much butter, salt, and pepper I put on, that sickening taste comes through. It's queer to eat things wondering whether they need salt or sugar, maybe lemon. I can only distinguish texture and temperature . . .

My hair is beginning to fall out where I had radiation. I'll probably get more radiation to my head and I'll lose more hair, but my main concern is that I have enough for Rick's wedding, that I look decent for that event, which is to take place two and a half weeks from now. I don't think there will be a dramatic change before that time. Perhaps this delay works in my favor in that respect . . .

I have had two roommates here, both for periodic chemotherapy treatments, both fine women, courageous, forbearing, and optimistic. So again it has to be emphasized, I am not particularly brave, as some of my friends imagine. People are brave. What a pity they have to be so much of the time.

May 14:
The latest news is not good, but I shouldn't be surprised. Of course, I knew the spread was extensive: new lumps appearing and growing noticeably daily, new discomforts, new sources of pain erupting all the time. I don't like knowing that the brain is affected. That has been my greatest fear. But the doctors say it is minimal and that radiation will very likely eradicate the problem. They give me broad assurance I can be helped; their words and manner don't convince me although I prefer kindness to brusqueness. I rely on fate's beneficence and my past experiences with a body responsive to medical procedures. At worst, if the body can't summon any more resources and gives up the struggle, I wish for a swift and easy end. That seems reasonable and hardly unusual. But maybe it isn't. No doubt, it's what anyone wants, not the modest supplicants but the most demanding and greediest of us . . .

Illness, especially serious illness, is . . . a leveller. When I went down for radiation this morning, I saw a woman in a wheelchair, her face marked up for treatment, waiting to be returned to her room. We talked a little; she seemed a bit dazed – as well she should have been, having suddenly and violently been newly struck by her illness – and I discovered she was the mother of a high-school friend of Rick. I had met her once before; she's attractive and chic, and I remembered her not fondly for having said something critical of Rick. It was dumb and insensitive and totally inappropriate, and naturally I would not forgive her. This morning she was my friend and I was hers. Three years after a mastectomy, without any clues of metastasis she suddenly became incoherent and lost her memory. Cancer cells were in the brain and within a day or two – I was surprised at the speed of diagnosis and the start of therapy – she was now undergoing treatment and evidently responding well. She remembered meeting me (probably not her comments; they hadn't meant anything to her at the time and less now, of course) and seemed perfectly normal, lucid, but clearly shaken by the events. She was a nice woman, no harm in her, no self-pity, no bitterness.

I see this kind of strength of character all around me. My friends think I am strong and brave, a non-complainer. I am usual, run of the mill. Most of the people I run into: roommates, clinic members, are like me. We take what has been handed to us (what's the point of wasting energy with grumbling and rage?); we follow orders because maybe the doctors know what they're doing, and if we're among the lucky ones we'll come out of it. There's nothing remarkable about any of us. It's a common quality: a refusal to surrender, a drive to go on, to believe in the efficacy of medicine. Clearly they have chosen: life is preferable to death. People can interpret that outlook differently: tenacity, courage, doggedness or wilful delusion. Those unfamiliar as yet with these challenges think it's bravery. Perhaps. But it's far from exceptional . . .

That was her last entry.

She went to Rick's wedding, her hair mostly intact, if now completely white, wearing an elegant blue linen dress, pearls, a bracelet of gold interwoven leaves, earrings of delicate, concentric gold circles, each piece of jewellery a gift from my father, and the diamond ring my father had bought her after they'd been married thirty-three years. Their fifteenth, twentieth and thirtieth anniversaries had passed without fuss. Ceremony wasn't his strong suit. One night as she served dinner he'd flourished a glittery circle from a snapping box. 'Now for the next thirty-three,' and he grinned at her stunned delight. Typically the box was second-hand, 'Tiffany's', it read, but that fooled no one. He'd got it for her wholesale.

The next day she was combing her hair, and out it came in thick clumps; within minutes she was half bald. I was upstairs with Adam and she screamed to me: 'Janet! My hair!' I grabbed Adam and leaped down the stairs. She was standing in the doorway of her bedroom, holding a fistful of hair. She pulled the comb through again. A large pink patch showed where the comb had been. Some Lou-like angel must have decided a bald mother-of-the-bridegroom would have been in bad taste.

She bought a wig, and we got used to her in it. One day Adam toddled in early to cuddle next to her in bed. He had surprised her and she was without her wig. 'Grandma,' he cried, 'you forgot your hair.' It became her joke. 'I forgot my hair,' she'd note as she met her bald self in the mirror. And then her hair, after the treatments ended, began to grow back, as if signalling she meant to carry on.

At the beginning of August her pain deepened. She underwent intensive radiation and surrendered to her bed. The rota sprang to life – her friends fell into step like a well-drilled troop, delivering food, checking up, reporting to me in Chicago and Gene in New York. Meanwhile, in Chicago, I recovered from my fertility surgery. After packing up our flat I was to go to Great Neck on September 1 for a month before joining Stephen in Cambridge. Gene, now an assistant district attorney and with a new baby and a five-year-old, lived an hour away but diligently stayed at weekends. Rick and Mark were away as planned. My mother's August was a blur of pain transmuting into oblivion from the painkillers.

And then, at the end of the month, she rose like Lazarus. What a model patient she was! What an advertisement for the doctors' arsenal! Our last Great Neck September was blessed: she was almost pain-free. In the balmy breezes off Long Island Sound it passed like a pleasant holiday, easy and affectionate. We kept strictly at bay all talk of my leaving and her dying. At the airport, saying goodbye, both surfaced. So in defence we planned my return, the coming January.

But at the beginning of October the pain re-emerged. She was given a new regime of medication. This time the doctors experienced her heretofore hidden steely side. She *would* go to

Cambridge and Boston, despite their strong misgivings. She *would* say goodbye properly to all her children. The doctors could time her treatments to her travel schedule and provide emergency instructions, couldn't they?

In mid-October, armed with her medicine, exhausted and irritable, she arrived in England. The visit began unpromisingly. Missing my work, friends and the rhythms of my life in Chicago, worried and unhappy away from her, I was quite hopeless at affecting joy. She spotted the drained energy and anxiety behind my smiles. We both strained to behave well and the very effort itself drained the visit of the peace it was meant to bring. By the third day I at last managed to focus on the enormous significance of this visit, remembering a conversation I'd had with my cousin Joyce, one of the triplets, a few weeks earlier. 'Janet,' she'd warned when I complained that I wished my mother would postpone her visit, as I doubted my ability to hide my growing depression, 'there's no real choice here. Try to honour that.' Who knew where the mending had started? Maybe I could at last honour her effort because she'd mastered her mood, made more extreme by jet lag, or maybe I did so first and she became more mellow. Whatever. We succeeded. She became again her gracious self, and I tried to respect her delicately wrought defences.

It was clear this was her last visit to me. I was back in England following what I knew, but didn't yet feel, had been good advice from her. The previous summer she, Adam and I had stayed at a friend's on Martha's Vineyard, while Stephen was visiting Cambridge. I'd put the phone down after he'd phoned with his news and went to join her on the shaded deck. Of course he was thrilled. And of course he'd said, 'We'll only go if you agree,' and of course we'd had that conversation – about whether I could go or he should stay, and in whichever direction, what possible forms our careers, our family lives, our finances and our futures might take – about a thousand times. I had hoped it would stay theoretical for as long as possible. My mother had heard both my end of the phone call and the snuffling following my tears. On the chaise lounge she stared ahead. 'Go, Janet,' she said, clearly, without rancour. 'You can't stay for me. I'm not going to be around for ever. And you know Stephen would be happier there.' She was right. Chicago had never suited him. It had been uncomfortable to hear her wryly and dispassionately voice her condition. But voicing it had made decisions around it possible.

Despite the short time allotted by her doctors for travelling, despite the wonderful time we did succeed in sharing in the end, my mother insisted on spending her two final days in London on her own, to visit museums and attend a concert. I was hurt. I wanted every last minute with her. 'No, Janet,' she explained, unyielding, when I begged her either to stay on in Cambridge or to let me join her in London. 'I want to be on my own.' I felt as if she were literally peeling me off her, like a clinging baby. But I guess she needed to be on her own to say goodbye to that wider world which had always drawn her.

On her last night in Cambridge she lay on her bed and cuddled me as I wept at her leaving. She had not held me like this for years. And then out of nowhere she whispered, 'I know you think I've always preferred the boys,' and she stroked my hair as if I were small again.

I didn't move; before she spoke I'd been transported back to the apartment in Manhattan, where she was telling me soft stories and crooning broken bits of show tunes, next to me in my narrow bed. But her words shocked me right back to Cambridge. Till she uttered them they'd never occurred to me. They were strange and unsettling. Briefly they seemed profoundly true, as if she'd spoken the secret that could only be uttered at the point of death. But they didn't fit. They were wrong . . . yet something about them was right. I realised afterwards – though I wish I'd known it then and could have set her right – that in them was a kernel of truth, but a far different one. My mother must have concluded that was how I'd felt: my fighting and opposition must have seemed to her like resentment, like a manifestation of a conclusion on my part that she'd given me a harder time than she'd given them because it stemmed from her loving me less. But I'd never thought that once. Never. I knew her passion for me came out differently from her passion for them. Just as I did not love her any less than I loved my father, though, in comparison, he and I had had an easy, almost friction-free relationship.

She went on. 'But I haven't. I have loved you as passionately as I've loved them. I love you so very, very much.' 'I know that, Mom,' I told her and hugged her hard. Everything was healed then. Absolutely everything.

She flew home, rested for a week, then took the train up to Boston, where she killed two birds with one stone: she visited Rick and Stephanie in their new house, and stayed with Phyllis and Irvin. Then she got on the train, went home and to bed.

There was one last thing to do: Thanksgiving was in a week; she wanted one last Thanksgiving. Everyone came: my brothers and their spouses, and Mark and his fiancée, Gene's baby Luke, born a month after Rick's wedding, Zack, Stephanie's parents and the triplets and Nina.

The next week, bed became the only place for her. Mark, by then a law student in the city, moved back to Great Neck. By December 22 the pain was unending. She became a patient of the hospice home-care team. Morphine was ordered.

Rick and Mark called me in England. Adam's first English birthday party (he was to turn three on Christmas Eve) was under way. We'd rented videos, strung streamers and balloons, and were cutting a big square chocolate cake decorated like a birthday present, the furthest reach of my cake-making talent, when the phone rang. Amid the festivities I heard Rick telling me firmly, 'Now. Come now.' We were leaving for Bath in two days, spending Adam's birthday and Christmas in England with his English grandmother and relatives. I had bought a ticket to go to New York in January. I didn't respond, stymied by the stupidest things. How would I return our rented video machine when I needed December 23 in Cambridge to do it? What was I to do with my non-refundable plane ticket? Understandably Rick became impatient. 'You don't have time to waste. Just get here,' he cried in exasperation. Shamed, I took in what he meant.

I asked if my mother could speak. Out of a rush of background whispers and prompts her very weak voice emerged. Her speech was slurred. She could hear the comforting sounds of small children squealing. I told her it was Adam's birthday party. We'd had *Mary Poppins* on, I reported brightly, trying to stir nostalgia for my own childhood. She sighed, 'Uh-huh,' politely. She was lost – neither Adam nor I could bring her back.

I told her Adam and I would be there as soon as I could get a flight; for various reasons Stephen wouldn't come. 'Can he come to the phone?' she asked.

'I have come to love you,' she told him, the words arriving slowly, halted by sheer effort, 'as well as respect you. Be good to Janet. Thank you.' As her illness had grown grave, and during her widowhood, Stephen's respect for her had overtaken his wariness of her changeability and sharp tongue. He wears his lack of sentimentality like a badge, next to his reserve. I heard him reply, 'It's been an honour knowing you, Regina. Thank you, too.'

My mother, unlike her sisters, was managing her death. Because of the hospice home-care team she could say farewells, heal wounds, and determine how to die.

I flew back with Adam on Boxing Day, the first day I could get a flight. My brothers and I, their partners, our cousins and her many friends kept a bedside vigil for a week. We read poems to her, including her own. In her room I found another journal she'd kept, this one from a trip she'd made with my father, Rick and Mark to Britain in 1965. I started to read it to her; it became like a chant. It brought her back, my father back, our family in its younger days. Over the days, as I read, she slipped more and more into sleep. In her last week she was never without us, her children, which is how she had always wanted it to be.

My mother died, at home in Great Neck, in the small hours of January 4, 1985. It was twenty-one years almost to the day from her first operation. There never was a Part II to her *Endings*.

PART III

DECISION

13
Facing Facts

If I hadn't had to be in America to help tidy and settle the remains of my parents' lives I would have stayed away. America was where I'd expected death to strike for so long that all I wanted to do was to turn my back on it.

It was icy, slushy, dark winter in Manhattan when we buried her. For two weeks I traipsed around in a fog of grief, joining my brothers in meetings with lawyers, estate agents and accountants, feeling as if the top had gone off my life, as if till then I'd been protected by an invisible layer above me which had now vanished. Stephen flew over for the funeral and took Adam back to Cambridge, to free me for the details and legalities of the ending of my parents' lives. When I returned to England the fog had transmuted into a constant ache, a rhythmic back and forth of pain as if it were physically inside me. When I thought of New York the icy, foggy state came sharply back.

Exactly one month after my mother's death, I found out I was pregnant. I cried not just in joy, but with bitter irony. This long-awaited birth would not reverberate in the hearts of either parent. It would seem like the sound of one hand clapping – and the hand wouldn't be my mother's.

A little over a year later I returned with tiny Daniel for a memorial reading of her poetry, organised by a group of her friends and given at the Great Neck Library. My grief was renewed. Then I did turn my back on America; I would plant myself firmly in Cambridge. I would try living without half listening for the phone to rouse me with terrible news, without my heart trained on Great Neck and the house, which we hadn't yet put on the market, and its emptiness. In this period I read my mother's journal and reread her poems. Doing so was a ritual to mutate her into a force inside me, to keep her voice with me. It has worked. I came to feel her as a dispersed presence inside me as I began to build a life in England. Eventually I knew I could return to New York without fearing I'd be washed away in a fresh wave of grief. For I've continued to keep her inside, even if I can no longer distinctly hear her actual, surprisingly girlish, small voice. She quietly observes me. She watches me in the same spirit she came to in the end, the same one she'd had in my childhood. She watches, that is, with a kind and tender eye.

Lexington, Massachusetts, August 1991

The English family (that's Daniel, almost six, Adam, nearing ten, Stephen and I) were back in America for the summer. The whole American family had got together, this time for a family wedding, and we were house-swapping in Lexington, a leafy, pretty suburb of Boston, where Rick and Stephanie and their son lived. It was a good base for my family to come to stay and for hopping up and around the east coast visiting friends and beaches.

In 1989 we began what became a pattern: every other summer we'd go to the north-east coast of America. We were fortunate to be able to take large chunks of summers here, living as we did primarily by a university calendar. Since we'd moved I'd built up a practice as a psychotherapist as well as becoming a senior research associate and part-time affiliated lecturer at the University of Cambridge in the Centre for Family Research. I'd also begun to do some occasional journalism and broadcasting. My research and teaching were on relationships – and within a year I had published my first book, co-written with Martin Richards, the head of the Centre. It was a study of extra-marital affairs. My mother would have loved to see it, hold it in her hands, see my photo on the inside cover. It was one of the ways I'd had to adjust to her death: the ambitions she'd had for me were now entirely my own. My achievements could not be reflected in pleasure in her eyes.

I was sunbathing with my triplet cousins on the beach at what Daniel called (and so now we all did) the 'reserpool', Lexington's reservoir, where the children were swimming. My cousin Nina was there, too. Nina does not resemble the rest of us; she has a different body type and colouring. But the triplets and I could be sisters. Given that they are about ten years older than I, they looked how I was likely to look like a decade hence. My mother, through much of her fifties and early sixties had become stretched and puffed by steroids. I observed their skins and bodies. I wouldn't be bad in ten years. They looked great. We seemed to have good skin, as a family – it didn't show our age. And their bodies were young, too. My mother had never made it to their age with breasts. Their mother never made it at all. So their bodies became my map for ageing.

Ever since I'd been diagnosed with endometriosis I'd nursed a possibly hare-brained theory that my particular hormonal imbalance, which is what may promote endometriosis, was a surfeit of oestrogen, and that that's what explained my young-looking skin. I wondered if that were true for them, too. I didn't ask. There were great walls of silence among the surviving women in our family, and one of them surrounded our bodies. Except our breasts. We didn't easily say the word 'breast' to each other, we gestured to our own as we asked the ritual question, 'Have you gone for your, you know, check-up?' We'd done that, this time. All checked out. I did not mention the operation.

A few years earlier, shortly after my mother died, Joyce had come to visit Cambridge en route to a business meeting in the Netherlands. I was pushing Daniel in the pushchair, Adam holding on to it, as we all walked into town. Joyce and I had already done our ceremonial gesturing and asking about check-ups. As we walked I asked, 'Have you thought about the operation?' Joyce was then in her late forties. She'd never had children. I was the only daughter of the Smith girls to have children and I'd finished having mine. She might lead the way.

'Yes,' she said, tight-lipped. 'It's not for me. I couldn't do it.'

I was startled at her clarity. 'Why? I mean, how can you dismiss it so totally?'

'I just couldn't face the surgery. I'm a coward about things like that, I guess.'

'But if it's the thing that will make you live—' I began, but she cut me off.

She gestured to the pushchair and then to Adam, walking alongside. 'That's why *you* should do it, Janet. I don't have that same need. I don't have that sort of reason.'

We walked on in silence. I hadn't raised the subject since then.

So there we were on the beach, in 1991, all whole-breasted and almost all past the age our mothers were when first diagnosed (the triplets were way past, I was creeping up). It was beginning to look as if our mothers' disease might have been a fluke of their generation. After all, as the geneogram showed, we knew no other women on our grandmother's side with breast cancer.

The explosion of interest in cancer in general had continued through the 1980s. There had been important research on the epidemiology of breast and other cancers, with funds for clinical and research development helped along by breast cancer lobby groups. Centres for 'alternative' complementary treatment had emerged on both sides of the Atlantic. As one result, people had become more aware of cancer and what caused it. They knew there were areas in which cancers seemed to cluster. In fact, northern New Jersey was now being referred to as a 'cancer belt', because of the density of cancers there.

So we daughters of breast cancer mothers were thinking: maybe not us. Maybe our mothers' deaths were a fluke of their Paterson childhood. Maybe their cancers were entirely environmentally caused. Maybe no faulty genes were involved at all. As we grew older and nothing affected anyone in our generation, it was a hypothesis that competed strongly with our original one.

I lay back in the hot sun. I wore a modest two-piece. My body hadn't changed all that much over my life – I was roughly the same size and weight I'd been in my teens. I tried not to think too much about my breasts, though I'd loved breastfeeding in a way that had surprised me. Once, when my mother was visiting in Chicago, she'd walked in while I was breastfeeding Adam. She stood, stopped in her tracks by the image before her. For a nanosecond the sublime connection between me and my baby and the utter peace it brought wavered. Then like a whisper it settled, and as it did my mother's silent watchfulness became a partner in the bond: mother and child and mother and child. Adam paused in his sucking and my mother said, 'I love to watch you.' I had loved, also, the feel of my breasts in lovemaking. And I'd liked their shape. I had taken it for granted that the shape of me would, for the most part, persist.

Those breasts encased in the stretchy red fabric of the bathing suit had played their part in giving me pleasure, both intense and ordinary. Twice a year I had to go into the clinic of 'high-risk women', and have my palpation by the breast specialist at Addenbrooke's Hospital. Once a year I went to the radiology clinic and got my mammogram done. Following each I would tear open the letter from the specialist: 'On examination your breasts are satisfactory', or 'The mammography records no changes of note.' Only on those occasions when the potential danger of my breasts was sharply focused and I had to consider them as things apart did I think, 'These may be bad things. I should concentrate on what that doctor said in Chicago. I've had my babies. I should think about – just consider – having them off.'

Mostly, I hadn't thought much about it. Then, in August 1991, I started thinking I might never have to. It might well have been New Jersey's fault all along.

Cambridge, September 1991

We were back now, slowly losing our jet lag. Daniel was in Year 1, no longer even in the baby class at school. Back in a routine: Stephen walked the children down the road to the local primary school, and I either saw clients straight away or turned to my computer, writing chapters of my book. After trips to America it usually took about two weeks until I felt at home again in England, with American life, its news, its politics, the details and dramas of my friends and relatives, fading away. On this day I tapped out the words of one of the interviewees for my book, and Lexington, New York, Cape Cod, Martha's Vineyard were back in a parallel world. It was early afternoon. The phone rang and I cursed it for breaking my concentration. It was Joyce, from New Jersey.

She sounded small and weak. She was phoning, she said, with 'bad news'. There was no one left waiting to die. The years of being so afraid of the phone's ring with its faraway voice setting off worry or grief had gone. I'd got accustomed to feeling safe. But I immediately knew what she meant. The alarm found its old home in the pit of my stomach. For we spoke in immediately decipherable codes: 'bad news' was *the* bad news we had been waiting to hear, the news whose absence had made us feel lucky up to now. We'd just been waiting to hear which one would be struck first.

I listened, knowing what she was going to confirm, but I found myself still disbelieving it. Hadn't we all reassured each other just a few weeks ago? But she told me that although she had recently had a mammogram – like me she had one once a year and her recent one had 'shown no changes of note' – for a few months she had been experiencing a painful pressure in her chest (like my mother, like me, she had kept the rest of us in the dark lest anxiety and hysteria mount). She couldn't feel anything like a lump, and her internist (the nearest US equivalent to a GP) had dismissed her. Joyce was loath to create a fuss but the pain did not go away. In this instance it was lucky that she was, by nature, a worrier; it drove her to insist on a further consultation. Finally, the week after our reunion in Lexington she visited a breast specialist. He'd examined her, listened, noted her family history, and immediately admitted her to hospital.

She was diagnosed with a malignant lump. It was neither invasive nor aggressive. She was about to undergo radiation. She was optimistic: 'We're lucky, Janet. I don't want you to worry. Because we have what we have – our legacy – we know to catch things fast. I did. I'm going to be fine. I know I am.'

I told her I was glad to hear she had had such a good prognosis.

She was not crying, so I knew I'd better not. I pretended I, too, thought she was very lucky.

And, in fact, she was. We daughters of the Smith girls were at the cutting edge of progress in treating and even curing breast cancer. Joyce actually did have a chance of cure. She had been monitored closely. Despite the failure of the main prong in our monitoring programme, mammograms, it was likely that her cancer was caught early. She had been referred as soon as possible to a breast specialist, resulting in faster, more expert decisions about treatment. That should mean that she had a good chance of catching her cancer so early that micrometastases from it hadn't infiltrated her blood stream. By now most people knew that some breast cancers can be cured if they are detected early enough. So women who had reason to fear breast cancer, or who had known sufferers, were being persistent, asking for early screening, diagnosis and treatment. Joyce had come that much further than her mother, Aunt Mary and even my mother.

Even though there would be a waiting period until in theory she could believe her cancer was unlikely to return – still the magic five years – Joyce was being assured that, given the early stage of her tumour's growth and its low-grade aggressiveness, she was likely to be cured. I did not hide from her the fact that I thought it was awful – we both knew it was – but I did hide the fact that I felt as if my house of cards was collapsing. I had the sick feeling familiar from when my mother reported her 'bad news' each time, and the time when she'd announced the 'bad news' about Aunt Mary.

I got off the telephone and as the early afternoon sunshine streamed through the windows of my study, far away from New Jersey, I sobbed. It was back, and it had got Joyce. Now I knew it wasn't just Paterson's environment.

14
Decision

My breasts gradually became my enemies. When Joyce's 'bad news' came I was well into the kind of middle-aged allure – I hoped – better described as dignified-and-attractive than as cute-and-sexy. I could, in theory, consider my breasts somewhat beside the point. They'd fed my babies, they'd helped attract men, they'd given me pleasure. Apart from a general desire to avoid further surgery, two reasons for keeping them remained: aesthetic and erotic. In theory, we could be creative about those. I could wear different styles, try different lovemaking.

Each time I visited my breast consultant the possibility of surgery arose. Though he never explicitly asked, 'How about the bilateral mastectomy, then?', there was a ritual ending to all our consultations: a summary of the facts as they stood at that point: 'So you have chosen the more conservative method of prevention, then – palpation and mammography – a perfectly safe option.' Then he dismissed me, put down my file, and that was it for the next six months, apart from written confirmation to that effect. 'Chosen' was inaccurate. It was a default option. I shied away from 'choosing'. Rather, my strategy consisted of blindly hoping that, as I moved up and past my mother's and aunts' ages at first diagnoses, and as my cousins also apparently avoided the doomed path, I wouldn't have to decide. So 'choice' rather dignified my fumbling along an undetermined route, imagining as I did a happier, luckier outcome, breasts intact, cancer-free. It really was wishful thinking.

Nevertheless, I had been making unconscious preparations for another journey. I had been distancing myself from pleasure derived from my breasts. I'd done so ever since I had reached the ominous age of forty, with all its implications for the end of fertility and the lengthening of the odds for breast cancer. At forty, my mother's age at first diagnosis (forty-three) loomed into view. Moreover, the incidence of breast cancer was certainly rising among women in their forties and fifties. I no longer wanted breasts to be a focus in lovemaking. I had also begun to dislike confronting other women's cleavages or naked breasts. I looked away from photo-spreads which sprang them at me and found myself irritated when leafing through fashion magazines at the growing trend among designers for transparency and peekaboo breasts. I preferred boyish, flat-chested figures – Kate Moss most definitely over Pamela Anderson – and came to believe that breasts, as a GP friend of mine remarked, are really very silly-looking things. 'You ought to see some of the ones I've examined,' she laughed. 'Pretty ones are like gold dust.' My observations from topless beaches on which I'd sunbathed, from Portugal to Greece to Martha's Vineyard, bore her out. Aesthetically I began to find breasts, in general, a turn-off.

But wrenching myself from an attachment to their erotic pleasures was harder. In time, as I came to dislike breasts in general, and mine in particular, that went, too. To help me think through my decision, Rick and Stephanie told me about two American friends of theirs who had had preventative mastectomies. One was a woman I'd known from Great Neck, who had been a friend of Gene's. Her mother had died when she was a girl; I remembered both her mother's death and hearing that her mother's sister had died soon afterwards. It took me two years to talk to the two survivors. To do so represented a major step towards my decision. If I talked to them I was facing it. I knew I wouldn't retreat from what they'd tell me, and I knew that what they'd tell me was that they did not regret their surgery. They were living proof of the good sense of having it. When I did eventually talk to them, they each settled the sex question, at least in theory. 'There are lots of different ways to feel loved and to make love,' one of them remarked. 'You just learn new ones,' the other reassured me.

In the end, I gave them up, those breasts, in my heart before I did in reality. They became untouchable. I had decided they would *not* give me pleasure.

Cambridge, February 1992

I was again in a doctor's waiting area. I had adapted to British clinics, in which I was not perceived as the valued customer I would have been in pay-as-you-use US medicine. After each visit I waited in the queue and was given a follow-up appointment, more at the clinic's convenience than my own. (My American friends and relatives found this primitive: 'Why can't you say when you want to be seen?' they asked, irritated that sometimes I had to arrange my trips overseas around clinic appointments.) The plan had been to see me in September and March of each year, but one year I went off pattern, and I began to come at odd times, sometimes not really six months apart. This year I was way off for a number of reasons and it was nearly nine months since I'd last been seen. During that time I had heard about Joyce, and so I felt that the picture had changed and that this time I wouldn't follow the usual passive-patient protocol.

Usually I stripped to my waist in a little cubicle, feeling ridiculous as I waited, topless, glancing through outdated and dog-eared, hard-to-believe-there's-a-readership-for-them magazines (*Knitting Quarterly*; *East Anglia Church News*). Then the consultant and his students would arrive. He'd announce himself gruffly and ask how I'd been. I'd smile and try to be chatty to no effect and he'd then begin to palpate – feel my breasts – firmly as I looked up at the ceiling. Then I raised my arms and he palpated again, while again I avoided all eye contact. Then he'd observe the breasts, with my arms straight down at my sides, as I gazed at the wall. Finished, he'd declare, 'Fine, fine' (and then slur my name, as he had trouble with the fact that I refused to be called 'Mrs Monsell', though he knew, because Stephen had come to my first appointment, that I was married. He did not know how, nor would he try, to pronounce Reibstein, and neither of us was comfortable with him using 'Dr' as my title. And he most definitely wouldn't be calling me 'Janet'). He'd announce 'You can get dressed now', and leave, examination over.

I had never warmed to this man. I doubt he ever warmed at all. But I'd been assured he was a first-rate breast specialist so, though seething inside, I put up with what I felt to be his outdated, patronising style. In our first consultation he'd addressed most of his remarks to Stephen, recognising a fellow soul in a male scientist across the desk. I'd considered asking Stephen to attend this latest session with me, then decided against it. I was gathering information in my own slow way. I'd talk about the operation and the decision when I was ready, and not before – not even to Stephen.

Normally I dressed hurriedly and made straight for the consulting room, careful not to keep the breast surgeon waiting. He sat at a large desk, his students on small chairs flanking him, and I sat opposite, alone. He'd peer at me and end with the ritual sentence about my 'choice'. Then I'd wend my way through winding corridors to the front desk, arrange for my next appointment, and on alternate visits I was given a slip to ferry on to Radiology down the hall, where I arranged my mammography appointment.

This time, because of Joyce's news, I was going to do it differently. I was going to be more assertive, ask questions and demand referrals. I sat in a crowded room, bleakly decorated in institutional cream and devoid of pictures, with old, torn copies of *Woman's Realm* and *Mail on Sunday* supplements stashed in compartments of plywood occasional tables mixed in among the chrome and plastic sculpted chairs. Most of the other women were elderly, though there were always a few of us pre-menopausals. I was going to tell my breast consultant about Joyce. This man was punctiliously non-committal – never once did he seem to take a position that either preventative surgery or careful examination would be the better option. We had discussed preventative mastectomy only once, at my first consultation with him after I had moved from Chicago, in 1985. I was aware that, even by now, a decade after the operation had first been mentioned to me, very few women had undergone such surgery in the US, let alone in the UK. I had in the past made unemphatic requests for an appointment with a plastic surgeon to ask about reconstruction following a mastectomy. It seemed these had fallen on deaf ears, though it was also possible I had been less than clear in my requests. But this time I was resolved to push. This time I would ask firmly and definitely for a plastic surgery consultation. I wanted a number of questions answered before I committed myself to undergoing such major surgery, such a massive self-mutilation.

But today something different was happening. Although the clinics were usually crowded and I often wasn't seen promptly (it could be an hour past my scheduled appointment) this time I seemed to have been overlooked completely. I was not sure how to behave. In the US, because I was a consumer of medical expertise, I could legitimately cause a ruckus ('What do you mean he can't see me for another two hours? I will refuse to pay. I'm a working woman. I have a life, you know'). I sat feeling stupidly meek and sure I was getting something wrong. I was alternately sure I ought to complain and sure I should sit tight. I did nothing. I still felt enough of a foreigner not to want to embarrass everyone by doing the wrong thing in a noticeable American accent.

Finally I noted with alarm it was almost lunchtime and the end of the clinic was near. I'd let it go too far, and by then I was enraged. I marched up to the desk, and tried to moderate my fury, masking it in extreme courtesy: strange, but it seemed that I'd been forgotten. A flurry of activity followed, in which a number of desk clerks consulted the files on their desks, then those on their computers. Then they disappeared behind closed doors, or whispered to nurses who suddenly appeared, and the whole process was repeated. I grew strangely alarmed.

Embarrassed apologies were showered on me and I was ushered (clinic was now formally over) in to see my consultant, skipping the undressing and palpation part. It seemed they could not find my chart. He was more than usually cold and clinical, clearly on the defensive, sniffing that of course my chart would be found, though unable to give an explanation of why it was mislaid. He would see me as soon as my notes were found. Another appointment would be made. I was dismissed. I felt bruised and stunned.

I left the clinic and walked to the car park in a daze. I didn't quite know why I felt like this, or how to understand what had just happened. I was vaguely aware that I would have to pull myself together, as I had to see clients in my consulting room all afternoon. I got into the car, put the key in the ignition, and suddenly collapsed into tears. The numbness had subsided. At first I panicked. I felt as if I were sliding down a long dark hole with no one to pull me out. That subsided and, ultimately, I simply felt forsaken, a complete stranger even to myself. Why was I so upset? I pulled myself together. I would be late for work. I started the car. I drove as if on automatic pilot, feeling empty and puzzled by my emptiness.

Time brought distance; later that day I got an image of myself, sitting in my car earlier, tortured and mystified. The veil lifted. I had been handing over control of the decision, of my fate and possibly of my very life to that medical team. Mislaying my chart meant they had lost the record of my body, lost the ability to track its changes, to watch over me and to tell me whether the premonitions of cancer were changing, moving, even invading. I had blithely handed over my care and control so that I could stop caring so much. So when the medical team lost my chart, I felt lost too. The consultant's iciness at our interview earlier that day had exposed the fundamental flaw in my design. I'd tried to make him my protector. He hadn't volunteered for the role. I was a medical file; I'd be tracked down in time. Panicked at the thought that my medical record was lost, I'd felt forsaken. Obviously there was no one behind the maze of medical office doors watching over me. Why should there have been? It was my body and life, not theirs. I had to be my own parent, not make them my surrogates. Only I could think, observe, monitor and, finally, take decisions. It suddenly became clear that I had to concentrate on the decision.

Lexington, Mass., November 1993

But taking control took time. I didn't even know how to talk to Stephen about it. I told him only what I knew for certain: that I was going to ask for a plastic surgery referral. I wanted him to come with me when it came through. When I knew something concrete, I could talk. But, though I was sure I wanted it, I still backed off from demanding a referral. There were so many strands to pick up and untangle. How much did I want to share with friends? Would I tell them before or after? When should or could I do it? Would I have the operation secretly, during the summer? If I did, few would ever have to know. How could I find out about how it might feel? About how I might look? What would the surgery actually be, and exactly how protected would I be if I had it? Who else had had it done – could I talk to anyone? Was this crazy? Where should I start? Though I did nothing I knew that something had shifted in me and I was edging toward some clarity.

Joyce sent me her pathology reports, which I gave to medically trained friends to interpret. They confirmed that her prognosis was good. Since doctors now knew breast cancer spreads into the bloodstream, in theory this should have meant that whole breast removal was not always indicated. Data were newly emerging that compared the effectiveness of mastectomy and lumpectomy. Because her lump was small and uninvasive, she had had a lumpectomy – by this time, research had concluded that a lumpectomy, removing only the cancerous lump, if done early enough, was as safe as removing the whole breast. Obviously, the change reflected the growing voice of women patients. It also reflected a change of consciousness in the medical profession, so that in general (my consultant, I realised late in the game, excepted) the field contained more sympathetic clinicians. They'd come to subscribe, mostly, to the view that the less invasive and disfiguring the surgery, the better psychologically for the patient. The important proviso was that the cancer not be too advanced. Joyce's cancer was at so early a stage, so unlikely to have shed micrometasteses, that she did not even need chemotherapy.

Lumpectomies are, of course, preferable. Who would want to disfigure herself if it weren't necessary? However, these outcome studies had not taken adequate account of the possibility of hereditary breast cancer. The triplets and I had been entered into genetic breast cancer studies, the triplets in Sloane-Kettering's and me at

Addenbrooke's. Both teams had our blood as well as copies of most of our aunts' and mothers' medical notes. On opposite sides of the Atlantic these teams were among those trying to discover a 'breast cancer gene' (or genes) – that is, a faulty one which predisposes a woman to develop breast cancer. Though surgeons ordinarily keep up with the latest findings, it apparently did not occur to those who treated Joyce that lumpectomy might not be as good as mastectomy in a case of potential hereditary breast cancer. Lumpectomy offers scant protection if other primary cancers are likely to arise or already exist in the same breast or the other one. As I've said, this is what happened to my mother. Despite her conviction otherwise for all those years, her first cancer was indeed cured. Her breast lopped off early, she was fine. But her other breast contained the same genetic material. Having a genetic predisposition to breast cancer means that every breast cell has the same mutation and so the same capacity to become cancerous. Eight years later lumps formed in my mother's second breast, and this time the timing wasn't good enough. Metastasis had already begun, cancer cells leaking, ever so slowly but surely, into her lymph system, then into her bloodstream, and on into neighbouring parts of her body. Cutting off her first breast hadn't been good enough.

Perhaps because she was motherless at sixteen, and perhaps shying away from making a difficult decision alone, because she had had neither a partner nor children – only her sisters, who had been as frightened as she was – Joyce, like me, had relied on her doctors. 'Lumpectomy's as good as mastectomy,' they told her. Frightened of deformation she'd complied.

Two years later I was on the east coast of America working on a programme for ABC Television which used chunks of my first book on affairs. I was visiting Rick in Boston and phoned Joyce. She sounded terrible. As soon as I heard her voice I had the sick feeling again. I knew what she was going to say before she said it. Another cancerous site in the original breast had been found, despite the most careful monitoring, the repeated mammograms, the examinations every few months. But I was confused. She was saying this new lump, in the same breast, was not secondary, or spread, from the first one, but a wholly new, primary cancer. 'It can't be,' I protested. 'They're just covering themselves. You should have been treated more aggressively.'

'I don't understand it either,' she replied, calmly but with resignation. 'But they're telling me it *is* a new cancer. I'm going to have chemotherapy.'

So I imagined another siege, another few years of focus and anxiety over the progress of another breast cancer, another few years of waiting for terrible phone calls, and the lifted then deflated hopes as each new treatment was tried, had success, then failed. I could feel the preparations begin.

Cambridge, December 1993

I went home and did some research. Joyce was right. Her second cancer was a completely new, primary site. She should have had a mastectomy. Her new cancer was like my mother's. This is why they do full preventative mastectomies, removing both breasts. If you're predisposed through heredity to have one cancerous cell – and it was a fair guess, even without any pinpointing of breast cancer genes, that Joyce was – so you can have another, and another, and another.

This time Joyce had a full mastectomy. I rang her just after her first chemotherapy session. She was in bed, and her voice was croaky and weak like a child's. 'Janet,' she implored – and as she did I heard my mother calling hoarsely to me from her bed, prostrate from injections which had made her vomit for hours after her clinic visits; I heard her whispers after her radiation, when her hair was gone, her skin mustardy – 'you don't want to go through this. Even if it saves you, even if you never get cancer again, you don't want to go through this. Have it done. Do it for your kids.'

And I realised, with crystal clarity, that I could not put my children through what I had endured, even should I survive. I could not bequeath them a memory of my vomiting; of my becoming bald, yellow and bedridden; of my becoming so twisted by thoughts of my own death that I would begin to hate my husband for bearing witness to my scarred body and the diminishing hope of survival; of my lurching from surgery to surgery, unsure whether this time I would be given a longer lease on life or would just endure more sickness and insecurity. I would not give my children what my mother's cancer gave me.

Lexington, October 1995

I was visiting Rick and Stephanie. I had made my decision, but it was not too late to recant. In six weeks I would enter Addenbrooke's Hospital. The previous year I had at last had my plastic surgery consultation, as well as a few sessions with my excellent, sympathetic GP, and one last one with my breast specialist, who would discharge me from his clinic after my operation. We had said goodbye, after a decade of twice-yearly brief encounters, with no feeling expressed. 'You have chosen the course of surgery. You will be in excellent hands. I wish you luck,' he announced in his clipped manner, and nodded at me in acknowledgement of my dismissal. I walked away relieved, thinking, maybe unfairly, 'And no thanks to you.' By his own conservative medical standards his treatment of me could not be faulted. But from my perspective, he had been the only glitch in my progress, a throwback to the generation that had treated Fannie. I had had the misfortune to land in his clinic, but the good fortune to be articulate, knowledgeable, and demanding in my health care. Most of his other patients were probably not so privileged. But he was near retirement. His kind was passing.

In late spring 1994 Stephen and I saw the plastic surgeon. It was very important that Stephen came. As he asked questions I felt that this was something we were doing together, a decision we were both taking. If my body did become grotesque he would be as prepared for it as I would be, at least. In fact, he was more prepared than I was. I hadn't believed his deadpan protests that it really, really didn't matter to him what eventual shape my breasts might take – he'd take them or, literally, leave them. They're gone, so what? Big deal, he'd said. He'd sounded outrageous then, but now, as I listened to him ask his questions, I was beginning to think he might eventually mean it.

The surgeon explained the operation and also my choices, which ranged from a radical mastectomy, of the sort Aunt Fannie had had, which no one performed any more – so 'choice' is not really the right word – to a subcutaneous mastectomy, in which about 10 per cent of the breast tissue remained, including nipples and some fatty tissue, the 'tails' extending under the armpits. This remaining tissue would round out the implants and add shape to the breast. Another option was to remove all possible breast material, but not surrounding muscle, as in the radical mastectomy. That would include nipples and extend to under the armpit, which would radically alter my appearance. Implants alone do not look as smooth and I would not have nipples. Because I am slim I could not, as some women can, have tissue taken from other, fatty parts of my body to pad my breasts. And because the instruments used in breast surgery are knives, unless you remove neighbouring tissue such as neighbouring muscles (as they used to do in radical mastectomies), a tiny percentage – it may be no more than about 1 per cent – of breast material always remains. But a full mastectomy would reduce my estimated chances of getting cancer by a further 9 per cent.

The thought of losing my nipples alarmed me. Couldn't follow-up check-ups immediately detect any cancer or precancerous growth in the nipple area anyway? In other words, wouldn't the risk of leaving 10 per cent – as opposed to only 1 per cent – be worth taking because early detection would be inevitable? The plastic surgeon, sympathetic and personable, agreed. We approached the problem scientifically: leaving 10 per cent of the breast material would reduce my risk by 90 per cent. I'd have much less risk of contracting breast cancer than most other women in the world. Setting that against a real cosmetic deformity and only a 1 per cent risk was a difficult decision.

'If I were your wife and she had this family history, what would you recommend?' asked Stephen. The surgeon replied immediately, 'I'd say have the operation. But you'd be the one undergoing the surgery.'

And which one would he recommend? The difference between

90 and 99 seemed miniscule. I could not go that extra inch: I opted for subcutaneous mastectomy. Stephen agreed. The image of breasts without proper nipples was scary. Not that we had any images to look at: at that time there were no pictures to help us decide. I shied from making myself unnecessarily ugly for both Stephen and myself.

We scheduled a follow-up consultation for the following year, and went away to think, to read and to let it gestate. But as we left it became clear I would do it, and Stephen's reaction was key. He'd asked penetrating questions during the consultation. He hadn't flinched from the sad truth that I'd be changed for ever. His attitude was 'Why should I love you less because of a change in your breasts? Especially if this is what is going to save your life – and put the fear of cancer to rest.' That fear had dogged our relationship: he'd observed its effect on us. He'd witnessed my mother's struggle.

I put my name on a waiting list, choosing a late-autumn 1995 date.

To put the finishing touch on the decision I went to Lexington. It was the peak of autumn when crimson, yellow and burnt orange leaves light hazy green hills, and Boston basked in balmy Indian summer. The main reason for my visit was to meet Stephanie's friend, another psychologist, almost exactly my age, whose own mother and sister had died of breast cancer, and who had had a preventative bilateral operation a few years ago.

A small but growing number of women in the US had chosen this operation. However, the sisterhood of prophylactic mastectomy survivors was secret. People remained revolted and confused by the notion that a woman would willingly undergo mastectomy without a definite diagnosis of breast cancer. Women with breast cancer had come out of the shadows, but what was done to them hadn't. Though breast cancer was the most common and feared disease in women, and though almost everyone knew someone who'd had it, details were sketchy. No one knew what happened during reconstruction, what took place during mammograms, what a mastectomy looked like, whether any sensation remained, or how a woman's identity or self-esteem fared after the removal of her breasts. The criteria for deciding whether to have a lumpectomy or mastectomy remained unclear. Moreover, most women didn't know they could choose from a menu of treatment options. There was a surgical choice – mastectomy or lumpectomy – and a choice in the type and timing of interventions: in some cases radiation or chemotherapy could be done first, to shrink your tumour, thus minimising the effects of surgery. In addition, most women still had not seen prostheses, did not know what a lump felt like, did not know that it was not only reasonable but advisable to see a breast specialist if they felt a lump. For there was still a cloud around breast cancer. Albeit no longer 'dirty' or the death of a woman's sexuality, it remained horrid and hidden because it might signal death.

The bad news was that more younger women were getting breast cancer – which made the widespread fear of it increasingly reasonable. The good news was that women's lives were being extended, particularly through advances in chemotherapy, and more were being cured through early detection. Early-screening campaigns had taken root. In Britain, women over fifty were routinely screened by mammogram, and women in high-risk groups at younger ages and more frequently; in the US the suggestion was annual mammograms from an earlier age. Health campaigners and women's groups were advising women to examine their breasts monthly in the middle of their menstrual cycle, to look out for changes in shape, discharge and suspicious lumps (though it was and still is the case that breast specialists are the only people you should rely on to distinguish dangerous lumps through palpation). Women talked about their breasts openly and discussed how to examine them. Magazines and newspapers ran regular articles and information boxes about breast cancer and self-examination. They published names of breast cancer campaign and support groups. Increasingly, famous women, ever younger and sexier ones such as Olivia Newton-John and Kate Jackson, announced they'd had mastectomies. They had survived. As a result more cancers were caught early and cured. There were problems, of course. Some screenings had resulted in false positives, which led in a small number of cases to women being told they had cancer when they did not. And, as with Joyce, mammography, was not wholly reliable (especially in women with particularly dense breast material, as women with the faulty breast gene seem to have).

I knew a lot more about breast cancer and mastectomies than most women did – and most women knew a lot more than my aunts had known – but I still lacked some vital information. I met Stephanie's friend at a party. We chatted politely, drinking wine, eating pretzels and making small talk. I had trouble eating. It suddenly felt real to me: a woman who'd done this was standing in front of me! She was pretty, slim and sexy. She was clearly thriving, the one who'd had the preventative surgery; her sister had died from breast cancer. That brought me up short.

She was courageous and kind, prepared to take me through steps to give me a frame for what I should expect. She could see I was adrift, even though I was already far down the road towards the operation. She understood that I needed to see what was likely to happen to me. If you have never seen a body without breasts or with breasts created from implants you have no idea what to picture, and that had been one of the most frightening aspects of the decision. (There had been no offers in Britain – presumably there was as yet no network of women willing to display their reconstructed breasts and discuss them with women like me.) I needed answers to questions like 'What will I look like?' and 'What will it feel like – if anything?' Because this was uncharted territory, I didn't even know that these were perfectly reasonable questions. Moreover, I was in not 'oncology' but 'plastic surgery'. There might have been some primitive form of advice or information in oncology, but thinking of what I was doing as 'prevention' rather than 'breast cancer' gave me tunnel vision: it didn't occur to me to turn to oncology. In retrospect, that was unfortunate.

With tremendous grace, she took me by the hand and led me through what I might look like and feel like afterwards. She asked the most helpful question for any woman at my stage: did I want to see what it looked like? I was tongue-tied by the generosity of her gesture and could only nod and stutter a thank you. Only later did I realise the profound importance of knowing what to expect.

We entered a bedroom, and she took off her shirt. To see something you have dreaded, but never actually pictured, is shocking. And I was deeply shocked. Breasts created after mastectomies are not perfect copies. Even the best – which I later realised hers were – are not quite right. If nipples are removed, their absence distorts the created breasts, no matter how convincing the implants or how small and hidden the scars. Pseudo-nipples can be created either from skin grafts (which are always too light) or from tattoos (which are too even and definite and which fade over time); neither looks precisely natural. In addition, scars cross the middle of the breasts, where the real nipples have been removed. If nipples remain, as mine were supposed to do, there are scars along the bottom of the breasts, where the tissue has been removed and the implants slipped in. And with little or no fat, the shape is not entirely convincing, either. I went white when she showed me hers; I hadn't really registered that I would indeed look different from the way I'd always looked – how could I have when there were no pictures? I'd even nurtured a fantasy my breasts would be improved – the sag lifted, the size perfect, much as my friend had suggested when this operation was first brought up in 1980. I must have registered my shock – I wish I'd been able to conceal it. She gently enquired if it was too much. 'No, no, it's fine,' I bluffed, hotly embarrassed. 'I've just never tried to visualise it before.'

And then I braved another question, one I'd been frightened, but needed, to ask: 'Can you feel anything?' No one had been able to answer this and it had been a sticking point for me: would there be any sensitivity to touch? Would the whole of my chest be a numb, unerotic zone, like a novocained mouth after dental surgery? 'No, not a whole lot,' she replied, unbothered. Clearly the human spirit triumphs over much: her response suggested that mine probably would, too. 'At first it was very strange; my daughters and I used to play a game, to gauge how much sensation I was getting. I'd close my eyes and they'd touch me and I'd have to guess whether they were touching me or not. I usually got it wrong. But it's better now.' She smiled reassuringly. I was upset to hear about the lack of feeling, but it was just as well to know beforehand. (In fact, women vary tremendously on this, and I found I did have quite a lot of sensation. It was not at all like going to the dentist.)

That night, I had vivid dreams about ugly and distended bodies, bodies mutilated. I'd tried not to think about this aspect of my decision, but now, with only six weeks till surgery, and a picture in my mind, I was having to do so. I was having to picture. My sister-in-law's friend, a pioneer of a sort, had taken me on to the next stage, readying me for the final step in altering my fate.

Before I went into hospital I told only a few people about my operation. Usually they commented, 'Oh, you're so brave.' I recoiled at the word, my mother asserting herself in me (like her cheekbones, her features, and the shape of her face, there she was in me), for she, too, denied bravery. I was surprised at my response. *She* was the strong, defiant one, not me. And there she was in me, recoiling at what was entirely inaccurate. She kept appearing, like a twin shadowing me – I'd spot her surprising me, and I'd happily figuratively embrace her. As I faced my operation my love for her leaped up a notch, as it had done after I became a mother myself ('Oh, yeah, Mom, *now* I know what you meant'). When 'brave' felt so jarring I heard a little 'Aha!' in my head – I understood what she'd meant: courage has nothing to do with it. You simply arrive at a point when you recoil from the horror of cancer – or death, in her case – and no other action seems available. You must sacrifice your body, or parts of it, in the greater cause of living. So what's the big deal? You literally give your pound(s) of flesh, for that's all they are, in order to live. There's no bravery, just a bigger fear.

Some friends were terribly shocked, even repelled, by my decision. That was much as I'd expected, but it angered me. For God's sake, what are a pair of breasts worth compared to survival? My peculiarity was brought home in the gulf between me and the repulsion. On one hand I was well inured to the idea of surgery, of having my body cut up, but on the other I had become particularly sensitive to the threat of illness and death. The gulf made me realise that I had had special knowledge and experience which set me apart. You don't realise as a child that your reality is not everyone else's. It was one reason why I told few people about my decision. It exhausted me to try to explain.

15
The Operation

Addenbrooke's Hospital, Cambridge, November 1995

I lay on the gurney shivering in my scanty hospital gown, a flimsy short-sleeved sack with loose ties at the back. Earlier that morning I had woken to a dry throat (nil by mouth since the night before) and then indulged in a final bath. Two hours later a burly man raised the aluminium tubing at the sides of my bed to form both barriers and handles and, like the transformer toys Adam and Daniel used to play with, my bed turned into a wheeled vehicle. He slid me down the corridor to the wide lift, where I avoided eye contact with fellow occupants ('Ooh, I wonder what's wrong with her?').

In the eerie quiet two images floated past. First, Sartre's bleak play *No Exit*, which I'd watched on TV as a child because my father's cousin was in it, the whole family gathered around the set to see her. It had been torturous, both inscrutable and endless; I grasped the tiny bit that now came back to me because my parents had primed me: 'It's about people waiting to get out of a room when they're really dead and in Hell but they don't know it.' Whatever that had meant to a ten-year-old, it had unnerved me – the claustrophobia, the impotence and the ignorance combined – and it was doing so now. The play's characters could not escape Hell; I couldn't escape my decision. I was here.

The second image before me was a scene from the TV series *The Twilight Zone*, in which, on a different planet, surgery was to be performed on a young woman who was grotesquely ugly. The twist was that she was perfect by earth's aesthetic standards but ugly by her own planet's. To many, perhaps most, people, in mutilating myself

I seemed cosmically misguided. On the gurney it occurred to me that I was entering simultaneously the Twilight Zone and possibly Hell. I had no doubts about my decision, though I acknowledged I was entering the unknown. First and foremost, of course, I did not know what it would be like to live without the shadow of cancer behind me.

In the room there was only me on my gurney, apart from the admitting nurse who, ignoring me, sorted through paperwork at her desk. The room was as featureless as the lounge in which the waiting souls sat morosely in *No Exit*. No paintings, no conversation distracted me. I wished the images would go away. I didn't want to remember *The Twilight Zone*. It brought back the funny old console television set, its front covered in brown fabric hiding the speakers, in our den. I could almost summon the itch from the wiry green sofa under my thighs as I watched. Remembering *No Exit* brought back my Great-Aunt Belle and Great-Uncle Ben, the actress cousin's parents, their flat on the Upper West Side and my father's extended family gathering there. Most dead, some disappeared, my childhood gone too. That made me think of my mother. For the first time fear gathered, for as I found her in my mind I found myself there, too, as her child. In an instant I was overwhelmed by my own fragility, by the realisation that in moments I was going to be cut and changed for ever. My body lying on the gurney could have been my mother's, or my aunts. They had once lain like this on gurneys, too.

I felt abandoned. I wanted my mommy! I wanted her so desperately the feeling was like a knife. I was astonished by its speed and intensity, and as it dissipated what remained was a clear desire: I did not want to be alone. The longing for my mother transmuted to wanting Stephen. I had just finished writing much of the first draft of a book and later TV series on couples called *Love Life*. Its central thesis was that everyone has an instinctive need for a secure partnership with one other. I'd just experienced emotional proof of my hypothesis. When I'd had my infertility operations I would awake in my hospital bed to find Stephen next to me, sometimes holding my hand, holding a vigil, and then, comforted, I would drift back into my drug-induced sleep. I wanted him there now. I glanced down at my taped-over wedding band. The symbol would have to do.

Much as this had been my decision, it had been shared by him. He had accompanied me to the key consultations, he had helped me think through the science of the matter. He also, I know, wished to ensure protection for me, his children and himself against the particular hell of cancer. Although like most people he could not really imagine reconstructed breasts, he knew they would not be beautiful. Nevertheless, his judgement was, like mine, unequivocal: I should have this operation. Of course I hadn't forgotten that my mother's flat chest and scars had turned my father off, or perhaps she thought they had. Whatever the cause, the upshot of her not having breasts was a deadlock in their marriage. I hadn't forgotten how ashamed she'd felt. But there were contrasts in our situations. I would be getting breasts of a sort. I also had forearmed myself to a degree, because Stephen and I had talked about it and about how it had hit my parents. Stephen had done his best to reassure me it was the me who mattered, the breasts a small if ornamental appendage to that me.

What the surgeons would do was this: with their scalpels they would scoop out 90 per cent of my breast tissue, leaving the nipples and some surrounding fatty tissue. The implants I had chosen were a type called Trilucents, made out of soya. At that time they were new, state-of-the-art implants, giving a better shape than saline ones and without the problems of leakage possibly attendant on silicone. My plastic surgeon, eager for a fine cosmetic result, had pushed for silicone, but I'd refused. The point of the operation was to eradicate anxiety, not to insert a new cause for it. Too much controversy still raged around silicone's safety. The implants would be slipped in through pockets of skin flapping from my almost emptied breasts, pockets created by slits made under the breasts. Sewn up again and healed, the incisions would eventually be barely visible. The look of the breasts would be quite even (though less smooth than before), because a slight amount of breast tissue would remain to surround and soften the implants.

While I lay on the gurney, another sort of comfort emerged: the wonder of the fact that I was there at all. It was almost magical that I was able to arrive here poised to attack the possibility of cancer, rather than submit to it. I'd arrived scarcely fifty years after Fannie had had no choice, yet until roughly the last twenty years the treatment for breast cancer had remained stuck, unchanged in principle from that of the ancients: cut, slash, burn, then wait to die. What I was about to do represented the cutting edge (literally) of what women with an inherited tendency towards breast cancer could do to prevent it. Not great, perhaps, and possibly not what would be done ten, twenty, thirty years from now, but so much better than waiting for the probable diagnosis one day. My operation also signified amazing progress for a far larger population than the relatively few of us with a wonky genetic loading.

This journey of mine was one strand in women's struggle to achieve control over the killer, breast cancer, either to tame or to defeat it. I now counted three friends who had over the years had a breast removed, each diagnosed in her thirties or early forties, one almost fifteen years ago, the others thirteen and seven years ago. All had had early screening and intervention. All remained cancer-free. In the next few years, through the network of women friends around the world, I would meet many more. All had seized control. Many – though sadly, still not most – like my three friends, will have been cured.

The boys knew. We'd been upbeat telling them: I would avoid what Grandma and the aunts they'd heard about, and Joyce, had had. They accepted it, apparently concerned only that I'd be uncomfortable from the surgery and would be in bed for a few weeks afterwards. Which was perhaps the only thing they could relate to. We brought in back-up: Stephen's mother was coming, and we had a wonderful au pair. Stephen and I hadn't shown particular anxiety, so I could believe in what I saw: the boys' uncomplicated reaction.

And we weren't particularly anxious. I'd had surgery before. I wasn't afraid of either the cut or the recovery. I wanted to get it over with and be free. In the days leading up to my personal D-Day Stephen was tender. He bought me a beautiful cloth-covered notebook and some pens, because I thought I might want to keep a journal myself. He brought home carrier bags full of novels and front-buttoning nightgowns. He would bring me home-cooked meals as soon as I could eat again.

The scrub nurses appeared. I was wheeled in for my pre-op sedation.

The following day, November 18, I woke in my hospital bed. After my surgery, the rest of the day before had passed in a haze, as I drifted in and out of a drug-induced grogginess punctuated by shooting pain, which I could ease by pushing down on a small tube which sent pain-killers through me and let me gently drift back to sleep again. Today the disabling pain of the surgery had eased, so I could think and feel with some degree of clarity. What broke through the discomfort of the bandages, the throbbing of the wounds, the unsightly bags of blood draining from them, and the tubes and posts holding fluids and medicines dripping into me, was a sweet euphoria, an unfamiliar freedom I had not known I'd been yearning for. Only with the removal of the shadow of cancer did I know how great that shadow had been, and how much of my life it had determined. I felt weightless; I fairly floated. Only the apparatus of surgery, and the drains, deep red and spilling my blood into their plastic containers (which my neighbour in the next bed dubbed her 'shopping'), kept me earthbound.

I wrote that day to one of my oldest friends: 'I'm free! I'm like everyone else – though I'm not sure what everyone else is like. Do I start watching my diet, monitoring for what – heart disease? What can I worry about now? Do I worry just as much? Is it just the kind of killer that changes? . . . I peek at life past my fifties. Here's a proposition: let's go around the world when we're seventy-five. Wow – just thought of another thing: I might have grandchildren. You know, I didn't realise that I had never imagined myself having them . . . but maybe that was normal. Who knows?'

I knew how right I had been to do this. For forty-eight hours I lived with a delicious lightness I had never before experienced.

The morning after this the doctors arrived on their rounds. My plastic surgeon, spreading his entourage of white coats and solemn faces around my bed, bustled up. Heartily he began his report. Having heard the parade of doctors rustling around the other beds on the ward, I'd feebly readied myself, combing my hair and sitting up, poised for my public exam. They'd check my blood drains and ask how the implants were feeling (crummy, actually: under the massive, bloodied bandages I could just about feel weights, like packages placed on my chest, unpropped and heavy). I wasn't expecting a report.

'You are one lucky woman,' my doctor began unexpectedly. I nodded in fierce agreement. I'd fooled the odds. I'd beaten my possible fate, cheating the Grim Reaper by being so clever. He took no notice. 'For it seems you would probably have been here soon, anyway. Yes, we were really very smart. The pathology department let us have a preliminary report,' he smiled, proudly. 'Yes, indeed. Very, very early. We got it.' I hadn't caught up with him; I was carried away both by his heartiness and by my grandiosity. What he had just implied took time to register. By then he and his students had left. Meanwhile, I'd vigorously shaken his hand and thanked him profusely. He'd departed pleased, his entourage sweeping behind him.

And then, in the emptiness behind them I grasped what he'd said. And I wondered how all of us had failed to note the obvious: that perhaps when they opened me up they would find cancer already there. But I had been going for a *preventative* operation. I was going to get that cancer before it got me. Besides, I'd been checked and checked again: I was going into this surgery clean. The 'preventative' label had marred everyone's vision. Never for a moment had it struck me or, apparently, anyone else, that I might already have had cancer.

But I had had it, in its tiniest, earliest form. It had been in me and I hadn't known it, even though I had done every possible thing to monitor my body. On both sides of the Atlantic there were fifteen years' worth of X-rays, taken once a year; on both sides master hands had palpated my breasts and experienced surgeons had given me the nod twice a year and written to tell me, each time, that I was fine.

'I am pleased to report that on examination and mammography your breasts are perfectly satisfactory,' they wrote – shrewdly qualifying their reports, I realise now, with 'on examination and mammography'. There was nothing to worry about. But at some point during those years, a disgusting, horrible thing had begun inside me, ready to eat away at me, threatening to grow. The one thing I had both dreaded and also expected had knocked on my door and announced, 'Hello. I'm here. I've come at last.' It had happened. Never mind the excellent prognosis. Never mind that I'd done the wise and lucky thing, had achieved what I'd set out to do, that is, survive. It had come to pass.

In fact, I *was* very lucky. The pathology report revealed many individual primary sites of carcinoma-in-situ, the very earliest stage of a cancer, the kind my mother had had in her womb. Like Joyce, I had had numerous ones in the same breast, and any or all of them could have grown into a malignant lump. Almost all the tissue had been removed, almost all the possibility now that any of my breast cells could do that. And because all had been 'in situ', none had spread tiny little micrometastases beyond the breast ('in situ' means all had been contained). Removing them meant cancer had been prevented.

But that explanation, while certainly an overwhelming intellectual comfort – and a validation of my actions – was a million miles away emotionally. I was shocked and confused. My earlier euphoria vanished. Would I never be free? Or was I really free, and this just a kink in the journey, a glitch which, once ironed out, would lead me back to that nice warm place?

The kink was a big one. I was put on a different path. From being a simple plastic surgery patient on a plastic surgery ward, on my discharge (check-up in two weeks, then again in three months), my label changed. Now I was an oncology patient. I remembered having gone with my mother to see her oncologist, sitting in the waiting room at North Shore Hospital, with hairless, emaciated people. What an irony. I'd been doing everything I possibly could so I would never have to enter an oncology clinic, and here I was, four weeks after my surgery, with Stephen at my side, at my first consultation with an oncologist. The plot I now found myself in was like a version of *Groundhog Day*. Just put in different faces – the protagonists in my version of the script change with each new decade – but we're back, waiting for the doctor once again.

Oncology meant I wasn't finished but, because mine was such an early stage, perhaps I wasn't really a 'cancer patient'. Post-mortem examinations of the breast tissue of elderly women showed that a relatively high percentage of them had had carcinoma-in-situ of the breast. They had not died of, nor were they diagnosed as suffering from, breast cancer. So is carcinoma-in-situ properly 'cancer'? It became important to name my condition: was it cancer, or had I caught it before it really was cancer? I needed to know what was facing me, as well as what my actions had prevented.

Carcinoma-in-situ is the very earliest stage of formation of a cancer, though cancerous development – the kind that is threatening – may take so long that it may never occur in a woman's lifetime: she may well die first, of something else. My oncologist reiterated, as he explained the basic facts to me, that many women do die with undiagnosed carcinomas-in-situ. But he also made clear that if they had lived, with time for the cells to grow, an oncologist might have encountered them as patients: in time, their 'in situ' status probably would have changed. At present I myself occupied something of a no-woman's-land. How should I think about what had happened?

He went on to talk now about me, in particular. In my case, since there were so many primary sites, and given my family history, it was almost certain that I was not going to be one of those women whose numerous in-situs remained tidily in place. Instead, mine were likely to be the growing kind. Moreover, I was pre-menopausal. I had enough oestrogen in my body still to make it likely that the oestrogen itself could stimulate the growth of at least one of those early cancerous sites – one or more of the in-situs would probably have multiplied and gone on to the next stage pre-menopausally. As I was now in my late forties, that would have meant that, as my plastic surgeon said, I would probably have been under the surgeon's knife in a short time, but at a later and more dangerous phase of cancer. I thought, fleetingly, of my notion that the particular hormonal imbalance evidenced by my endometriosis was an excess of oestrogen.

One of the most confirming aspects of this consultation was the fact that it was practically conclusive that I'd had a breast cancer gene mutation. When I had decided to have the surgery, no gene test had been commercially available. Before deciding on this surgery, I'd tried unsuccessfully through the auspices of the genetic study based in Cambridge of which I was a part to obtain an early version of the test. It might well have told me nothing useful, because it tested only for the one or two known mutations associated with breast cancer (BRCA1 and BRCA2). There were certainly other mutations waiting to be discovered in other genes, or I might have had an atypical sequence of unknown significance, in either the BRCA1 or BRCA2 genes. However, I learned in our consultation with the oncologist that it would be extremely unusual for a woman without the genetic kind of breast cancer to have more than one primary site of cancer – in my case, carcinoma-in-situ – in the same breast. With my family history, the explanation that these were cells which had genetic mutations was a much more likely one. So I didn't really need a genetic test to confirm what I'd already concluded was likely to be the case.

But therein lay the problem. Every remaining cell – the 10 per cent I'd elected to keep – would have the same genetic mutation, so I might be harbouring primary sites either now or in the future. Clearly, mammograms would be useless. Moreover, I now had breast implants, which would make monitoring more difficult. Looked at purely statistically I still had reduced my chances of breast cancer by 90 per cent and had rooted out the beginnings of the cancer I'd had. But statistics did not tell my particular story. I still had breast cells, so the chances for more cancer were still the same.

The oncologist laid out the upsetting choices. I could take Tamoxifen (the hormone therapy my mother had thrived on in her advanced stage). That might reduce the chances of any remaining breast tissue becoming cancerous (because Tamoxifen is believed to work by blocking the take-up of oestrogen by cancerous cells). Or I could have more surgery to remove 99 per cent of the remaining material (and there's the tiny rub: without scooping out neighbouring tissue some tissue remains. A scalpel cannot remove absolutely everything). Finally, I could just wait and consider my options.

A friend's mother had had a family history much like mine. At the age of forty-five, she had had a preventative mastectomy, and all that could be was sliced and removed. Five years later she was dead.

The story didn't make sense. I probed further. Was it a different cancer? 'No,' the friend maintained. 'Secondaries from breast cancer.' But how could that be? They'd removed everything, hadn't they? 'Yes,' he replied, 'so they said. But they actually hadn't removed it all. All it takes is one rogue cell, spreading, undetected.'

I recounted his story. 'He must have had it wrong,' I said, 'don't you think?' The oncologist was direct. 'No,' he replied. 'It's happened – I've heard such reports. You see, you can't actually humanly get all the breast tissue out – not unless you do a deforming operation which would remove tissue surrounding the breast tissue, including muscle and other non-breast material. No one does that any more. It leaves women deformed and in constant pain. It would be extremely unlucky, but it's possible that that story is true.' So nothing could be guaranteed. I'd have to settle for very close.

Stephen then asked the gold standard question, the one that had cleared the way for us with the plastic surgeon: 'If this were your wife, what would you recommend?' The oncologist didn't hesitate: 'I'd tell her to have another operation. But I'd tell her to do so when she felt comfortable doing it; with Tamoxifen, there is no hurry.'

His response was like crystal, sharply etching clarity on to the mass of data we'd been given. We were reeling from all we'd heard, but we shook his hand and made our way down the twists and turns of the hospital corridors, a journey which before the appointment had seemed a baffling maze. Now we slid along easily, its confusion paling in comparison to the emotional labyrinth we were in. In the muzzy rain, as if on automatic pilot, we walked towards the car. Across the street, through the black feelings, I caught sight of a colourfully dressed, boisterous woman I knew from a university women's group. I mustered every ounce of my draining energy to avoid catching her eye.

I also felt the weight of the numb packages on my chest. At that moment they were hateful. They'd betrayed me, those balloons of soya, leaden underneath the mass of bruised skin and wounds. Tears formed, of frustration, of exhaustion. We reached the car, wordless. I wept silently all the way home. Stephen made me tea. We couldn't talk yet. He went back to work, while I obsessively ruminated. Then I went across the street to my great friend Fiona, whose clear brain and immense heart were exactly what I needed, and by the time I got home again I knew what I'd do. I would wait. I would take Tamoxifen in the meantime. I would seek more opinions. I would recover, reflect. And at the bottom of my consciousness I knew that I would almost inevitably go ahead with more surgery and finish the job.

The problem, after the first few weeks, when exhaustion gave little room for contemplation, was inaction. I lay upstairs in bed recovering, those packs of implants, swollen and still numb, plopped on my chest, making sleep as much a problem as it had been during the last months of pregnancy. I couldn't sleep on my front, and if I turned on my side one implant would be crushed. I had to lie on my back, not my normal sleeping position. I tried to plot courses of action. I'd done the major thing (even though that was maybe insufficient), but now I needed to move forward, to give a form to my recovery. Instead of breaking through to a life free of anxiety, I found myself covered in a new kind of fuzziness. I still didn't know how to think about myself. I couldn't say I was cured. If I had had – or, indeed, still faced the chance of – cancer, I might have found a clue to a way forward. If I'd needed, like Joyce, further treatment, which would move me towards cure, I'd have had some way of thinking about myself, though I didn't wish for this particular scenario, it's true. But I had decided I would take Tamoxifen. Maybe that signified I had 'cancer'. On the other hand, who wanted to be a member of that, to paraphrase Kurt Cobain's mother, 'stupid club', women with breast cancer.

It wasn't clear whether or not I'd joined or even whether they'd have me.

One day, a few weeks after I had left hospital, I was walking in town and a young boy not much older than Adam was standing in front of the shopping mall, shaking a collecting tin. 'Would you like to make a contribution to support Breast Cancer Research?' he asked as I approached. He wore a pink ribbon. He proffered his tin. I grew flustered, seconds away from blurting out, 'Do you realise you're asking someone whose breasts have been chopped off? I am – or maybe I'm not – one of those women you're collecting for.' A kind of unwelcome pride filled me: a member of that club, if only a subsidiary one. But the pride wasn't about that – that would have been twisted. It was that I wanted to let that boy know I was a pioneer, that raising money was a noble cause, and I was a sterling example of the women who benefited (the Greeks were right – pride is a sin for which even at that moment I felt soiled and guilty). My toes curl as I recall the blood rush to my face as I thought, 'I was *helping* women!' 'Look at me,' I wanted to crow. 'Look at me, I'm an example of how raising funds for breast cancer helps.' I reached into my wallet and fumbled for change, feeling a solidarity with the women who were indeed victims, but at the same time conscious that I was not. I dropped the money into the tin. He was almost certainly a student. Perhaps his mother had had cancer. 'It isn't so bad, now, you know,' I wished I could say. 'Not everyone dies.' 'Good luck,' I said instead, and he smiled and thanked me warmly. Where did I fit? Was I a 'victim' who was now saved?

For much of that first year I told only a select few about what I'd done and what I'd been told by the doctors; I cannot pretend any nobility in this. So much of it was not being able to give a coherent story, especially now that the story wasn't over.

Indeed, a few months later I had visits from two of my closest American friends. I usually see them on visits to America; we are in regular phone and e-mail contact. Neither had visited England for years, yet suddenly both were making time, clearing spaces in schedules so crowded that normally each flew over England, unable to detour on their way to France, Israel, Spain or Africa, all of us too busy to meet halfway. None of us spoke of why they came now. But I knew. I reassured them with facts. I gave them as clear an account as possible of the science of my condition. But I still think they thought I had 'It'. I tried to explain my grey area. 'I'm not really ill,' I kept telling them. I burdened them with detail. Nevertheless, both were dismayed by the story. Maybe it was enough for them that the bad fairy, in whatever infant form, had knocked on my door. I hoped that that was what brought them over to me, and not a misplaced worry that a real question mark hung over my lifespan.

I'm glad they came, still a little embarrassed that they did. I felt a bit like the boy who cried 'Wolf!' OK, it was sort of breast cancer. But only a little bit.

I thought of myself as similar to other women with a cancer diagnosis in the sense that those remaining cells were potentially cancerous. That way, especially in those early weeks when I tried to plan how to cope, I could do what women like that are advised to do, how they are supposed to live. I needed to know how to live internally, how to shape myself to the things the doctors could do for me. Living with It – the curse I'd feared – is not just taking the medicine or going in for the surgery. Or waiting. As my mother's journal showed, how you thought about It – this thing both apart from but also inside you – *that* was the key to whether It would get the better of you and shape you, or whether you would shape It. To that extent, thinking I had been given a 'cancer diagnosis' helped me (though it also felt wrong). It meant I could trade on what, so I'd read, women with cancer diagnoses benefit from. It is important, first, that they feel 'in control', and, second, that they begin to lead a healthier life. For the genetics are only a piece of my family's story: the gene is simply a predisposition. Environmental and lifestyle factors, such as diet and smoking, are probably just as important in determining whether any woman, gene or no, develops breast cancer.

Lying in my bed I resolved I would give up chocolate, coffee, high-fat and processed foods – all known or suspected to be carcinogenic (the processed foods bit lasted about two seconds; self-control was one thing, complicating my life beyond the limits of my sanity was another altogether). And I would exercise. Exercise is correlated with health in general, and with not developing cancers in particular. It helps your immune system. So instead of my paltry stop-and-go efforts over the years to keep in shape, this time I would exercise regularly. All I needed was the right exercise machine. I would tell Stephen, and he would, of course, immediately praise this life-affirming step. We'd rush out to buy the machine. Up till then I had felt a renewed closeness to him, starting at that moment on the gurney, then intensified by our shared shock. His calm, reasoning attitude towards the news when it came, in turn, had calmed me.

Fired by determination, I dragged myself downstairs and sat next to him as he listened to music. Perhaps it wasn't the right moment. Perhaps I should have waited until the CD ended. Perhaps if I hadn't been so buoyed by a foolish omnipotence ('I can defeat this. I can eradicate anxiety') I would have waited. Instead, I blurted out my plan to take control over my body. Actually, whatever I'd said, however I'd presented it, the result would have been the same. He looked at me as if I were mad. For even in phrasing it that way – 'control over my body' – I was describing myself as if I had cancer, and needed to fight. Stephen, a rational pessimist but emotional optimist, had been content to take home the comforting statistical message of our oncology consultation, which said I was at the moment 90 per cent tissue-free and soon might be 99 per cent free; that women with carcinoma-in-situ may never even receive a diagnosis. Therefore, with mere carcinoma-in-situ, there was no need to give me a cancer label. To call what I'd had 'cancer' meant summoning the demons of my mother, her dark moods and suffering. And here I was behaving as if I'd been labelled as she'd been.

I am a psychotherapist to couples. I know that couples need to respect each other's defences. It's bad strategy to attack them straight on. But I could have been an astrophysicist at that moment. Just when I needed professional wisdom I reverted to primitive emotions, and sounded, I think, just like my mother had to my father. Clinging to my own new, bright defence, I attacked wholesale with precisely the words that would divide us: 'You can't understand, that's clear. You've got no right to judge. *You've* never had cancer applied to *you*.' A line of battle was drawn.

We began to avoid each other. I was so hurt by his response that I turned to friends, who, as my mother's had done, supported me abundantly. Cancer was dividing me from Stephen, even in this infant form, despite our careful preparations. Like a malign octopus it gripped us in ways we had not seen coming. Perhaps what I was experiencing was just what my mother had felt. Perhaps she had felt that my father, once her soulmate, after cancer could never really know her again. Perhaps that's part of why they drew so much closer together once he had cancer, too.

Our breach was clear. I felt that Stephen refused to understand what had happened to me, this unsuspected, problematic and rather disgusting outcome. He felt that I was over-dramatising my actual condition. A wall built up between us. Each had expected the other to be the pivotal, key support, yet instead each felt wronged and misjudged by the other. Resentment grew as the months of not speaking about it mounted. When we did speak we were nasty – each dropped wet towel, each forgotten message, elicited a snide remark. Friends who visited watched in distress. 'Do something. Get a grip,' they warned. I saw our relationship disintegrating, but my resentment paralysed me, fuelling my inaction, and I willed Stephen to be the one to make amends. Bitterly, ironically, I thought about my work. I had completed *Love Life*, and it was being made into a television documentary series. How could I pose as an expert on strong and resilient marriages when mine was so broken?

The question of whether or not Stephen could ever love my body again hardly presented itself. I hated it. I hadn't much reason at that point to think it ugly. In fact, the implants weren't so bad. Since I'd kept my nipples they looked pretty normal, though a bit lumpy and uneven. You couldn't see the scars below. But they were hard and numb, and felt constantly heavy, reminders that they weren't me. And reminders that they'd probably soon be gone. I didn't want him to touch me there – I didn't touch myself – I wouldn't let him; he knew that and didn't try. Besides, by then we were hardly speaking about anything.

The *Love Life* project was our turning point, at least for me. It reminded and showed me, through observation of the happy couples we were filming, that strong relationships have weak times; they weaken further if couples let them and if one partner forgets the other's vulnerability. That meant me, and it included my numbness to Stephen's fears. Forget about my obvious vulnerability. Stephen, like all main players in a breast cancer scenario had his, too. He, like most partners, was afraid for my health, but he also had his particular fear: I'd become twisted. Watching those couples make efforts to believe in each other's goodwill even during desperate times, I began to trust that Stephen knew I wasn't mad or stupid, that I knew the difference between cancer as my mother had had it and the diagnosis I had received. Perhaps it would help if I could show him I believed that.

This was the beginning. I'd gone to enough doctors over the previous few months. What was one more expert opinion? 'Physician, heal thyself,' I thought ironically, and lifted the phone to make a difficult call: I asked another therapist to help us. He did. Gingerly, sometimes angrily, we started to talk. We'd been wounded in just the ways we'd been trying to avoid but therapy helped us come back together. Eventually, he could make jokes and I could tease, the little pleasures returning. We actually enjoyed each other again.

At the same time a close friend gave me a book on Tamoxifen, which by the end of December, just after my oncology consultation, I had begun to take. It was written by Yale scientists involved in its development. In it, in black and white, carncinoma-in-situ was classed as 'earliest stage cancer'. I knew this book, a proper, scientific text, was respectable so I gave it to Stephen. It became our acknowledged, neutral common ground. There, in unambiguous terms, we shared an interpretation of my present condition. We were connected again.

My mother's legacy to me came through, again, in my struggle to understand this unimagined aftermath: I would live through it, as if, whatever the case, it was moving forward that mattered.

And then, every so often I'd feel differently.

On the beach in Cape Cod that summer, surrounded by family and friends, and feeling again robust and energetic, I lay reading an article my friend Janet had given me, summing up advances in breast cancer. Again I was confronted with the ugly fact that nothing could assure me 100 per cent that I would be breast-cancer-free for ever. One single rogue cell could kill, with no way to detect its spread until it was too late. The oncologist had told me there were no tests to tell whether I had more cancer. Once I had had all possible breast tissue removed, should the histology on that tissue prove cancer-free, I would be discharged as a cancer patient. There would be nothing more the clinic could offer me. Only if I turned out to be one of the unlucky ones, like that mother of forty-five, dead five years later – that is, only if an undetectable cancer had flourished in another point in my body and become invasive, only if I became symptomatic – would I know. In other words, only if cancer returned at a more advanced stage would I be able to get help. I would have to be vigilant, my oncologist said. 'Do you mean monitor every ache and pain?' I asked with growing dismay. I always had aches and pains – a bad back, a bad neck, a pulled muscle, a sore hand. Was I to become a neurotic hypochondriac?

'Within reason' was the reply. Back to monitoring. Back to not relying on doctors.

Very infrequently, as on that day on the beach, I would metaphorically slap myself into grim attention: perhaps I was being smug, assuming I would defeat my family killer. Perhaps I should feel doomed by my family history, as that dead mother had been by hers. Reading the article that day on the beach I felt my vulnerability, all over, in my bones – small, frail and destructible. I balked at imagining not seeing, knowing, being, especially with my sons. 'The children have always been foremost in my life,' wrote my mother in her journal. In this regard, also, I have found her in me. I gazed at the boys plunging into the waves, joyful and vigorous, tanned and strong. I turned from them in sharp pain; the tears rolled down, dried, rolled down, dried and rolled down again.

And then I came up short, face to face with my self-pity. I drew in breath sharply. Of course I'd be there. Of course I wasn't going to be the one-in-a-million unlucky one. Stephen's rationality kicked in: 'You're not a victim; you reduced your chances to 10 per cent, better than the woman on the street. You can hardly even say you had cancer. You're more likely to be run over by a bus.' That sent me veering in another direction: 'You're an over-dramatic, maudlin fool. You're healthier than almost anyone else your age.'

Mostly I carried on mundanely, slowly adapting to having these hard, unfamiliar appendages on my chest. They remained hard because it turned out I had a tendency to form scars very quickly. A hazard of implants is something called 'capsulisation'. The word describes what happens – a capsule of scar tissue forms round the implants and a hardness, painless but uncomfortable, results. As the new breasts became more familiar, and as I lost the memory of having ordinary ones, I came to ignore, rather than have any feeling for, them. They would almost certainly be gone soon, anyway, and eventually be replaced by others. I did not feel them to be me, but over the course of the year, knowing I'd be rid of them soon, I did not feel them to be enemies, either.

As the year wore on the skin on my chest became itchy and then settled down. I was left with small patches of numbness amid an expanse of normality; on the whole, the skin of my chest restored itself to something like the skin elsewhere on my body. Luckily, I was not inordinately desensitised. But as the implants were not likely to stay, and as I still did not know how to feel about my chest – it was not yet a cancer-and-anxiety-free zone – I still refused to let myself be touched; I disliked looking there. It became a no-go area. An off-limits department. A wait-and-see place.

I was nearing the end, close to completing the task I'd started, but not yet there. There was little I could do about that; I'd chosen to wait and recover, to get second and third opinions, to take the Tamoxifen. My next surgery was to be almost a year after my first. So life, which I ventured into with less unconscious anxiety about what might befall me, if more dismay at what had, than before my surgery, went on. I got on with appointments and got back to work: I saw clients in psychotherapy, wrote articles, worked on the TV series. I re-entered domesticity: I cooked meals, enjoyed and got cross with the boys and Stephen, went to school meetings, saw friends, went to films, plays, dinners, read novels. In other words, life slid back to normal. Only when I went for my numerous medical appointments, sometimes as often as a few times a month, did the fact that I was an oncology patient, that I had joined my mother, aunts and Joyce in being – perhaps – one of the black 'Cs' on the geneogram on a geneticist's chart, did it really penetrate, sitting there, strangely and uncomfortably, with the other outpatients.

'This Tamoxifen is wonderful' came back to me, with my mother looking eerily radiant months before she died. Tamoxifen had come to me with a good press. We now know my mother was right: its side effects are comparatively minimal. Tamoxifen, now commonly used in breast cancer treatment, is giving many women longer leases on life. The only real drawback is the increased risk for endometrial cancer, which my mother had had, but which did not supposedly carry a hereditary risk. I wouldn't be taking it long enough to create a risk for myself. It seemed the most sensible route.

I did have minor, annoying side effects, such as frequent hot flushes and disturbed sleep, and it brought on the menopause. These were relatively easy to bear. Harder were the heightened and unpredictable emotional swings. After a few months I asked my doctor to put me on anti-depressants, to stop me feeling as if I barely had skin to cover my nerve endings, to plug up my overactive tear ducts, to make life easier for Stephen and the boys. It was worth every swallow of every pill: I tolerated Tamoxifen with much greater ease. I didn't like the tiny disruption Tamoxifen had imposed upon my life; my mind boggles at how legions of breast cancer sufferers have tolerated the unimaginably worse effects of other treatments, especially earlier, during my mother's and aunts' illnesses.

And our children? They were ten and fourteen at the time of my first surgery. What message should we give them, when I had had something which was cancer, the thing they knew was the family killer, but only its beginnings? Should I name it for them, risking that I bequeath them the shadow I lived under, or should I tell them nothing, and risk their anger and bewilderment if my health did at some point get worse? How could I do it differently from my mother, yet not fall into different traps? After all, a major point of all this surgery had been to spare my children. I now found myself in what was admittedly a pale shadow, but nevertheless a shadow, of my mother's situation. My parents would have talked about what to tell us, their children, and how to tell it as Stephen and I were doing now. Experiencing the pale shadow was humbling. I could imagine my parents' moment of reckoning when they had to face each of us in turn with what was so much worse to tell. There were moments over those months when I shook my head in disbelief. How did I end up in this surreal state, rehearsing what to say to my sons, when just months earlier I'd had every expectation of saving both myself and them? Still, each step of the way I understood my mother better. Each step of the way I reflected with a new understanding on my younger self, this time seeing her through the eyes of a mother. And there was one piece of unshakeable wisdom I'd gained from my history. I knew that whatever and however we told the boys it would be stupid, cruel – and in a deep sense inaccurate – to give what I'd had a killer name. For, unlike my mother, I was for all practical purposes assured it would never be *my* killer.

So Stephen and I fumbled about and arrived at words, principles and timing for telling the boys. When a surgery date had been agreed, we would broach it. We'd avoid words which caused fear – such as 'cancer' – and use words which made sense – such as 'further prevention' – for why I would be going back.

I didn't gain the clarity I needed to tell them until a few months before the date of the surgery. Up till then I'd entertained a different course: to live with my 10 per cent tissue and place my faith in Tamoxifen. But I decided against that in May after a second opinion, at St George's Hospital. The consultant there echoed the oncologist at Addenbrooke's but was more definite. So in June I put my name down on the waiting list for more surgery. This time both the plastic surgeon and the breast surgeon would be there. This time they would remove more than was strictly necessary, including tissue from my lymph nodes. This time a breast surgeon would be on hand to spot any questionable tissue. So now I had certainty. Now I had to tell my children.

That summer on the beach on Cape Cod, I said goodbye to my youngest brother, Mark, who was off to Thailand. He hugged me long and hard, knowing that he would not be seeing me again until months after my next operation. 'You'll be fine, Janet,' he said. 'It will all be over soon.' We suddenly saw that Adam was standing near us. He was just within earshot, catching the shreds of Mark's blessing with what must have been astonishment. He concealed it. I couldn't know whether he'd heard. Time had run out.

One balmy day in Cambridge, soon after our return home, Stephen asked the boys to sit down with us. We had something we needed to talk about. My doctors, we said, recommended I should reduce my risk further; they'd found and removed cells which could have developed into cancer like the other women in my family had had. *Everything* possible that could be removed now should be removed, to make me as safe as possible. And then I'd be finished. The boys seemed to take it in so effortlessly that there was a slightly unreal quality to the moment, as if they wondered why we thought they'd have any trouble with it.

I guess they had understood more than I realised. No one used the C-word, but months later each told me he'd understood that those 'cells which might have developed further' were in some way the beginnings of cancer.

Daniel, full of passion and energy, adept at expressing and describing his and others' emotional states, and, as a friend once described him, with feelings worn on his sleeve, asked many questions, hugged me a lot, and let the subject come up freely. Adam, reserved, his feelings held in, attuned but cautious in his expression, listened hard but, over the months, when asked if he was all right or wanted to know anything, was quick to reassure me: 'I'm fine, Mum. Really.'

They both were trying to believe we were telling the truth. They also tried to reassure us by not showing us their doubt and fear. I'd seen this time and again when working with families undergoing divorce. 'The kids are fine,' parents often reported. 'They didn't cry when we told them. They play with their friends as normal. Everything looks fine.' As if children aren't smart enough to know their parents are suffering and conceal their own pain. So when both the boys seemed eerily unconcerned about my going back for more surgery, we ought to have known there might be something wrong with this picture. In their separate ways both were covertly upset. Sometimes I would catch it in a worried glance at me. Other times, from teachers' reports, it came out as trouble concentrating in school, or being too quiet and good, or more anxious about friendships than usual. I remembered Hennie, the stupid nurse and my horrid displaced anger at her. I remembered being the best sixteen-year-old daughter in the neighbourhood. And I remembered crying into my pillow, door closed, alone.

When Daniel walked into my hospital room for the first time after my first surgery, I had forgotten to warn him what I'd look like: I, like my father, had become so inured by then to the sight of patients that I'd forgotten my shock at seeing my mother after surgery. He froze as I had frozen. He stood on the spot, his lip quivered, and he closed his eyes when he hugged me. Then he said he didn't want to come back until the drains with my blood in them had been removed. A few months after my second operation I realised with a shiver that Adam was almost exactly the age I had been when my mother was first diagnosed. His reassurances to me summoned ghosts of the obedient way I had behaved with her. I had tried to protect my mother by not talking about her condition unless she did, and he had been doing the same thing. My 'forgetting' of the parallels was telling. Freud got this one right: the power of the unconscious to shut out pain is awe-inspiring.

My mother kept rising up in me. '*I gave you bow-legs and a fear of failure*' ran the first line of a poem she wrote for me. And the gene. And my bone structure. And very, very much more. I have her voice in me, both when I'm too stern and also when I tell my boys not to worry about me. I have her fears for us in me as my anxieties for my children. Even though I'd advanced much further to evade her killer, and was almost out of its sight, even though I suffered in that post-operative twilight year just a smidgeon of what she, her sisters and my cousin had suffered, I felt I'd joined them, had them in me, in many and surprising ways. The jolts of recognition and identification with my mother kept coming throughout that between-surgeries year, from my temporarily ruptured marriage to my label in Oncology, to my flock of nurturing friends, to my faltering wisdom with my children. I saw, I felt, I *knew* now why my mother did not want to talk about her cancer with me. But to be silent is to be gripped by cancer, it would seem, just as it is to talk too much.

At the end of September 1996 I would enter hospital, intending to finish the enemy off. I would have everything possible removed. I would go off the Tamoxifen, as it would no longer be necessary: no need to prevent oestrogen feeding non-existent breast cells. I would live for a few months with a scarred and flattened chest, without any implants, without any nipples. The chest skin, diminished further by this next surgery, would be 'prepped' over those months, stretched by gently, increasingly expanded temporary implants. When I left hospital two valves, one on each side, just under my armpits, would be inserted, along with temporary implants filled with only a tiny bit of saline. Tubes from these valves would connect to the implants. I would visit the plastic surgeon's outpatient clinic every few weeks and more saline would be added, gently stretching the skin. In the final visit the skin would be over-stretched to make it easier to accommodate the permanent implants and for the necessary give for sewing me up. In February 1997 I'd re-enter hospital for a few days – around five, I'd been told – to have the final ones put in. Skin grafts taken from my thighs would serve to create nipples. Bogus breasts, but safe ones. I would at last be finished. I would walk free.

16
Almost There

Things went awry. On paper the formula for beating cancer – you remove the breasts and voilà! you're free! – was simple. In real life it was more complex. I hadn't admitted that yet. Surely after I cut out everything my story would end?

I'm wiser about bodies now. I've learned that, no matter how sturdy a body is on the outside, delicate and complex things are happening inside. I didn't understand that, because I'd done so much to compromise it, my body had begun to run down. I'd always had trouble with my chest: my colds seemed never to run a simple course or be bog-standard. Ever since I'd arrived in the UK they had burst into more serious infections: bronchitis, sinusitis, tonsillitis. Every winter I'd stagger through weeks with blocked nose, hacking cough and scratchy throat. The winter prior to my first surgery a cold became bronchitis, which turned into pneumonia. Clearly my whole chest, inside and out, was a weak point. I'd become phobic about colds, trying to keep a distance from coughs, hoping against hope that sneeze droplets would miss me. A month before I was due for my final surgery I caught the first cold of that winter. I was probably less likely to fight off infections after having had two major operations within a year of each other, the last only a few months earlier. Within a week I had pneumonia again. But it didn't occur to me to postpone surgery; antibiotics were ordered. A clear X-ray was my goal. In my compromised immune state I should never have proceeded with surgery a few days after the X-ray, but I did.

After what was not a small operation – another major anaesthetic, skin grafts and major cuts – I was anxious to get home. Hospitals are at best boring, at worst depressing. I'd seen a body removed, met women in their twenties with a second breast gone, been shouted at across the beds in the middle of the night by a demented eighty-nine-year-old woman. Staying only five days became an *idée fixe*: I was going home by the fifth day, no matter what. My book and TV series were being launched at the beginning of March. I wanted to rest for two weeks and then get on with the publicity I'd committed myself to. It sounds mad now. But I had been told it was a straightforward operation, less than a week in hospital, one week bed-rest, then take it easy for a third week and presto! Done!

On the morning of the fifth day the bleeding hadn't stopped. At noon it was still trickling. By three o'clock it had slowed to a tiny dribble, and it looked as if I could be discharged. By six o'clock it had stopped. I called Stephen and was soon on my way home. Within a day I was back in hospital with a high fever. For a few days it wasn't clear what the source of the fever was, but then it became all too clear: my right breast grew bright red and hot and began to swell and throb. I had an infection on the site of my right implant, the kind of scary post-operative infection I'd read about, for which normal antibiotics are useless. I spent three more weeks in hospital. None of the drugs worked, not even the ones locked away like diamonds, as they cost practically as much, stored away for the use of burn victims. Finally, defeat: there I was, again on the gurney: my right implant, the new, supposedly safe soya implant, would have to be removed.

I left hospital with a flat right side and prosthesis. At least, unlike my mother, I didn't have to skulk around shops whispering to sales assistants. The nurses at the hospital fitted me, gave me names of suppliers of mastectomy bras and swimsuits, and steered me towards shops which had trained assistants.

I was a citizen of a new world, the world of the one-breasted. I'd joined the Smith girls again, though fortunately minus the threat of death. It was as if I had to go through what they'd gone through in order to grasp what that had been, but without the distortion of fear, so I could observe the battle in the fine detail; I could report back from the front.

I pictured my mother's strangely static, rigid chest – a chest of prostheses just a bit too high and a bit too rounded – the first time I wore mine. Mostly it was fine; apart from some clothing restrictions, it generally made no obstrusive demands on me. The only problem occurred with bathing suits, which could not hold the prosthesis firmly; I had to perform an underwater adjustment each time I surfaced.

Some implants can look better than others, depending on which kind you have, how large they are, and whether or not you can have fat tissue grafted from other parts of your body to cushion them. Silicone offers a better cosmetic result than either saline or the Trilucents I chose. I also decided to have small implants to suit my small frame. I made an informed decision not to look better than before, or even as good as I could. It is true that implants do not sag as much as real breasts. That was some comfort: perhaps I'd look more youthful – or at least while fully clothed.

During the months I'd had my chest expanded clothes had been a problem. I kept changing shape. One week I was almost flat. Six weeks later I was a Dolly Parton parody, with giant hard balloons curving out comically directly below my collarbone. I had a formal ball to attend that November. I couldn't plan what to wear, not knowing what shape I'd be. In the end I wore a dress with a shawl arranged like a cowl all across my chest, a brooch anchoring it, to conceal my ridiculous proportions. Now, with only one breast I faced the same problem, having to dress artfully, and would do so until I decided to have another implant. Or not. When I left hospital this time I did not want to contemplate further surgery. Maybe I'd do it, maybe not.

Ironically, I now had a body almost as misshapen as my mother's after her first operation, a body which had caused her such shame. Actually, in some respects mine might have been worse. The surviving implant was ripply and uneven, and the 'nipple' looked like one on a rubber doll (if they make dolls with nipples). Still, in clothes the implant was perfectly acceptable. Like my mother I avoided looking at my naked chest. In fact I didn't think about it much, except when, inadvertently, I caught sight of my lumpy and scarred left side, next to the flattened right. I didn't like it but I had no regrets. My chest did remind me it existed when it came gradually itching back to life again. The welcome itch signalled that underneath the skin nerve cells were engaged in regeneration. It's still happening, years on.

I'd decided one thing after my February in Addenbrooke's. I would think about whether to go back for another implant only after I'd spent at least one winter without succumbing to either pneumonia or bronchitis – or, for that matter, any other illness. I'd be fighting fit before I entered any hospital again. If I decided to. Perhaps by then I'd have got used to my new body.

It was a wiser decision than I knew: I had a few more illnesses to endure post-operatively. I launched my book and series, and an infection set in in the wounds where the skin had been grafted from my thighs. Soon afterwards came another upper respiratory infection.

My friend Jane brought me cups of tea as I lay in bed one day honking and coughing. 'I'm calling Caroline, my acupuncturist,' she declared, and she dialled the number and made an appointment for me. I let her. Previously I'd smiled sceptically over her alternative therapies. I don't know why or how, but it worked. I felt well and energetic after five sessions. I also started taking vitamins and echinacea for my immune system – all things I'd formerly dismissed. Finally, I did take up exercise, just as the magazines and health pages I'd had so many hours to read in hospital had exhorted. Moderate – I don't like to sweat. And I got my exercise machine. That and jumping around to aerobics tapes for twenty minutes a day – twenty not so terrible minutes – have become routine. That summer on holiday in France we swam and hiked. My energy surprised and delighted me.

I achieved my goal: to get through a winter with just a simple cold. Four days and the cold was over! I felt stronger and fitter a year beyond that awful February of 1997. And I could turn to the question: did I want more surgery?

I'd begun to adjust to this new body of mine. I didn't love my chest. One of my friends, a doctor who's seen war in Kosovo, called my scars and funny-shaped new breast 'honourable' – as if it was itself a battle scar. I began to feel respect for my chest. Not pleasure; and pride would be too strong a word.

Clothing remained problematic. So was sex: I didn't want my chest touched. But the words of those two wise pioneers came back to me, and they have helped: 'You find other ways.' Yes, you do. And if you're all right with that, so is your partner. I think that's the answer to the question about my parents: I think if my mother had been all right about her flat chest, so would my father have been.

I'd always been able to wear what I wanted; I'd developed a style. I didn't like having to discard clothes I liked because the implant might be obvious. Or having to wear a careful scarf arrangement above a low neckline, or a vest underneath. These were minor irritations but they were nagging reminders that I hadn't completed what I'd started. Perhaps I couldn't shake off my mother's shame. Whatever, I decided I'd try one more time.

At the end of June 1999 I re-entered Addenbrooke's. But not before one more twist in the tale. A few weeks before my scheduled operation I got a form letter from my plastic surgeon. It said that the Trilucent implants, filled with soya, which I had been given, and of which one remained, had become problematic. Apparently they had not been sufficiently tested. Though no one told me, I felt as if I had been a guinea pig. The soya had leaked in some of my fellow guinea pigs, just as silicone had in earlier implants. Newspapers published reports of foul-smelling leakages. Although no woman had suffered harm or damage, we were advised to have soya implants removed. So, as well as having a new implant inserted on my right side, the Trilucent implant on the left would have to be replaced. My plastic surgeon recommended silicone over saline implants for cosmetic reasons. While he again reassured me that there was no proof that silicone was risky, I chose saline. I'd live with the lumpy result. A suit has now been filed on behalf of women like me who have had to remove Trilucent implants.

There was one last scare. The day after my implants were inserted in late June 1999 my right breast blew up again. I watched it expand and redden; in the space of a few hours it became the size and shape of a small pink balloon. That was it. God was getting me for my pride and vanity. Why couldn't I have lived like my mother, with a fake pink insert which didn't threaten my health and which fooled most of the world most of the time? I endured another day and night of uncertainty, another antibiotic, and then another anaesthetic while the infection was treated, and under surgery the swollen area drained. The swelling shrank, the infection cleared, though it has left underground scars which I can feel and which shift the implant slightly upward and off-centre. War wounds, as my friend said, lest I forget. Still, it does fool most of the people most of the time. Even myself, as I hardly think about, much less am bothered by, my consequent loss of symmetry.

17
Staying Alive

Sardinia, August 1999

I'm on a beach again, this time staring into the blue-green Mediterranean. I'm wearing the same red stretchy two-piece I wore years ago on the beach in Lexington. It is a small secret pleasure for me to wear it again: it means I no longer need a mastectomy bathing suit. For two years I wore one, alternating the same design in black and navy blue (from a catalogue: the simple, stolid style nesting among splashy floral prints, smiling blonde models echoing the false sunniness of the prints – as if both could cancel out the truth: these photos lay in a catalogue for women with breast removals). No more secret underwater adjustments to secure a prosthesis before I surfaced.

Under my stretchy red top lie two breasts fixed inside me under my skin. Saline-filled, safe ones. They do the job. Under clothes, they are just fine.

Three weeks post-surgery I watch Stephen sail and Daniel bodysurf. I like my shape. These breasts are neither beautiful nor grotesque. They are neither me nor not me. Because I will almost definitely experience some capsulisation and numb patches, I will always know something 'not me' is there, but these are minor sensations. Mostly the new breasts blend well into me, and so become me. I am grateful for them. I swim and exercise a bit each day, and each day I feel stronger. I eat healthily. I feel I'm in control, just as the books and studies say I should. This is it. It's over.

Around me on the hot beach women are sunning their bare

breasts. I observe them critically. I no longer resent boob-fixation, cleavage and transparency in fashion in the same way as before: it's only silly and/or exploitative now. (In an ironic twist my photo appeared in British *Vogue* a few months after my failed implant operation, under a full-body shot of a model covered in sheer chiffon: 'Transparency' was the title of the page, and I was in there because my TV series was supposed to represent 'emotional transparency'.) I regard the breasts of the sunbathing women of varying ages and sizes with no longing but also with little identification. I am beyond breasts. I find it strange they hold such fascination for so many. I'm aware, of course, that this is my defence, to look at breasts from a Martian's point of view: funny-shaped, funny-sized hanging appendages. Martians have never experienced pleasure from them, never had them as part of who they've been. It's a good defence.

When it gets hot I do wish I could take my top off, simply for comfort. I can't. The world – and I – are not ready for the exposure of wounded breasts which tell such a story as mine, though an episode of *ER*, to my grateful astonishment, showed a fleeting, blurred glimpse of Rebecca de Mornay's supposed single-breasted chest. And a recent ad campaign for a breast cancer charity attempted to show models with apparent, though not actual, mastectomies: focus groups joined in a single negative if sympathetic voice to protest. That campaign, so far, remains unaired. Almost there, but not quite. These surrogate breasts of mine are not beautiful. They must remain private.

And then I muse that I'm not likely to be the only woman at this resort in this position: statistically it is now likely that some women, probably in their forties or early fifties, here have had breast cancer. At least one of the women lying on the deckchairs near me or sailing on the boats in front of me is likely to have one breast, or no breasts, or one implant, or two implants. I play a guessing game but there's no way I can know. Just as there's no way they can know about me. That makes me feel good. Normal.

On this holiday I've met a few people with whom we share friends and acquaintances back in England. When I get home I phone one of them. My friend laughs at the coincidence of meeting her friend, and then confides, 'I don't know if I should tell you this. Well, actually she is very open about her condition – in fact, she feels it's important that people should know that women with breast cancer survive and remain productive.' I know what's coming: I just hadn't guessed that she was the 'at least one' woman like me at the resort. 'I'll bet you didn't know that X has had a mastectomy, too?' Snap. I knew I was right. I wasn't the only one. I'm part of a growing crowd of healthy, recovered or recovering women who've endured mastectomies, faced varying forms of breast cancer and are out there, engaging with life every day.

We know a lot about breast cancer these days, and among the things we know is the fact that it needs the right conditions to develop. We know that even women like myself, who have a genetic mutation which sets the scene for it to grow, do not necessarily develop cancer. Joyce has an identical triplet sister, so their genes are exactly the same. Only Joyce has developed breast cancer. Barbara has chosen not to have the operation. They're doing well, and living with less and less anxiety as they grow older and survive, and do so with their bodies robust enough to enjoy exercise, to feel well, and not worry that they will die in the lonely, grotesque way their mother did.

Breast cancer develops and grows if its growth is fostered. That is where environment and lifestyle come into it. Women without a faulty gene have a lower risk, of course, but being exposed, through lifestyle and environmental factors, puts all women at some risk. If we smoke, if we take pills with high oestrogen content, if we eat high-fat foods, if our diets contain a high concentration of preservatives, if we fail to take exercise, we may be preparing the ground for breast cancer (and other cancers) to develop. But we don't yet know enough: plenty of women don't develop breast cancer who do smoke, do eat high-fat and preservative-studded foods, do live in unhealthy environments and do not exercise.

Breast cancer has become, over these last fifty years of huge change in lifestyle, environment and medical knowledge, a spectre hanging over the industrialised world. In a large ongoing epidemiological study of general health in Britain being carried out at the University of Cambridge, a great proportion of the women – a normal population drawn from across England – report that their major health fear is breast cancer. Everyone knows someone, often someone close to her, who has had it. Often they have watched their mothers suffering; now they are also watching friends, cousins and sisters. They ask, quite understandably, 'When will it be me?' or 'If not, why not?' or 'If me, will I survive?' and 'If me, what will I have to endure to survive?'

Breast cancer has become *the* disease of modern Western women at the beginning of this century, much as tuberculosis was *the* disease at the beginning of the twentieth. Formerly a disease of old age, in Western industrialised nations breast cancer has moved down the life cycle. Its increase in incidence began after World War II as women reached their sixties and seventies in larger numbers; in this bulge in the female population a relatively large number develop breast cancer. More recently we've become aware of a rise in pre-menopausal women being diagnosed. It is occuring even in women in their thirties: women like the young journalist Ruth Picardie, who wrote a deeply moving book recording her last months. Her cancer was apparently misdiagnosed, and she therefore lost the opportunity of early treatment and potential recovery. Ironically, it marks women in the developed West, breast cancer rising in numbers and lowering in age as these women have crested through the advances of feminism, healthcare and contraception.

There are several hypotheses about why this is happening. One is that carcinogens are multiplying in the environment, due to industrial processes, vehicle emissions, factory farming, food technology and packaging, and so on, not to mention smoking as well as a diet rich in fatty foods. This greater load of carcinogenic pollutants presumably increases the probability of cancer being triggered earlier. Other hypotheses point to changes in the typical life cycle of women in the industrialised world. For one thing, we are less likely to die in childbirth or of infectious diseases than our great-grandmothers were and our counterparts in less developed countries still are. This leaves more of us available at any age to get cancer. In addition, we have fewer children. It is thought that the development of breast cancer is facilitated by the presence in the bloodstream of oestrogen, produced especially during the first half of the menstrual cycle. Oestrogen production is suppressed during pregnancy and breastfeeding. The fewer children a woman has, therefore, the larger a proportion of her reproductive life she is awash with oestrogen. Cells which become malignant are helped to multiply by oestrogen; hence the effectiveness of Tamoxifen.

By the time a typical Western career woman – especially if she has inherited a breast cancer genetic mutation – who has put off having children until at least her late twenties or into her thirties and even forties, who then has only one child more three or four years later, or even, extravagantly, a third a few years after that, who commutes to her stressful and demanding job in an urban sprawl in which the air is filled with pollutants, serving convenience foods wrapped in chemically treated packaging to ensure longer shelf life and sterility, reaches her middle to late forties, she has become a more likely candidate for breast cancer.

And so breast cancer has now become emblematic of the progress women have achieved as we begin the twenty-first century: no longer felled by our wombs – dying in childbirth, burdened by continual childbearing – we now have our breasts to remind us of our limits, of our mortality.

This is not to scare women but to validate their reading of the facts: breast cancer is very much around. But my family's story presents another aspect of the facts. As women have become active in the development of a breast cancer 'industry', creating changes in medical and nursing practice, pushing developments in treatment, and educating themselves, they have reached a point at which they do not necessarily die from cancer. I am extremely unlikely to do so. Stephen, the rationalist, is right: 'You have a hugely higher chance of being hit by the proverbial bus,' he pronounces, 'than dying from breast cancer.' My children believe it, and so do I. I have prevented it. I am cured.

My friends treated for breast cancer in the 1970s and 1980s –

who all caught theirs early, had surgery and other treatment, and have had no recurrence since – were non-genetic cases. They will undoubtedly die from something else, but probably not until old age. I now have numerous other friends – and keep hearing of more and more women, most non-genetic – who have been diagnosed more recently and who are now either out of the magical five-year period, or edging towards it. Again, a sign of changed times: the word catches like fire on the wind of women rushing to help each other; I am now contacted by women with either breast cancer or a family history of it whom I've never met but whose friends of friends have heard a version of my story. I am not alone in this: informal, impromptu networks now routinely supplement helplines and support groups. My mother might not have used this network, but I like the fact that women I've never met can phone and we can share the details of our experiences, and each take away a helpful piece of the other's story.

My friends have had drug and/or radiation therapies as well as surgery. Many have explored alternative healing practices, even with the encouragement of their breast cancer treatment teams. Some have had massage during and after medical treatments. Others have taken nutrition and vitamin or homeopathic advice to boost their immune systems and restore energy, or acupuncture to do the same; yet others use meditation or have taken up exercise or yoga. Many use a combination of these things. I am one who does; I feel that, though science does not yet conclusively back my feeling and so it may be a placebo effect, my confidence, energy and immune response have all been boosted. I have completed three full winters without illness. Many friends in the breast cancer network lead comfortable lives, their periods of medical treatment relatively short and compassionate, despite inevitable suffering and discomfort, in comparison to what Regina, Mary and Fannie endured twenty, thirty and fifty years ago.

Since the late 1980s, when my blood was first drawn for the study of breast cancer families being conducted in Cambridge, and then, a few years later, for the study in New York, knowledge of the genetics of breast cancer has exploded. It is sometimes said that 'breast cancer genes' have been found. This is not only inaccurate but misleading. I waited, hoping, for this miracle discovery to guide me in my decision, but in fact the genetic advances so far would not have helped me.

To talk about breast cancer genes makes no more sense than talking about homosexuality or schizophrenia genes. No gene in itself produces either of those, and nor does it produce breast cancer. The gene plus other factors is the important combination. Every gene contains a complex set of instructions which normally guide our bodies to work but also can be faulty, giving the wrong information and possibly causing defects and disease. That is what happens in the two 'breast cancer genes' marked so far. Two sections of the human genome (the entire set of human genes which has been 'mapped'), named BRCA1 and BRCA2, show certain mutations (atypical variations in the sequence of the genetic codes) which are associated with a high risk of cancer. These atypical variations, or mutations, are more common in Ashkenazi Jews – Jews from eastern Europe, where the Smiths came from. The association of the mutations tell geneticists a number of things. First, that these sections of the genome are genes (much of the genome is 'junk' – with no effect); second, that they are involved in some way in the manufacture of breast tissue, or with substances that affect breast tissue; and third, that these mutations somehow increase the chances of a faulty manufacture or maintenance of the breast tissue, which increases the chance of cancer. However, there is not just one mutation found on BRCA1, for example, but many. Some seem to be associated with a greater risk, some not, and most are of unknown significance (there are no, or too few, data). It is this type of mutation that our family has: 'BRCA1 (but) of uncertain genetic mutation' read the printout when our blood was finally examined.

As further work is done it may become possible to differentiate the role of different segments of the code and the effect of different mutations at these locations. It is also possible that future research might find that BRCA1 and BRCA2 have more muted roles in cancerous growth than we think. Scientists have based their current calculations of very high risk on studies of women like me, who have attended breast clinics. We are women with reason to worry; usually we're there because we've encountered breast cancer in our family. But it's possible that random samples – i.e., genetic data from women in communities rather than in hospitals – might yield a weaker association between these genes and cancer. However, at the moment, my family history and the histology of our tissue (that is, the fact that our breast tissues contained many primary sites) indicate only that we almost certainly have one or more faults somewhere in our genome, in genes responsible for making or maintaining breast tissue, but we don't know where. Yet.

Any genetic consultation, though, still starts, as mine did, with a family geneogram – a chart on which the generations are mapped, and the people who've been affected are pictorially shown. Our map suggests that our gene came from my mother's father. He may have had sisters in the Old Country, or their daughters, who would have died from breast cancer. My grandmother had two sisters; they had daughters; these daughters themselves had daughters, of my generation or older. None that we know of has had breast cancer (one died recently, but it looked as if the primary site of her cancer had been the lungs). Men can be carriers. Genetics, in general, is a hot branch of medical research, with continually unfolding discoveries. With the full map of human genes completed, in theory mutations should be easier to identify. And so, perhaps, genetic treatments might be on the cards.

When my operation was first suggested twenty years ago it seemed crazy and freakish, if also logical. In January 1999 one of the most influential and respected medical journals ran an editorial stating that the best practice for women with the breast cancer gene or with a clearly high incidence of breast cancer in their families is to have a prophylactic bilateral mastectomy. It's not fringe any more. It's the recommended way to save lives.

Treatment of breast cancer has been changed enormously by the use of Tamoxifen, which is extending women's lives with relatively little discomfort and may (the research is still ongoing) be curing more. Almost weekly the press heralds new developments. Taxol and other drugs are also helping advanced-stage sufferers achieve longer lives – and, again, opening up the prospect even of cure for some, especially as they live longer and longer and more treatments and breakthroughs may be achieved. The toxicity of these drugs still causes terrible side effects, but alongside the development of new cancer treatments the industry now at least also tries to develop ways of combating them, rather than turning its back on sufferers as it did in the past. Perhaps most promisingly, new ways of destroying cancerous cells without killing healthy ones are being researched, along with trying to prevent cancer from the outset. New treatments in all forms of cancers are multiplying. There is cause for much hope that breast cancer, as one of the most public and feared kinds, will benefit directly from the new developments, and its treatment become swifter, gentler and more effective in the near future.

Though there is debate about how extensively and frequently to provide screening, most practitioners in most countries agree that the present system of prescribed periodic mammography and educating women to examine themselves is catching more cancers at earlier stages of development and significantly saving lives. The next step of the current design in the UK – fast-tracking of women with suspicious mammograms or lumps into specialist clinics so that specialists examine their breasts at the earliest possible moment – will also probably net more women with cancer at potentially curable and treatable stages. Hopefully, fast-tracking will become both standard and standardised so that women can rely on getting the best treatment available, no matter where they live. For there lies our best hope: that women can rely on being helped by both governments and medical establishments in their quest to take informed care of themselves.

Breast cancer still kills. It should no longer occupy first place in the league table of women's killers, but it does. The more aggressive breast cancers may be temporarily stunned in their growth but they still elude treatments and kill in too short a time. It is still the case that you can squeak through that supposedly safe marker of five years with no recurrence, yet it can still get you later, even much later, the cells mutating and growing at a very, very slow but still lethal rate. The length of survival from breast cancer, though, has been stretched and the treatments within that period are often more tolerable.

Some unlucky women have particularly vicious forms of breast cancer. They can extend their lives even so. Doctors can now make differential prognoses and women therefore receive differential and better-targeted treatment: some women with particularly aggressive tumours now can have healthy stem-cells harvested for use after aggressive treatment, and their lives are being extended for years in some cases. It would be better, though, if we no longer had to talk in terms of life extended, even for those with aggressive tumours, but instead talked in terms of cure.

Exeter, Devon, May 2001

In March last year we completed the sale of our house in Cambridge and the purchase of the one we're now in, in Exeter. I teach at the University of Exeter, part-time. I'm expanding the teaching part of my life. The family has moved on. Adam took his A levels. He's completed his secondary education. On his gap year, before going to University of Edinburgh in the autumn, he has worked and lived independently. As I write he is deep in Central America, on a six-month community and environmental project. He has moved out and on, to a life largely apart from ours. Daniel is at a new school. He's in his first year of the GCSE course, which signals the beginning of the end Adam has reached. They both dwarf me now. I have become my mother again: baffled by and marvelling at these large, gorgeous boys I love so desperately, whose independence is beautiful yet painful, as mine was for her. Now I know how she felt.

But the beauty and pain are entirely normal. Cancer does not intervene and twist them. It doesn't hover in the background. It's no longer part of us. It no longer comes between Stephen and me. It no longer grips me.

I will have grandchildren some day, I hope. If I don't live to see them, it's more likely to be because my sons choose either not to have children or to have them late in life, when I will be dead in advanced age of something other than breast cancer. (I *think* I hope for old age – now without breast cancer I'm finding myself glancing sideways at reports of Alzheimer's, a smaller but still ugly spectre forming somewhere in the corner of my consciousness . . . But that's normal, too.) But whether or not I see any grandchildren, I have a hope for them, as I have for any child of the next generation who carries genes from the Smith girls: I hope they'll be able to take what I've done a step further.

By the time a putative granddaughter or great-granddaughter grows up I hope she will *know* she will live. Maybe she will be able to march confidently to her doctor's office, have her gene blueprint taken and read back to her, and then, if necessary, unfazed, swallow a pill or have a jab, and painlessly erase or control the curse of the family. I went one better than my mother. Because of her I fought. Because of her I was vigilant. Because I live when I do, I stopped it, caught it quickly, and survived. I had the chance to defeat the thing she tried to defeat and, in her way, did defeat. I know she would have been proud of me. I have imagined her loving me through this very strongly. I can almost see her crowing down from an imaginary Heaven, shouting, 'That's my girl!' It would be great if the next generation could go on to be free of the shadow, free, too, of the knife. Now *that* my mother, and her sisters, would have loved.

Reading in the Early Years Handbook

Reading in the Early Years Handbook

Robin Campbell

Open University Press
Buckingham · Philadelphia

Open University Press
Celtic Court
22 Ballmoor
Buckingham
MK18 1XW

and
1900 Frost Road, Suite 101
Bristol, PA 19007, USA

First Published 1995
Reprinted 1995, 1996

A catalogue record of this book is available from the British Library.

ISBN 0 335 19309 9 (pb) 0 335 19310 2 (hb)

Library of Congress Cataloging-in-Publication Data
Campbell, Robin, 1937–
Reading in the early years handbook/Robin Campbell.
p. cm.
Includes bibliographical references.
ISBN 0-335-19310-2 (hardback) ISBN 0-335-19309-9 (pbk.)
1. Reading (Primary) – Handbooks, manuals, etc. I. Title.
LB1525.C217 1995
372.4044–dc20 94-40594
CIP

Typeset by Type Study, Scarborough
Printed in Great Britain by St Edmundsbury Press Ltd,
Bury St Edmunds, Suffolk

Contents

Acknowledgements

The writing of this handbook originated from two main sources. First, there were the direct discussions that John Chapman and I had about such a text. Those discussions considered how such comprehensive material might best be presented to the prospective audience of teachers, student teachers and interested others. Second, there were the frequent enquiries that I received from students, on initial teacher education and in-service courses, which suggested that a general text in a particular format might be helpful.

The actual writing of the handbook was made easier by the support and comments that I received from colleagues around the world, who also have an interest in early years reading. More especially, I had support from nearer to home, and at home. The teachers and children who I have observed in classrooms engaged on literacy activities have guided the writing of this book. And, more directly my wife Ruby, as a nursery/infant teacher, informed me, regularly and frequently, about classroom practice. Then my children, and subsequently my grandchildren, taught me daily and very directly about the process of becoming a reader.

Introduction

There are many books on the teaching of reading and very often they are contentious because there are protagonists who would wish to argue for a particular method or the benefits of a new set of materials, etc. Most recently, but in many ways reflecting the debates of the last 100 years or so, there have been debates about phonics teaching and the whole-language and real books approaches. Such issues are not neglected in this handbook. However, the book attempts to be much wider in scope and deals with numerous aspects of the teaching and learning of reading with young children. The reader will find that recent research as well as somewhat more dated references are provided as an aid to understanding both historical and contemporary issues in the teaching of reading.

How can the information be presented? Most usually books on the teaching of reading follow one of three formats. First, some books deal in considerable depth with a very specific aspect of reading. For instance, Alison Littlefair's (1991) book on *Reading All Types of Writing* deals very specifically with issues of genre and register and the implications for reading and writing across the curriculum. Second, some texts are somewhat broader in their scope and deal, perhaps, with an approach to the teaching of reading. My own book on *Reading Real Books* (Campbell 1992) provides us with an example, where an approach to early reading teaching is addressed. Third, there are also texts which attempt, comprehensively, to provide an introduction to a wide range of ideas, topics and approaches to the teaching of reading. John

Chapman's (1987) *Reading: From 5–11 Years* is, perhaps, one example of such texts, which typically have the broad titles that one might expect (e.g. 'Reading', 'The Teaching of Reading', etc.).

This *Reading in the Early Years Handbook* is a text that belongs to the third category. However, there are some differences. First, the text deals more specifically with the early years of reading development, which might be thought of as being from birth and through the nursery years to school age, and therefore Reception to Year 2 in the UK and Kindergarten to Grade 2 in the USA. Second, rather than following the usual chapter format, the book has been arranged rather differently, which it is hoped readers will find helpful. It contains numerous short sections under a wide range of headings which are arranged alphabetically.

Each section is designed to provide an introduction to a particular topic, to provide some debate and to signal connections with other headings in the book by indicating in italics (e.g. *shared reading*) where there are further details relating to the subject. Then following each section there are some suggestions for further reading where the particular subject can be considered in greater depth or from another perspective. A number of sections in addition have a short passage – 'In the Classroom' – which highlights the debate with a practical example. It is expected that the handbook will be used either as a conventional text and read from cover to cover, or utilized as a reference book where a particular topic can be found with ease without the need for an index and where some important insights are provided about subjects which are of particular interest to the reader.

The entries

apprenticeship approach

An 'apprenticeship approach' to reading was given considerable impetus by the publication of a small text by Liz Waterland (1988) entitled *Read with Me: An Apprenticeship Approach to Reading*. That booklet was developed from Waterland's dissatisfaction with the teaching of reading in primary classrooms. In particular, she was concerned that there appeared to be many children who could read but in practice seldom did so. Or, the children could read but did so hesitatingly and with little apparent sense of making meaning. Such concerns led her, in her own infant classroom, to move away from reading schemes and a skills model of early reading teaching.

Instead, she proposed a move towards a recognition of language as a whole, where the text to be read is vitally important and the adult acts as a guiding friend. In making these suggestions, the apprenticeship approach demonstrated its links with *whole language* in the USA (Goodman 1986) and *real books* in the UK (Campbell 1992). The approach also emphasized the links with parents, who have contributed so much to their children's *emerging literacy*, and who are encouraged to maintain that support in tandem with the school. And much of that support for the child as a developing reader is based on the *shared readings* between the child and the teacher/parent/adult.

Such *shared readings* are based on a notion of the children contributing what they are capable of at that moment. Initially, therefore, the role of the child may be to listen to the story being read by the adult and making few contributions to the reading. But, with a growing knowledge and increased confidence, the child gradually takes on a more prominent role (as described in the section *shared reading*). Importantly, as Waterland has indicated, the child is encouraged to read with, rather than to, the adult. And that is a reading which allows the child to take on the role of an apprentice who gradually does more as learning takes place.

However, just because the child is reading with, rather than to, does not mean that in the classroom the teacher is no longer assessing the child's growth as a reader. Observations of the child as a reader (and writer) are made and recorded so that the teacher is aware of the child's development as a reader. And in that analysis a note is made of the child's growing knowledge of letters and sounds, because, Waterland argued, being able to check on the initial letter (or initial letter combinations) in a word is helpful. But that skill of knowing the letters and sounds develops from the child's meaningful readings and is built upon by the teacher. It is that way round rather than the letters and sounds being the starting point out of which eventually comes reading.

Of course, the approach does not just use shared readings with real books. The children in the classroom listen to *story readings*, have periods of quiet reading, engage in *paired reading*, use sentence makers, as in *Breakthrough to Literacy*, and they write. And the expectation is that the children will be learning as apprentices supported by the person who at the time knows more about reading. Therefore, the teacher, parent and other adults have an important role in this approach.

Further reading

Coles, M. (1990) The 'real books' approach: Is apprenticeship a weak analogy? *Reading*, 24(2): 50–56.

This article considers the analogy with notions of apprenticeship and concludes that the analogy is safe providing it is seen as suggestive rather than exact. Coles emphasizes that apprenticeship implies observation, but also coaching and practice, and that (as Waterland had indicated) the role of the teacher is not to be *laissez-faire* but requires skilful teaching. Coles also emphasizes the social context in which learning takes place, with teachers having to ensure that there are many opportunities for the children to see many 'experts' at work with literacy.

Waterland, L. (1988) *Read with Me: An Apprenticeship Approach to Reading*. Stroud: Thimble Press.
This short booklet describes the events which led Liz Waterland to change to a different form of teaching and instigate what she refers to as an apprenticeship approach to reading. She indicates in the booklet the influence that other writers such as Goodman, Smith and Meek (as well as Huey 1908) had upon the changes she made. The booklet, of course, gives a more detailed account of the approach than is provided above.

Waterland, L. (ed.) (1989) *Apprenticeship in Action: Teachers Write about Read with Me*. Stroud: Thimble Press.
This text demonstrates that Liz Waterland is not alone in her attempts to develop apprenticeship-type approaches in primary schools. The text brings together the experiences of a number of teachers, headteachers and advisers who, at these various levels, have provided more holistic learning experiences for the children in their classes, schools and districts. These various contributors indicate not only what they perceive to be the benefits of the approach, but also the problems encountered as they changed their practices.

assessment

It is inevitable, and appropriate, that teachers of young children will make assessments of the children's reading and writing in the classroom. Why inevitable? Well, because the very nature of teaching involves the observation of children, an assessment of what is being achieved, an evaluation of that achievement, and a subsequent teaching based on that cycle. As Robert Anthony and his colleagues (1991) indicate, assessment and evaluation are closely integrated and are an integral part of classroom life. So, as teachers, we make assessments daily and they inform our on-the-spot teaching. However, the assessments also have a more long-term effect, because on the basis of the evaluations that we make, there may be more major alterations to the classroom organization for literacy teaching and learning. Furthermore, we also have to think about collecting together those assessments in order to inform other teachers and parents about the progress of children. Such a bringing together of evidence implies some form of *record-keeping*, so that the information can be given in a detailed and systematic manner. For some teachers, in addition, the assessments and records are required in a particular format in order to meet the demands of the National Curriculum.

How might the teacher of young children set out to assess the diverse literacy achievements of the children in the classroom? Yetta Goodman (1989) provides a useful framework by suggesting that the teacher might informally and formally observe, interact and analyse the literacy activities of the children. We can put that in the context of some of the sections of this book. First, the teacher will observe informally throughout the school day; as the children engage in *play activities*, the teacher will note which children are involved in such activities and the range of writing being produced by the children in that context. Of course, such observations may tell us about the organizational needs of the play area as well as informing about the children's use of literacy. More formally, the teacher might decide to collect the writing from the play area for a period of time in order to make a more complete evaluation of the extent to which the area is encouraging writing and the nature of that writing.

On occasion, the observations will lead the teacher towards informal interactions with the children. For instance, the teacher might observe a child writing in the play area, or elsewhere, and during that observation a particular aspect of writing might be noted. The teacher might then stop to have a short interaction with the child, centring the discussion on an aspect of writing (e.g. content, development of the writing, etc.) or features of transcription (e.g. letter formation, spelling, etc.). But the teacher will not just wait for opportunities for informal interactions to occur, but plan formally for interactions to take place. So *shared readings* require a careful *classroom organization* in order that they can proceed satisfactorily. During such interactions, the teacher has an opportunity for the regular assessment of the progress of each child's reading. With a five-year-old, it might be that the teacher will assess the way the child handles the book and uses the illustrations and print in order to construct the story. With older or more advanced readers, it might be that the teacher makes a note of the miscues in order to determine the language *cue systems* being utilized and/or concentrates on a discussion of the book in order to consider the child as a reflective reader of the book.

The interactions, and the observations, include to some extent analyses of the children's literacy. The shared readings do provide the opportunity for the teacher informally to collect and analyse the miscues of a child. Although the procedures suggested for a *miscue analysis* (Goodman *et al.* 1987) would not include teacher support – which clearly *is* the case in a shared reading – nevertheless as a child produces miscues a teacher with a knowledge of miscue analysis is bound to analyse those miscues and the child's use of the language cue systems. More formally, the teacher might have a system for analysing the literacy progress of each child. With writing, the most common feature in the busy early years classroom is for a collection to be made of the child's writing. That collection, as part of a portfolio, enables the teacher to analyse the child's writing development and to pick out particular aspects for a detailed assessment of development. So the child's growth as a conventional speller can be noted and, perhaps, features of spelling which might be creating a problem detected. And many other aspects of writing can be analysed from that collection, as well as during the writing conferences which are arranged by the teacher.

Although assessment is part of teaching, it has been highlighted in recent years when teachers have had to consider the attainment targets of the National Curriculum. And although teachers have been critical of the time demands placed upon them by the assessment procedures of that curriculum, in another sense those assessments have been insufficient in that they occur at the age of seven and at one set time in the year, whereas assessment and evaluation have to be part of everyday teaching and learning where reading and writing occur in real situations. Fortunately, parents can give some support in the assessments made of early literacy. For instance, when reading cards are passed from school to home and back again, both teachers and parents are likely to comment upon the children's reading. Comments from the parents can give insights into the reading strategies and interests of the children as well as giving the parents' perspective on reading growth. And children can be involved in the assessment procedures. They can be asked what they need to do to improve a piece of writing, and although their answers may initially be limited, nevertheless it is an important step along the path towards self-evaluation. And that self-evaluation will be a key feature of the children's future literacy learning.

Further reading

Goodman, Y. (1989) Evaluation of students. In K. Goodman, Y. Goodman and W. Hood. (eds), *The Whole Language Evaluation Handbook*. Portsmouth, NH: Heinemann.

The first chapter in this collection of papers is by Yetta Goodman. It is an important chapter because it provides the framework of literacy assessment and evaluation for the subsequent sections in the book. In it, Yetta Goodman outlines the notion of informal and formal observation, interaction and analyses and gives some suggestions for each of these. The subsequent chapters in the book extend that introduction and frequently provide classroom examples.

audience

In Denny Taylor's (1983) book on young children learning to read and write within the context of the family, she noted how the children would often write notes to other children in the family or to their parents. Of course, with the youngest children those notes might be difficult to decipher – although children receiving such notes might claim to be able to read them. But an important feature of that writing was that the notes were being written for a real purpose and with a genuine audience in mind. Such opportunities for writing may arise naturally within the home. Nevertheless, the teacher in the nursery or infant classroom will try to replicate these natural writing occasions. Therefore, the teacher will attempt to provide opportunities for writing where there is an obvious audience and a purpose for communicating in print.

The writing which can occur during *play activities* is one example where children find it natural to write notes for an audience of other children. The nature of the play will determine the purposes for the writing, but messages, instructions and letters are all likely to be produced for other children as well as notes for oneself. Such natural writing will be assisted where the teacher has arranged the play area for a particular activity and with numerous materials for writing and reading. The writing for other children can be encouraged at other times by the teacher. So letters to children who, for example, are absent from school or are in another class enable the children to write with a real audience in mind. The children can also write books, with varying degrees of support from the teacher, for other children. Frequently, such books are to be found in the library corners of infant classrooms. This writing of books also encourages children to consider the conventions of print, such as *punctuation*, because they will want the books to look like the printed commercial texts available in the library. So the influence of the audience is not only to provide a real purpose for writing, but also to encourage the writer to consider the needs of the reader during the production of that writing.

The teacher can suggest further audiences for writing in addition to other children. Parents are an obvious example. Letters informing about activities in the classroom, or used as invitations to events, can be commonplace. But there are many other occasions to write to, or for, parents. Margaret Lally (1991) describes how in one nursery classroom the teacher and children worked together to produce a notice to remind the parents to close the high latch on the nursery gate. The children contributed to that notice and also received a demonstration from the teacher about the construction of print. A further outcome, as we might expect from three- and four-year-old children, was that many other notices were produced by them over the next few days as they imitated the behaviour of their teacher.

The writing by the children can be extended outwards from the parents to the wider community. So a letter to a policeman or policewoman, or other guest, after a visit to the school can be viewed as writing for a real audience. However, the audience can also be imagined (although perhaps real to the children). Jeanne Price (1989) describes how the children in her nursery classroom became involved in writing letters to a ladybird after the reading of Eric Carle's (1982) *The Bad Tempered Ladybird*. The return letters from the 'ladybird' ensured that the children remained interested in writing to that audience. However, these letters also helped the children to begin to perceive some of the conventions of letter writing and to begin to produce the salutation, closure and signature that are typically evident in a letter. In addition to extending the audience out beyond the classroom, there are also opportunities for the children to write for themselves. For older infants, this might include a diary or journal, but the younger children also write for themselves. During play activities, for instance, children write lists for their own use – a shopping list is an obvious example, which the children might have rehearsed at home after seeing their parents prepare a list before a shopping expedition.

All of these examples are merely indicative of the ways in which the teacher can attempt to provide a variety of audiences for the children's writing. Of course, the teacher can also be the audience for some of the writing. Connie and Harold Rosen (1973) suggest that young children assume that their teacher will be interested in their writing. Therefore, the teacher can act as an audience for some of the children's writing. However, the aim will be to create a diversity of audiences because that will encourage the writer to consider the reader as he or she writes and therefore to match the writing to the purpose and audience.

Further reading

Hall, N. (ed.) (1989) *Writing with Reason: The Emergence of Authorship in Young Children*. Sevenoaks: Hodder and Stoughton.

The subtitle of this book indicates that it has as a central purpose the consideration of the child as an author. For a child to act as an author, it requires that that child has the responsibility for selecting what is written on the paper. And that means that he or she needs to be aware of the audience for whom he or she is writing. The twelve chapters in this book are written mainly by classroom teachers, and provide examples from nursery and infant classrooms where the children were writing to a variety of audiences (e.g. writing dialogue journals with their teacher, contributing to the classroom noticeboard, writing book reviews for the other children, as well as writing to the ladybird that we noted above).

big books

At the simplest level, 'big books' are those large books which teachers of young children use with a group or class of children. Most frequently, they are story books and the print is large enough to be visible to the children from a distance of fifteen to twenty feet. Initially, such big books were developed by classroom teachers so that the story reading experiences of home could be replicated in the classroom. Of course, teachers of young children do read stories from normal-sized books to the class, but, as Holdaway (1979) argued, in such story readings the children cannot see the print in the way that they can at home in one-to-one interactions with one of their parents.

Big books were developed, therefore, so that teachers could model the reading process in front of the class. By pointing to the words during the reading, the teacher enables the children to both hear the reading and to follow the print. In doing so, the children can learn about the left-to-right and top-to-bottom orientation of print, the separation of one word from another by a space and other conventions of print. The print is large, therefore, so that it can be seen, but also so that it can be shared and discussed.

As noted by Holdaway, big books were initially constructed by teachers. Subsequently, however, many publishers began to produce big books and a large selection is now available. But, importantly, because teachers want the children to join in with the reading, the books that are made, or acquired, need to be predictable books. Such books are helpful if they contain patterns of repetition (phrases and sentences rather than single words), which the children can recognize, learn and repeat. The books are also helpful if they have a rhythm that supports the children in the reading of the text (Rhodes 1981). In addition, predictable books should be written in a natural language (that is, they sound sensible and real when read aloud), with pictures that support the text and with stories which reflect happenings in the real world.

Such books allow the teacher to provide support initially by reading the whole story, but subsequently, during re-readings, the teacher can read in a way which encourages the children to join in with a reading of key words or repeated phrases and sentences. So the use of big books provides the opportunity for a 'shared book experience' (Holdaway 1979). (At times, the phrase 'big books' is used simply to describe books with large print. However, it is also used in a more global sense, as a shorthand for the interaction of 'shared book experiences'.)

Although stories form a major part of the big books in the classroom, nevertheless there are other possibilities. Holdaway (1979) also constructed big sheets of *nursery rhymes*, songs and poems. These were used as part of the extended shared book experience, with the children joining in as the rhymes and songs were recited or sung. As the children's knowledge of the sheets increased, so they were able to anticipate the language and join in more frequently.

Shared book experiences are also discussed by Judith Slaughter (1992), who suggests that a range of events might be used by the teacher during this literacy activity: a discussion of aspects of the story before it is read in order to develop a background knowledge; using the title and the cover picture in order to encourage the children to make predictions about the story; using questions after the reading to extend the children's understanding of the story; encouraging choral reading of part of the story (or more frequently with poems and songs); and discussing the *illustrations* and thinking about authorship.

Teachers working with very young children will find big books and shared book experience a useful activity to get children involved with, and interested in, books. And it will provide important learning experiences about the conventions of print, the structures of stories, and the nature of books and authorship. In particular for those children who may not have experienced frequent story readings at home, the shared book experience with big books appears to be beneficial (Combs 1987). Furthermore, as Judith Slaughter notes, teachers find that children who have had many experiences of story reading will begin to use elements of the stories, that were used during shared book experience, in their writing. So the children's learning during big book interactions forms a basis for learning about reading, learning to read and as a support for writing.

Further reading

Holdaway, D. (1979) *The Foundations of Literacy*. London: Ashton Scholastic.

This book is widely regarded as having introduced the idea of big books and the shared book experience. And both of these were introduced by Holdaway as he tried to replicate in the primary classroom context the individual book experiences of story reading at home. Because he felt that story reading in the classroom denied children the opportunity to see the print and join in with the story, so he developed his own big books for group and class readings. In the *Foundations of Literacy*, there is a vivid account of his initial attempts to develop big books and to use them in the classroom.

Slaughter, J.P. (1992) *Beyond Storybooks: Young Children and Shared Book Experience*. Newark, DE: International Reading Association.

This book develops the ideas first suggested by Don Holdaway in considerable detail. Judith Slaughter writes on organizational features, such as selecting and making big books, and displaying them by means of an easel. However, she also considers the way in which the use of big books and shared book experience can be extended. Follow-up work, including writing, is debated through the use of some classroom examples. The appendix provides a list of predictable books and comments on each.

Breakthrough to Literacy

In primary classrooms in the 1970s, many teachers were using a *language experience approach* with very young children (and, for good reasons, some aspects of that approach are maintained in infant classrooms today). The emphasis of that approach – to get children to talk, write and read about their experiences and interests, with support from the teacher – was also the basis for Breakthrough to Literacy. Indeed, in paragraph 7.14 of the Bullock Report (DES 1975), where it advocates a language experience approach for the youngest children in school, a link is made to 'Breakthrough' (the shorthand term used by many teachers for the materials and approach) for reasons we shall explore in a moment. But, first, what is Breakthrough and what are the principles on which it is based?

The teacher's manual (Mackay *et al.* 1970) indicated that Breakthrough integrated 'the production (writing) and the reception (reading) of written language', and furthermore that written material 'should from the very beginning be linked to [the children's] own spoken language' (p. 3). Therefore, as with a language experience approach, the children were to use their own experiences and interests to form the basis for their reading materials. However, with Breakthrough, the children were aided in this task by the provision of some materials. In particular, the sentence maker (a card with slots to allow for the insertion of smaller printed inserts), and the smaller word inserts and blank inserts (for the children's own special and personal words), were a major feature of Breakthrough. These materials enabled children to compose sentences and longer pieces of prose by inserting the words into the sentence maker in the appropriate sequence.

There was also a word maker, which looked like a smaller sentence maker, with letter inserts that encouraged the children to build up unknown words. Additionally, there were some Breakthrough books, nursery rhyme materials and a magnet board for language demonstrations. However, it was the sentence maker and the word cards which were argued to be central to the process, because they helped overcome two difficulties that the authors perceived 'small children have when they attempt to write: their lack of manual dexterity in handling a writing tool and the difficulty they have in spelling words' (Mackay *et al.* 1970: 3). Therefore, handwriting and spelling were key reasons why teachers wishing to use a language experience approach adopted Breakthrough. However, these supposed difficulties might be viewed differently now.

'The difficulty that children have in spelling words' would now be seen in the context of children's own *invented spellings*. During the process of writing, children have to consider each word on the basis of their knowledge of that word, their developing awareness of English phonology (Read 1971) and their increasing familiarity with the letters of the alphabet. And in the process of attempting to construct the word, children are engaged actively with literacy and, with support from the teacher, gradually become more proficient users of written language. Furthermore, such an engagement with writing, letters and sounds helps children in their reading development. Therefore, children's unconventional spellings (rather than incorrect spellings) are viewed as a developmental process leading towards literacy rather than as a difficulty hindering writing. As much as anything, such a view now requires a change of attitude on the part of the teacher, especially in relation to the spellings produced by young children.

Similarly with handwriting, children need to write in order to develop their motor skills related to writing – although, in the future perhaps, skill at the keyboard may be more relevant than handwriting. And children will, of course, already have been scribbling, which leads to drawing and writing, before arriving at school. As teachers, we need to support that handwriting by guiding, instructing and encouraging individuals, groups and the class as needed. The Breakthrough manual recognized that need, and devoted a chapter to the teaching of handwriting but away from the process of composing.

The perceived difficulties that in part led to the development of Breakthrough might not, therefore, be seen to be so relevant today. And other concerns have been expressed about the materials and their use. First, at a practical level, the maintenance and storage of the materials is not unproblematic; and unless the teacher is very organized and careful, pieces can be lost on a daily basis. Second, as the Bullock Report (DES 1975: 103) noted, 'whether or not the knowledgeable teacher needs this particular material once the [language experience] approach is well established is open to question'. So, Bullock was suggesting, it might only be those teachers who are not yet confident enough to engage in a language experience approach who need to use Breakthrough to Literacy.

Nevertheless, when Jessie Reid (1974) conducted her evaluation of Breakthrough to Literacy, she noted a number of positive features that were linked to that usage. In particular, she indicated that it made the children 'progressively aware of the way language works' (p. 92): the existence of words, the structure of sentences, the nature of bound morphemes (-s, -es, -ed, -ing) and the terminology of language (e.g. letter, word, sentence, etc.). Waterland (1988) adds that it provides an opportunity for children to play with writing independently of the teacher, and she therefore advocates its use as part of an *apprenticeship approach*.

Therefore, given these positive aspects, whenever a teacher decides that Breakthrough will not be part of the provision in the classroom, then thought will need to be given to the ways in which *writing* will be facilitated and an awareness and *knowledge about language* and its terminology encouraged.

Further reading

Mackay, D., Thompson, B. and Schaub, P. (1970) *Breakthrough to Literacy: Teacher's Manual*. London: Schools Council/Longman.

The teacher's manual for Breakthrough to Literacy was first published in 1970 and provides a most useful guide to both the theory and practice of the materials. There are very detailed suggestions for the use of each of the materials in the classroom, as well as chapters on working with parents and record-keeping. In a number of ways the manual not only describes the materials, it also provides an introduction to aspects of linguistics, because the purposes for the materials are outlined.

Reid, J.F. (1974) *Breakthrough in Action: An Independent Evaluation of 'Breakthrough to Literacy'*. London: Schools Council/Longman.

In her evaluation of Breakthrough to Literacy, Reid indicated a number of positive features linked specifically with the use of the materials (these were noted above). However, her evaluation also noted some of the practical problems which teachers face when using the materials. Examples of children's writing, some interviews with children and an awareness of the classroom at work, enable the reader of this book to gain a good insight into the use of this material with young children.

Bullock Report

The Bullock Report (DES 1975), as it became known, was the Report of the Committee of Inquiry set up under the chairmanship of Sir Alan Bullock in 1972. The inquiry was set up as a response to concerns derived from an NFER Report on reading standards in England from the 1950s through to 1970 (Start and Wells 1972). Reading standards, it was suggested, had risen steadily throughout the 1950s and 1960s with a slight decline in 1970. Although the Bullock Report also noted this decline, or levelling out, it questioned the validity of the tests used and noted the problems encountered with the sampling procedures in the NFER study. Nevertheless, despite these caveats, the Bullock Report (DES 1975) advocated a number of measures for raising reading standards.

However, raising reading standards was seen in the context of the complexities of language and literacy. So the committee, as reflected in the report, moved from a narrow analysis of reading to a larger consideration of language. Reading, writing, speaking and listening were suggested to be associated abilities and teachers had to ensure that throughout a pupil's educational life attention was paid to this crucial aspect of learning. 'Literacy demands a continuity and community of endeavour' (p. 26) stated the report, thus emphasizing in one sentence the need for teachers of all subjects to attend to literacy from five to sixteen or eighteen years of age.

The report was very influential within the UK and was used to develop language policy in the majority of schools. However, the report also had an international audience. Goodman (1986: 60) noted that the report called for major changes in the curriculum 'based on insights into the relationships among language, thinking and learning'. And he noted that the report elevated the issues of language and thinking to the level of policy, where they became a topic of debate in many English-speaking countries. However, we need to consider the ways in which the report had an influence upon reading in the early years classrooms, an influence that was both general and specific. Let us look first at its general influences.

We need to recall that the recommendations that were being made were based in part upon practice that was observed in schools and on developing theories of language and literacy. A major thrust of the report, as noted above, was to ask teachers to think of reading development within the context of a more global view of language, thinking and learning. The influence of James Britton, a member of the Bullock Committee, and his colleagues is apparent in that part of the report (see, e.g. Barnes *et al.* 1969). Arguably, this view has become more firmly established in ideas such as *whole language*. And there was an emphasis upon the use of literature, or story, in classrooms, as would be argued now for whole language. However, the report did not argue specifically for story in early years classrooms in the way that it is advocated today.

Two other general features of interest were related to the organization and promotion of literacy in schools. The first suggested that each school should have a policy for language across the curriculum, a policy to be developed from discussions between all members of staff. Although in the UK this might seem obvious in the 1990s, in the 1970s this was not the norm. The establishment of language coordinators in schools, with responsibility for advising and supporting colleagues in language and reading development throughout the school, provided an extra impetus to the development of a community of learners – among teachers as well as children.

Other suggestions were more specific to the early years. As a starting point, considerable weight was placed upon the opportunity to develop complex language patterns at home, in the nursery classroom and in the infant school. In schools it was suggested that a framework needed to be developed, and time made available, for one-to-one interactions between adults and children in order to facilitate the children's language development (the work of Joan Tough, 1973, underpinned these suggestions). Such an emphasis upon activities and interactions that encourage language development would be regarded as a basic element of early years classrooms today.

With regard to specific comments about literacy activities, the report emphasized *home–school links* and the value of *story reading* and interactions with *environmental print* at home. Furthermore, in a manner which preceded the most recent writings on *emerging literacy*, the report saw little value in notions of reading readiness, suggesting 'there is no virtue in denying a child access to early experience of reading, provided that it carries meaning and satisfaction' (p. 100). Although we have mainly considered comments on reading, this does not mean that *writing* was neglected. For instance, the report suggested that children should make their own books, largely derived from personal interests, which is akin to a *language experience approach*.

The report suggested that new *reading schemes* should demonstrate that they considered the vocabulary and syntactic structures of the learner, as 'reading schemes which present highly contrived or artificial sequences . . . lack predictability. They prevent children from developing the capacity to detect the sequential probability in linguistic structure' (p. 105). Such views indicated a need for reading materials written in a natural language, and hinted at subsequent developments towards *real books*. Because the report attempted to deal with all aspects of classroom practice at the time, there were suggestions regarding *phonics teaching*, though they indicated that 'the phoneme–grapheme relationships should be self evident, and readily acquired by inductive learning with the absolute minimum of formal instruction' (p. 109).

The practice of *hearing children read* was recognized as widespread in infant classrooms and the report suggested that such one-to-one interactions provided the opportunity for the teacher to make qualitative observations about children's reading progress. Many aspects of the interactions described would suggest that reference was being made to what many would now call *shared reading*.

From the very brief summary given above, it might appear that the report largely comprised a number of suggestions for literacy activities. Yet that would only be part of the story, because a very strong emphasis was placed on the *teacher's role*: 'The major difference between teachers lies not in their allegiance to a method, but in the quality of their relationships with children, their degree of expert knowledge, and their sensitivity in matching what they do to each child's current learning needs' (p. 106). So, the quality of literacy activities is determined by the skills, knowledge and enthusiasm of the teacher.

Further reading

DES (1975) *A Language for Life* (The Bullock Report). London: HMSO.

The obvious suggestion for further reading in this section is the report itself. I am acutely aware that my summary above, of a text which is over 600 pages long, cannot do justice to such a major piece of work, which has been so influential on classroom practice in the UK and elsewhere for nearly twenty years. Furthermore, I have only concentrated upon part of the report. We need to recall that the report extended its brief in two ways: first, by dealing with language rather than more narrowly, and inappropriately, with reading alone; second, by dealing with language and literacy from the home to school leaving ages. In that way, the report attempted to present a picture of a language for life.

Even though the report was very wide-ranging in its scope, one of the members of the committee, Stuart Froome, felt a need to write a note of dissent. He questioned the emphasis upon talking and writing, rather than upon listening and reading. He was concerned by what he saw to be discovery methods being promoted and a denial of didactic teaching. Readers will not need to be reminded that such debates remain today, and Martin Turner (1990) in his argument against real books continues in this vein, arguing for formal teaching and for the teaching of phonics.

classroom management

Before the children reach their classroom, the room will have been organized by the teacher as a preparation for the activities that will take place. But, in many ways, that might be regarded as the easy part. How will all the activities be managed once the children are in the classroom? Many teachers find that creating a structure or framework to the day is the first part of classroom management.

The school day is already defined by start and finishing times, and the inclusion of the lunch break and other breaks during the day. Linking literacy activities to these boundaries is a relatively common practice. *Story readings*, for instance, are often placed at the end of the school day (Trelease 1989). Placed there it brings the school day to an enjoyable, quiet and reflective finish. Yet, many teachers of very young children want to use stories as a stimulus for drawing, painting, play activities, drama, movement and writing. Therefore, having the start of the day devoted to story reading begins to be attractive. Some nursery and infant teachers find it easy to reach a compromise – they place story readings at both the beginning and the end of the school day. They do so because of the benefits which are derived from engagement with stories.

Sustained silent reading, when used in early years classrooms, would also appear to be best placed alongside one of the natural breaks in the school day (Campbell 1990a). In part, this is because it involves the whole class and making arrangements for it is logically linked to the lunch break, for instance, when the children have to be brought together anyway.

But that merely allocates two major literacy activities to the structure of the day. What about the rest of the day and the other important literacy activities? Many teachers of young children create a structure in which a number of activities are available for the children throughout the school day. The children then move between these activities, which include other curriculum areas as well as literacy, so that there is always something worthwhile available for them. Ideally, the children do not have to wait for the teacher in order to become involved with an activity, as the teacher's prior preparation ensures that there are interesting, worthwhile and appropriate activities readily available. And because the children do not have to wait for the teacher to tell them what to do next, there are less likely to be problems maintaining order (Goodman 1986).

However, other modes of structuring the school day are possible. Cambourne (1988) describes one such structure, in which the first two hours of the school day are devoted to language. (This amount of *time for literacy* demonstrates the overriding importance of language and literacy in the school day.) These two hours are divided into four main components and each is described by Cambourne in some detail. The first component is described as a whole-class focus time lasting approximately ten minutes. This time might be used to read to the class, write in front of the class or to demonstrate to the class some new language activity – and the emphasis is upon an open sharing of a process, a demonstration rather than direct teaching. Next, for a period up to twenty-five minutes there is sustained silent reading, or for reception or kindergarten classes perhaps ten minutes when the children are involved with a book if unable to read in a conventional sense. Then, for up to an hour there is a period of elective or compulsory activity time. In the former the children are free to choose from a range of options, whereas in the latter the activity of the group is chosen by the teacher in order to emphasize or introduce an aspect of language learning. However, once a compulsory activity has been organized, the teacher will need to move around the classroom to interact with the children and offer support where required. In the final part of the language session, there are twenty-five minutes of sharing time. This is a whole-class period when children report on their reading and writing and others listen and question. The teacher can help to develop the sharing time by providing a model of the kind of questions that might be useful.

Neither of the structures suggested above may suit you and your classroom. But what each teacher must do, probably in consultation with others in the school, is to provide a structure to the day which supports children in their learning and allows the class to be managed effectively. Of course, even when a structure is in place, the teacher still has to manage the moment-by-moment happenings in the classroom. As Cambourne (1988: 95) notes in relation to the activity time, the teacher needs to move around the classroom to 'observe, evaluate, interact, teach, redirect, refocus, demand, pursue, question, clarify, analyse, support, celebrate, coerce, coax, cajole, sympathise, and empathise', and although we can debate whether some of these suggestions are fully appropriate, nevertheless the quotation neatly indicates the complex task of managing in the classroom.

The list provided by Cambourne provides an insight into some of the strategies that teachers use to manage the classroom, maintain a good working atmosphere, and keep events and the children quietly under control. Holdaway (1979) indicates that it is useful to think in terms of positive teaching as a principle for governing teacher–child interactions. So, in relation to making predictions during shared book experiences, it is possible to say 'Yes' or 'It could be' rather than being negative and corrective. Such a strategy would appear to be helpful in aiding the management of a busy classroom.

Finally, all teachers know how difficult it is at times to manage transitions – for example, into the story reading at the end of the day. Yet here, too, the positive principle might be applied. Wherever possible, teachers need to use interesting and beneficial activities to bridge the gap from one set of activities to another: 'They didn't settle easily so we sang a favourite song and a nursery rhyme or two' (Holdaway 1979: 66). So, the two or three minutes that it takes to tidy and get ready for story reading can be filled in part with *nursery rhymes* or other worthwhile literacy activities. This is not to understate the difficulties or to fail to recognize the demands placed upon the teacher. However, the transitions which can create disorder can instead be transformed into short activities. And these are activities which aid the management of the class and contribute at the same time to the children's literacy development.

Further reading

Holdaway, D. (1979) *The Foundations of Literacy*. London: Ashton Scholastic.

Don Holdaway's book is part of the further reading suggested in the section on *big books*, which is appropriate because of his influence on the development of those materials and the ideas associated with them. Although there is no substantial or specific section in the book relating to classroom management, nevertheless aspects and insights into that important part of the teacher's work do permeate the whole book. His vivid accounts of classrooms in action contain many suggestions for daily management.

classroom organization

The discussion throughout this book of various literacy activities is important. We do need to think carefully through the reasons for such activities, the principles that lie behind the practices, the way that they fit into an overall plan, and the benefits that they bring to the children. All of this is self-evident. And yet in the reality of the classroom the teacher is responsible for twenty, thirty or more children. In such circumstances, the literacy activities can, occasionally, seem to be more problematic. However, such literacy activities can flourish where the teacher has devoted a good deal of attention and effort to the prior organization of the classroom, and subsequently to *classroom management, time for literacy* and the *teacher's role.* These are key, albeit basic, issues for the teacher. For the moment, let us consider the organization of the classroom.

A starting point for that organization is the physical arrangement of the classroom furniture. Because literacy activities require individual interactions, groupwork and whole-class sessions (as do other areas of the curriculum), the tables, benches, chairs and mats, as well as the partitions, cupboards and boards, need to reflect that requirement. The teacher needs to ensure that there is a sufficiently large space for whole-class sessions, including the very important *story readings,* where the children can sit in comfort without being too close to one another. Often, the overall organizational requirements will be reflected in the grouping of the children's tables and chairs into blocks catering for four to six children, of a number of bays or areas to cater for specific purposes (e.g. the library corner), and some small bays to allow for individual work. And, hopefully, the organization of the furniture, and the size of the room, will ensure that there is space between the blocks of furniture. Those spaces help the children to work undisturbed next to other activities being undertaken in the classroom, as well as allowing the teacher room for movement between the activities.

Ease of movement for the teacher is important because it enables him or her to support, guide and encourage the children in the various activities. It also enables the teacher to find a space to interact with an individual child before moving on to another area. How the furniture is laid out can also encourage child–child as well as teacher–child interactions.

Space between the blocks of furniture also allows the children to move from one activity area to another as they complete their work, to collect materials from clearly labelled drawers, boxes and cupboards, to consult charts among the *classroom print,* and to consult dictionaries or information books as necessary. It is part of the management of the classroom by the teacher to monitor the movement of the children and to ensure that such movement is purposeful.

The furniture in nursery and infant classrooms is arranged in a general manner but is also arranged very specifically for a number of areas more clearly designated for literacy activities. The teacher will need to determine how best to organize the classroom for the *library corner, listening area, writing centre,* and a play area or home corner for *play activities*. This makes a very considerable demand upon the space in the classroom, as well as on the ingenuity of the teacher. But such efforts are worthwhile, because each of the areas provides many opportunities for literacy involvement which contributes to the children's literacy development.

The library corner is a focal point for early literacy development. This being the case, many teachers make it their first priority when organizing the classroom furniture. We shall explore the internal arrangements of the *library corner* elsewhere, but the teacher will want to ensure that the corner attracts the children and is arranged in a manner which enables the children to engage with books in comfort and undisturbed by other children. This can be organized, even though some teachers find that limitations on space mean that the *listening area* might also need to be sited within the library. However, the use of headphones should minimize any interruption from that source.

The establishment of a *writing centre* in the classroom, with a wealth of materials to encourage writing, might only require a few tables and chairs together with a store for the different sized paper and writing tools. However, the benefits of having an area always available for children to write are considerable. And the home corner or play area will almost certainly be one of the teacher's priorities – with or without an emphasis upon literacy. Increasingly, however, teachers attempt to develop the *play activities* in that area, so that it is used for a variety of sociodramatic activities, each with numerous opportunities for literacy (e.g. Hall and Abbott 1991).

Occasionally, new developments in the teaching of literacy lead to accusations of poor teaching or even of non-teaching. Phillips' (1990) criticism of real book approaches as a non-teaching movement is a case in point. Yet the reality is that child-centred methods, like other methods of teaching, require complex and sophisticated skills on the part of the teacher. And a first part of that teaching requires the careful organization of the classroom, which provides the foundation for the establishment of worthwhile literacy activites.

Further reading

Burman, C. (1990) Organizing for reading 3–7. In B. Wade (ed.), *Reading for Real*. Buckingham: Open University Press.

The chapter by Chris Burman is one of ten contributions in this very helpful book edited by Barrie Wade. There are two strands to the chapter. First, there is a case study of the organization, teaching and support given to six-year-old Kevin as he developed as a reader in an infant classroom. Then, there is a debate on the classroom environment which provides the context for that learning to take place.

Cambourne, B. (1988) *The Whole Story: Natural Learning and the Acquisition of Literacy in the Classroom*. Auckland: Ashton Scholastic.

Brian Cambourne's book is 'about children learning to read and write' (p. 1). In the text he explores a model of learning as applied to literacy learning. However, his exploration of the theoretical is related very closely to the events of the classroom. And the analysis of the classroom includes sections on the organization of space and of resources. He makes the point that even an average-sized room can be organized so that it is not overcrowded. Although we would all probably prefer to have a classroom with plenty of room, nevertheless, with planning, the classroom can be organized for the spaces that are required for literacy learning – and that is demonstrated in this book.

classroom print

Teachers of young children will be aware that the majority of them – whether three, four or five years of age – will arrive at school with some awareness of, and knowledge about, environmental print. That being the case, teachers will want to capitalize on that knowledge by bringing some of that *environmental print* into the classroom for displays, *play activities* and discussion. However, teachers can also extend the use of contextualized environmental print by developing various examples of classroom print.

Teachers will not want to develop classroom print simply for its own sake. Instead, classroom print will be such that it can be seen to serve real purposes. Furthermore, teachers should not be content just to provide meaningful classroom print displays, but should also ensure that time is spent discussing the print with the children and responding to their enquiries about it.

So what forms of classroom print might be made available? In part, of course, this will be determined by the age, and experience with literacy, of the children. Nevertheless, lists of various types of classroom print are given in a number of texts (e.g. Cambourne 1988; Campbell 1992). However, a starting point could be environmental print. Goodman (1986) suggests that children might be taken for walks to look for environmental print, and such questions as 'Why is the print there?' and 'What does it say?' can be raised. This can then lead to the development and display of environmental print in the classroom. For instance, the children could collect pictures or examples of road signs – or make their own – and display them. Their discussion of these signs with their teacher can lead to aspects of road safety as well as encouraging literacy development.

With the very youngest of children, attendance charts can be used, which they are asked to sign each day. This is an important task for young children, because of the considerable interest they have in beginning to recognize, and have control over, the production of their own names. Harste *et al.* (1984) describe with examples the development of children's writing of their own names in a context in which a teacher of pre-school children has asked them to sign in each day. Although the teacher was concerned whether the activity was successful, the examples of the children's 'scribbles' indicated differences between scribbled writing and scribbled drawing. The examples also demonstrated how the children were gradually developing more sophisticated and conventional representations of their names. All classroom print activities have to be as meaningful as this, because contextualized environmental print is being replaced by decontextualized classroom print.

A daily message board can be used to inform the children about important happenings during the day, as well as indicating the activities that are immediately available. And this can work as well for children emerging as literacy users as for children who are beginning to gain some independence with reading and writing. For those children who are not yet able to read in a conventional manner, the teacher will have to spend some time talking about the messages on the board and perhaps reminding the children of those messages throughout the school day.

A bulletin board can be used to extend the usefulness of the message board by telling the children about other events later in the week or in the very near future. And this separation of function can be useful, as the children's attention will not then be distracted from the daily immediacy of the message board. Regular, albeit short, discussion of the contents of the board will be needed, especially with the younger children.

Functional labels can supply important information to the children. Drawers, cupboards and boxes of equipment can be labelled to inform the children of their contents. The children have a real purpose for reading the labels and this enables them to work with some degree of independence from the teacher. Furthermore, the teacher is able to engage in important literacy interactions, rather than spending time supplying pencils, paper and other materials. But we need to remind ourselves that the functional labels must serve a real communicative purpose. Simply attaching a 'chair' label to a chair serves no real purpose; however, a 'pencil' label on a drawer containing pencils can be useful and is functional (Donaldson 1989).

Nursery school and reception/kindergarten children love to sing short songs, recite *nursery rhymes* and poems, and partake in language games, some of which can be displayed on large charts. These then form part of the classroom print, and the teacher and the children can engage with them on a frequent basis. During such activities, the shared reading/singing begins to resemble the interactions that occur with big books and the children will gain similar benefits from the experience. In particular, the children will begin to note some of the conventions of print (e.g. left-to-right directionality, top-to-bottom reading, space either side of a word, etc.) as their teacher links the oral words to the written print.

Birthday charts are also significant to young children, as they indicate the timing of a very major event in every child's life. And such a chart can be used to relate an individual child's birthday to the birthdays of the other children in the classroom. They can also be used to teach sequences of time, including the months of the year, the days of the week as well as the numbers from 1 to 31.

A weather chart can be linked to the daily message board on which a child might be nominated to record the weather. Children will enjoy having the responsibility for recording the weather. And with the very changeable weather in the UK a morning and afternoon recording would not be inappropriate! This activity also brings together a number of areas (e.g. reading, writing and science) in a natural way.

Although the message board can be used to nominate children for particular responsibilities, this can lead to the board becoming overcrowded and therefore less easy to read. Some teachers, therefore, prefer to have a separate chart of job responsibilities, with the children's names changing on a weekly or even daily basis. And because of these regular and frequent changes, it will form the focus for brief but regular teacher–child interactions.

Around the room may be hung charts which tell the children about the activities available in a particular corner or centre. For example, in the *listening area* there might be instructions about the number of children who can use the area at any one time, as well as informing the children about the use of the equipment and the tidying up procedures at the end of the day. Another more general chart might list the classroom rules and expectations. The children can contribute to these rules and expectations as the teacher debates the list with them and reminds them of expected behaviour and responsibilities.

Among these different wall charts and displays will be some derived from the children's own work. In the *library corner*, for instance, might be displayed the children's book reviews. This might seem more appropriate for those children who have developed their writing; however, a picture of a main character with just the name underneath can also enliven the corner. And alphabetic friezes and sources of reference can be part of the classroom print. Furthermore labels to describe and explain the displays and exhibitions as well as graphs, derived perhaps from the birthday or weather charts, all add to the classroom being rich in print.

So to use Brian Cambourne's (1988: 101) phrase, teachers need 'to flood the classroom with useful wall charts', and having done so they need to use the charts, update them on a regular basis and discuss them with the children. These discussions give the children the opportunity to reflect on the messages and to learn about literacy.

Further reading

Cambourne, B. (1988) *The Whole Story: Natural Learning and the Acquisition of Literacy in the Classroom*. Auckland: Ashton Scholastic.

In this book, Cambourne stresses how important it is for the teacher to organize time, space and resources in the classroom. And one of these resources is classroom print. He argues that the classroom should be flooded with useful print and that the teacher and the children should talk about that print on a frequent basis. He provides a list of wall charts that might be usefully displayed and discussed.

computers

There are a number of problems in writing about the use of computers with early years classes. First, the technological advances that are being made in both hardware and software, as well as the possible uses of CD-ROM in the classroom, make anything written about computers today out of date by the time it is printed. Certainly, it is hoped that the software intended for young children will increasingly require thought from the children themselves rather than a series of conditioned responses, which was the case with some of the early materials (Wray and Medwell 1991). Second, one is unable to tell whether enough resources will be made available for the ample provision of computers in classrooms of thirty or more children. One computer per classroom, which can then be integrated into the normal daily literacy activities, might be as much as most teachers of young children could expect. Nevertheless, a single computer, used as a word processor, can be put to good advantage. Moore and Tweddle's (1992) case study of year-2 children writing 'Badger Stories' provides an example of the benefits which can accrue.

Most frequently, computers are used in early years classes as word processors. It is not difficult to see why, especially when using a word processor is linked to the notion of process writing. Using a word processor, the children can draft, redraft, edit and produce a final good copy without constantly rewriting the story or other piece of work by hand. Or, the children might just engage with one aspect of that process and be supported by the teacher more directly at other stages in the process. For instance, when Moore and Tweddle's year-2 children wrote their 'Badger Stories', they began by working in small groups and uttered their stories directly into a cassette-recorder. Subsequently, the teacher produced a transcribed story for each of the groups. The children in each group then read their story, debated it and amended or redrafted it as necessary. Finally, an edited copy was produced, which the children illustrated and developed as a book. Each of the books was then read out to the other children in the class. The production of such books, some of which may become part of the classroom library, is a major benefit of using computers as word processors. The children enjoy seeing themselves as authors, like to read their own books and the books add to the print resources in the classroom.

Many teachers encourage children to work together at the word processor. The stories that are then drafted, for instance, are debated as part of a collaborative exercise within a small group. Such discussions involve children talking about language; for example, spelling and punctuation are discussed directly and features such as story structure are discussed implicitly as the story is produced. Sometimes, however, the reason for grouping the children at the word processor is to make best use of limited resources. Nevertheless, the outcome is often that the children benefit from the discussions about language. Indeed, it is such collaboration when working at a word processor which many teachers in the National Writing Project (SCDC 1990) saw as the central advantage of such work.

Further reading

Moore, P. and Tweddle, S. (1992) *The Integrated Classroom: Language, Learning and I.T.* London: Hodder and Stoughton.

This book is one of a series, produced in the UK, which deals with 'Teaching English in the National Curriculum'. Moore and Tweddle focus on the use of computers to support language development in both primary and secondary classrooms. Nevertheless, a number of case studies are presented in the text, one of which explores a year-2 class writing stories, with the aid of a word processor for the production of final copies. It is recognized that many classes have just one computer and that the use of that computer has to be integrated into the daily events of the classroom.

SCDC (1990) *Writing and Micros*. Walton-on-Thames: Nelson.

This text, a product of the National Writing Project in the UK, is full of very practical suggestions for using computers, especially when used as word processors, in the primary classroom. The many examples provided of teachers and children writing with a word processor will be valued by classroom teachers wishing to explore this area.

Wray, D. and Medwell, J. (1991) *Literacy and Language in the Primary Years*. London: Routledge.

David Wray and Jane Medwell include a chapter on 'The use of the computer to develop language and literacy' in their general text on literacy in the primary years. Naturally, they write about the benefits of word processing, but they extend the debate by considering adventure games, information handling, text manipulation and using logo. And they provide a timely warning about the didactic teaching and stimulus–response–reward basis of some of the less helpful software. This reminds teachers of the need to evaluate the materials being used in the classroom.

conferencing

Teachers always respond in one way or another to the writing of the children in their classrooms; at times, this response may be of a very simple kind. As the teacher moves informally around the classroom, comments might be made about the children's writing in order to support and guide each child's efforts. Then, as a child completes a piece of writing, the teacher will often give a response – frequently one of encouragement to the youngest children. Other teachers working within a more formal perspective might pay greater attention to the mechanical aspects of writing by correcting at least some of the children's spellings and punctuation. Conferencing might be linked to each of these simple procedures, but in reality it is a more in-depth consideration by the child and the teacher of the child's writing. So the child and the teacher meet, albeit sometimes just for a minute or two, to discuss the child's writing and determine how it might be developed. This notion of conferencing evolved substantially from the process writing model argued by Donald Graves (1983). Given that this model suggests that writing, in many circumstances, moves from rehearsal, drafting and redrafting to editing, then the question might be how can teachers support that process of writing? Conferencing is an important part of the answer that Graves puts forward.

Conferencing is not unlike *shared reading* or *hearing children read*, for in both of these the child is the reader and the teacher follows what the child is attempting and gives support, rather than answers, in order to guide that reading. Conferencing is similar, but now the child is writing, or has written, and the teacher guides the child's endeavours. As Donald Graves suggests, the child should lead the discussion about his or her own work, with the teacher reacting intelligently to what the child has to say. If the teacher talks more than the child, it could be suggested that the teacher is adopting too active a role, as would also be the case if the teacher attempted to redirect the writing to another topic, or aspect of a topic. Supplying catchy words or phrases for the child to use or teaching skills too early in the conference might also be viewed as negative features of this interaction. So what might a teacher do during a conference?

Graves emphasizes that the teacher should encourage the children to talk about their writing, because as the children talk they also learn about what they know – they make explicit their implicit knowledge of the writing and about writing. But the teacher also learns about what the children know and, based on this knowledge, the teacher is able to offer more effective help. So if we need to encourage children to talk about their writing, we need to open up the conference with questions that invite them to indicate what they are writing and where they are in the process, and later enquire if they need any help. But the teacher will be trying to encourage the content of the writing because many of the spellings and other conventions can be left until the editing stage. And an important strategy for the teacher to use, as when *responding to miscues*, is to wait, to give time for the children to think and then to talk about the writing that they have produced. Initially, this is not easy for the child or the teacher, but most children soon realize it is a time for them to talk about their writing and they accept the opportunity.

The teacher, of course, has to organize carefully for the conferences to occur. The other children need to realize that while a conference is taking place they should not interrupt, and that is helped by knowing what materials and activities are available in the classroom and being able to access them without teacher support. The teacher and child need to conduct the conference side by side, which encourages collaboration, rather than sitting opposite each other, which suggests a more adversarial interaction. The first conferences may not be particularly successful, often because the children do not understand fully the opportunity that is being offered to them to talk about their writing. And as teachers we might be tempted to teach too much: the notion of emphasizing content, and teaching just one element, in any conference might be appropriate.

Most conferences are conducted on a one-to-one basis between a child and a teacher. However, peer conferences, in which two children share their writing with one another and raise questions about how the writing might be improved, have the effect of requiring the children to reflect upon their own and other people's writing and to learn from that experience. In small group conferences, the teacher works with a selected group of children in choosing a topic, developing a main idea or considering some of the conventions, such as capitalization and full stops. Occasionally, whole-class conferences are conducted, in which the children are able to share their writing with the whole class and one particular aspect might be highlighted by the teacher.

It is important to remember that not all writing needs to be redrafted and edited, and here a conference would have little place in supporting such writing. Furthermore, for the very youngest of children who are producing a line of writing, a conference (if that is the right name for it in these circumstances) might be a very brief indication of support and an encouragement for future writing. Nevertheless, these teacher–child interactions, with careful planning and thoughtful execution, can be supportive of children's writing.

Further reading

Graves, D. (1983) *Writing: Teachers and Children at Work.* Portsmouth, NH: Heinemann Educational.

This book devotes five chapters to conferencing, and the chapter titles give some clue as to the content: 'Help children speak first', 'Ask questions that teach', 'Let the children teach us', 'Work with children at different draft stages' and 'Answers to the toughest questions teachers ask about conferences'. Throughout these chapters, there are numerous transcripts of child–teacher conferences and they serve to illuminate the points that are stressed in the text.

Temple, C., Nathan, R., Temple, F. and Burris, N.A. (1988) *The Beginnings of Writing.* London: Allyn and Bacon.

A whole section of this book deals with conferencing and there is discussion of individual, group and class conferences. A list of questions that might be used are provided; these are not to be used within every conference, but they are an indication of the areas that might be covered. This list, and other guidelines, provide some suggestion as to how to proceed with writing conferences.

cue systems

When listening to children read aloud within a *shared reading* or as part of a *hearing children read* interaction, a number of miscues will be noted. These deviations from the text can be examined in detail using a *miscue analysis.* And it is this analysis that will provide information about the language cue systems that the children might have used. Such information, built up within an extended read, or with a young reader over a number of occasions when he or she read aloud, tells the teacher about what the child is attempting to do during the reading and it can provide insights into which cue systems the child might be using effectively or not so effectively. In order to gain most benefit from a miscue analysis, therefore, it is helpful if the teacher has some knowledge of language cue systems.

Language cue systems can be considered at two levels. First, we can explore the graphophonic, syntactic and semantic cue systems in a relatively simple way, as might be the case in a miscue analysis in the busy classroom. Second, these systems can be explored in far greater depth, in which a detailed analysis of the language cues might indicate the complexities of the systems that the young child utilizes.

It is often easy to recognize when a child is using the graphophonic cue system. In particular, we might expect young readers to pick up on the cue provided by the first letter of a word. They see that first letter, recognize it, and then produce the sound that is often associated with it. Attention might also be paid to the final letter(s), the length of the word, or a cluster of letters in the middle of a longer word. Comparing miscues with text words enables us to detect the graphophonic strategies of children. Second, children also use the syntactic cue system as they read. They may not be able to articulate their knowledge of sentence structure, but their miscues often demonstrate this implicit knowledge. We can analyse these miscues to see the way in which children try to keep their reading in organized sentences. Most usually, for instance, the miscues will be of a noun for a noun, a verb for a verb, etc. Third, children try to maintain a meaningful read when involved with a book. The miscues that are produced will demonstrate the use of the semantic cue system, as words of similar meaning are offered as substitutions. Such an emphasis upon meaning may sometimes lead the child to ignore the graphophonic cues. Of course, it is not the case that children simply use one or other of the cues. In many instances, it is apparent that children make use of all of the cues in order to read a text and that the miscues produced have some degree of graphophonic, syntactic and semantic similarity or appropriateness.

However, using language cue systems is more complex than the above might suggest. The graphophonic cue system provides readers with the orthographic written symbols of the alphabetically written English language and these symbols indicate the conventions of our spelling. And the sound or phonological system enables us to turn these written symbols into oral language. But it is not just the letters and words which are represented graphically, as punctuation is also represented on the page; apostrophes in particular are represented as part of a word and have to be dealt with by children. Next, the syntactic cues deal with the ways in which words, sentences and paragraphs are brought together within a text. Although we tend to study syntactic cues by considering the complete sentence, it is possible to consider the child's awareness of word features, in what Kenneth Goodman (1994) refers to as the lexico-grammatical language cue system. So although the syntactical feature of sentence order might be of prime importance, we can also look at the way in which children use the inflection system of bound morphemes (-ed, -s, -ing) and the function words (e.g. 'the') that carry less meaning but are instrumental in creating sentence patterns. Finally, the semantic cue system is used to create meaning and children demonstrate their attempts to maintain that meaning in the miscues that they produce. However, Goodman (1994) refers to the semantic–pragmatic cue system, which serves to remind us that a reader has to consider the context in order to extract the fullest meaning. A text might be written straightforwardly to convey a particular meaning, or it might be written to convey a more subtle message. The use of words in the text and the context in which they are written are important pragmatic features.

A knowledge of the language cue systems used by children enables the teacher to be more reflective in terms of the support that might be given during a shared reading interaction. And on the basis of the diagnosis made during a miscue analysis, it also helps the teacher to determine which literacy activities might be developed further.

In the classroom

Six-year-old Alan, while reading with his teacher from a book, demonstrated his understanding of the syntactic cue system. The text sentence to be read was:

> The giants live in the castle.

However, Alan read it as:

> The giant lives in the castle.

So having miscued 'giants' and read 'giant', Alan was confronted with a difficulty with the word 'live'. He either had to self-correct and read 'giants' or he needed to produce another miscue of the verb so as to maintain his reading as a sentence. Alan changed the verb ending, therefore creating a miscue chain, and in so doing he demonstrated his implicit understanding of sentences.

Further reading

Gollasch, F.V. (ed.) (1982a) *Language and Literacy: The Selected Writings of Kenneth S. Goodman. Vol. I: Process, Theory, Research.* London: Routledge.

Gollasch, F.V. (ed.) (1982b) *Language and Literacy: The Selected Writings of Kenneth S. Goodman. Vol. II: Reading, Language and the Classroom Teacher.* London: Routledge.

Fred Gollasch has collected together a number of Kenneth Goodman's articles in Volume 1 of this text. The main sections are concerned with the reading process and miscue analysis. Therefore, not only are there some key articles which address the cue systems directly (including 'Reading: A psycholinguistic guessing game', pp. 33–43), but also most of the articles contain some reference to the language cue systems. Although Volume 2 does not look at the language cue systems in any detail, nevertheless one of the articles, 'Behind the eye: What happens in reading' (pp. 99–124), is useful.

Goodman, Y., Watson, D. and Burke, C. (1987) *Reading Miscue Inventory: Alternative Procedures.* New York: Richard C. Owen.

This book is referenced in the section on *miscue analysis* and the main emphasis of the book is to provide the details of that means of exploring a child's reading. However, the second chapter of the book explores the theoretical understandings of a holistic view of reading, and includes a good introduction to the language cue systems. It serves as a useful starting point for an exploration of this subject.

discussions

In her short booklet, *How Texts Teach What Readers Learn*, Margaret Meek (1988) retells how she read *Rosie's Walk* by Pat Hutchins together with the young reader Ben: 'First we looked at the cover and talked about the hen, the fox, the bees, and the trees with apples and pears. Ben was the leader in this discussion' (p. 8). And there was far more to that discussion, as the teacher and the child explored the title, author, dedication and illustrations, as well as the characters and setting of the story. So by the time the actual words of the book were to be read, Ben had an awareness and understanding of the story which facilitated his reading. Such discussions can play an important part in the reading of stories with young readers. Furthermore, these discussions can take place to good effect not only before but also during and after the reading. And they can occur in a range of literacy activities, such as *story readings*, *shared reading* and *hearing children read*, all of which involve the teacher interacting with the child (or children) centred on a book.

Marie Clay (1991) argues that introducing a new storybook to young readers by means of a discussion is important as a means of enabling them to read the book with some fluency and independence at a first reading. The discussion can achieve that because the children's background knowledge is brought into focus, and perhaps some new knowledge is introduced by the teacher. But the children have to be active participants in this discussion, drawn into the interaction by the skilful questioning and prompting of the teacher rather than being told about the book. Furthermore, the discussion should be like 'an easy conversational exchange which does not dismember the story' (Clay 1991: 266). So the teacher and the children discuss the story in a relaxed but informed manner, which provides a foundation for reading the story and leaves the children with an interest in doing so.

Also, there are often short discussions during the reading of a book – in particular, children often comment upon the story as it is being read. The teacher should respond in a way which requires the children to predict or speculate on their comments or questions. But the teacher will also wish to get the reading back on track, but without doing so in a heavy-handed way which might suggest to a child that his or her comments were unwelcome. Sometimes the teacher might instigate a short discussion during the reading, but this is usually done during a natural break in the book (e.g. as a page is turned) because the teacher does not wish to cause anything more than a minor disruption to the story.

At the end of the reading, the discussion is often used to clarify aspects of the story or to contextualize it for the children by making *text-to-life connections*. However, as Jim Trelease (1989) notes, we need to engage in these discussions with care, for it is not the purpose of the discussion to prise every detail of the story from the children as though it was some form of quiz. The notion of an easy conversational exchange is a useful one to adopt here. Teachers usually also try to get the children to reflect upon the story that has been read and perhaps express their feelings towards the story or its characters (Mason *et al.* 1989). Such a strategy helps young children with their reading, but it also encourages them towards reflective reading.

So discussions are an important part of these storybook

interactions, and we might have included the shared book experiences with *big books* as part of that debate. But this omission reminds us that discussions about literacy occur in many other contexts. For instance, in the section on *classroom print*, it is suggested that it is not enough just to flood the classroom with print, important as that may be, but the teacher needs to bring the children's attention to the print and to discuss it. Such discussions can clarify the messages and help the children to learn about, as well as through, literacy. And within *play activities*, the teacher can provide demonstrations, which Cambourne (1988) argues are an important feature of the classroom. Often these demonstrations lead into a discussion of some aspect of literacy.

Discussions about literacy are a part of most literacy activities that occur in the infant classroom, as the children seldom work in isolation but instead are supported by an adult. Therefore, discussions enable children to articulate queries, comments and uncertainties with the expectation that the teacher will guide and support them towards an increased understanding of some aspect of literacy.

In the classroom

When six-year-old Leah shared her book, *Good-Night Owl* (Hutchins 1972), with her class teacher there was a brief discussion before Leah began to read:

Teacher: So what is it about?
Leah: Good-Night Owl.
Teacher: Good-Night Owl.
What's owl doing?
Leah: Trying to sleep.
Teacher: Is he? When is he trying to sleep?
Leah: Mmm, during the day.
Teacher: Is he? And that's when he sleeps is it? We'll have to find out.
Leah: Owl tried to sleep.
Teacher: Oh, where's he trying to sleep?
Leah: In the tree, in a hole in a tree.
Teacher: That's right. He is isn't he?

In part, this discussion is about the title of the book. But it is also about the main theme of the book, that the owl is trying to sleep during the day. The teacher also uses the first sentence of the book to extend the discussion. This first sentence is the only writing on the first two pages, so the discussion at this point could take place while the page is being turned. Although the discussion is very brief, and led by the teacher's questions, seen in the context of a teacher working with a large class of children, it demonstrates how even a brief discussion can be woven into the interaction between a teacher and a child with a book.

Further reading

Clay, M. (1991) Introducing a new storybook to young readers. *The Reading Teacher*, 45: 264–73.

In this article, Marie Clay suggests that if an adult reads a storybook aloud a number of times, it enables children subsequently to read the same book more easily and with greater understanding. However, she also explores those occasions when it might be regarded important for a child to read a new text independently – part of *reading recovery* would be an example. In such circumstances, the prior discussion might be important as an aid to the child's reading. This article explores the nature of such discussions and provides some transcript evidence from teachers and children working together to help describe such discussions in a practical way.

emerging literacy

Teachers of young children, whether in the nursery, pre-school classroom or the reception or kindergarten classroom when the children start school, have to consider how to help the children develop as readers and writers. In part, that consideration will be based upon views that the teacher has about children as learners and the extent to which each child is perceived to bring to school knowledge and skills about literacy. In recent years, the notion of emerging literacy has developed as a way of viewing children as literacy learners, as intensive – and often longitudinal – case studies have produced evidence about children's learning to read and write at home and at school. And the evidence from these studies has suggested that children are engaged with literacy in many different ways during their early years. This engagement provides the basis for literacy to emerge from each child.

But why use the term 'emergent'? Nigel Hall (1987) suggests that there are four reasons for doing so. First, the term indicates that the

development of a child as a literacy user comes from within. It is children who make sense of all the print data which surround them during their early years, albeit supported by interactions with adults about that print. Second, emergence implies a gradual process which takes place over time – literacy development does not wait until the school years in order to begin. Literacy emerges while the child is at home engaged with print in a variety of ways. Third, emerging literacy recognizes the abilities that children have to make sense of the world. It perceives children as active learners constructing a sense of their environment, an environment which includes a substantial amount of print. Fourth, literacy only emerges if the conditions are right, so there has to be meaningful print and engagement with adults who support the child's enquiries. There also has to be respect for the child's literacy performances. So when children produce their emergent readings (which might be meaningful but not yet constrained by the conventions of the print) of a story book or they begin to write with *invented spellings*, adults need to accept and support such efforts.

These reasons for using the term 'emergent' help to demonstrate key aspects of the role of the child in the learning process. Teale and Sulzby (1989) develop this further in their consideration of emergent literacy. They suggest that a portrait of young children as literacy learners should include a number of features, some of which can be linked directly to Hall's (1987) list. First, they indicate that learning to read and write begins very early in life. Of course, it is not easy to determine the extent of such early learning or when it begins, but we do recognize the encounters that very young children have with literacy, and we can speculate on the learning that might be taking place. Children in the first year of life are often read to by their parents and grandparents and often informed of print in the environment. Each of these interactions will help children to learn about literacy. And opportunities to write, even though they may at first only appear as 'scribbles', also help children to emerge as literacy users.

Second, children learn about literacy from real-life settings. In part, this is because of contact with *environmental print*, but it is also derived from their observations of adults using books, newspapers and magazines. Many children, therefore, see adults using print for real purposes and they begin to see the ways in which literacy can support particular goals. Third, it is literacy that emerges rather than reading or writing; as Teale and Sulzby (1989: 3) indicate, 'reading and writing develop concurrently and interrelatedly in young children'. They extend this to argue that

oral language proficiency is also related to growth in reading and writing. Finally, they emphasize that children emerge as literacy learners through their active engagement with written language. And, we recognize that young children need the support of adults who can facilitate such learning by demonstrating, suggesting and guiding the children's efforts. (Teale and Sulzby refer to literacy as a complex sociopsycholinguistic activity, which emphasizes the role of parents and others, and subsequently the teacher, in helping the child to emerge as a literacy user.)

Emerging literacy may well appear to place the emphasis on learning rather than on teaching, but it does not deny the important role of the adult. So what does emergent literacy suggest for practices in the classroom? Teachers will want to build upon the literacy that has already been learnt at home and in many instances replicate some of the practices which the children have already experienced. Therefore, a classroom should be rich in print, most of which serves a real function and some of which is drawn from the environment, thereby creating a link with the reading with which the children are familiar. Teachers should read stories to the children on a daily if not more frequent basis, and use such story readings to develop activites of drama, painting and writing which are stimulated by the stories. Additionally, the *play activities* that are provided should be developed to encourage the children to engage with literacy and again this will reflect some of the experiences the children will have had at home. Partly, the play activities will encourage the children to write, as will some of the story readings, and the teacher should encourage meaningful writing knowing that the children's involvement with letters, words and sentences will help them to develop further their emerging literacy.

Further reading

Hall, N. (1987) *The Emergence of Literacy*. Sevenoaks: Hodder and Stoughton.

Nigel Hall's book, as the title indicates, is about the concept of emerging literacy. It provides a good deal of theory to substantiate what he refers to as the rediscovery of emergent literacy. It is a rediscovery because, as is presented in this book, there is a historical background to these ideas. Emergent literacy is contrasted with other literacy assumptions which, for instance, might have emphasized reading readiness – where the role of the teacher might have been to get children ready for reading, therefore denying many of the experiences that the children brought to school. The final chapter in the book is devoted to 'emergent literacy and schooling', in

which practices to be developed by the teacher to support emergent literacy are suggested.

Strickland, D.S. and Morrow, L.M. (eds) (1989a) *Emerging Literacy: Young Children Learn to Read and Write.* Newark, DE: International Reading Association.

Reference was made above to the work of Teale and Sulzby, the authors of one of the twelve chapters in this book. The authors of the other eleven chapters are also considered authorities on the topic of young children learning to read and write. Reference to another one of the chapters, by Lesley Mandel Morrow, is made in the section on the *library corner*. The book should be very useful for teachers of young children, as it provides many practical ideas, as well as a theoretical background, related to the encouragement of an emerging literacy in children.

environmental print

Most children in the developed world are surrounded by print in their homes and immediate environments. Importantly, this print is contextualized. For example, when a child sees the word 'cornflakes' it is likely to be on the cornflakes box, and the pictures, colours and writing on the box as well as the contents of the box immediately assist the child in determining the connection between the word, or initially the logo, and the product. So the contextualized nature of environmental print supports the child's learning.

In the home, children's toys are often labelled with their 'names', and the boxes the toys were purchased in are covered in print. Print also appears on the labels of their clothes and, more directly, as writing on the T-shirts they and those around them wear. Many children also see a wide variety of printed materials brought into the home – newspapers, magazines, cookery books, telephone directories, etc. And TV programmes, especially during the introduction and conclusion, include a lot of print, as do many commercials – to which children often appear to pay a good deal of attention.

Outside the home, there are street names and road signs, and the names and notices on and in buildings. Then there is the wealth of print which confronts children in supermarkets: the print on labels and boxes again, the signs on shelves, the special-offer posters and the directional signs.

Children are aided in their search for a meaning to such print by seeing adults responding to and using the print and talking about it. Even more directly the adults might talk with the children about the logos and the print. Where that happens, the children will be helped to understand the nature and message of the environmental print.

Case studies of young children learning to read and write help us to see the way in which environmental print, and parental comment about that print, supports the child's learning. Baghban (1984) provides an example in her book, which details the growth of her daughter's reading and writing. Giti was able, we are informed, to identify the broad yellow 'M' for Macdonalds by the age of twenty months. Furthermore, she was able to do so whether the 'M' was outside of a Macdonalds, on an advert or on a cup. As we might expect, children do appear to be able to recognize environmental print and to do so with a confidence which enables them to read that print with the contextualized support gradually reduced. So, initially, children might be able to recognize the logo together with all the background features, then there is recognition of the logo alone and, finally, recognition of the logo, as a word or letter(s), written with normal script letters and without colour (Goodman and Altwerger 1981).

Laminack (1991), in his study of his son Zachary, also provides many examples of contact with and recognition of environmental print. These began at the age of thirteen months with Zachary's recognition of a 'Stop' road sign, when he responded to his father's question 'What does it say?' by replying 'Stop the truck'. At the age of three years and eleven months he was able to indicate how he worked out some of the subtle differences in signs, when he was able to discriminate between the drinks available from a vending machine: 'The diet Sprite has two yellow words and the regular Sprite just has a red dot'.

Another way of considering children's growth in their understanding of environmental print is to note how they are able to recognize a label or logo with a gradually developing accuracy and appropriateness. Harste *et al.* (1984) found that when asked about logos, children might first provide a functional response (e.g. 'a toothbrush' for Crest toothpaste) that might later become a categorical response (e.g. 'toothpaste') and finally a specific response (e.g. 'Crest'). And that development they argue is very much related to the opportunities and experience the children have to transact with the print and to be supported by an adult.

Because many children start school familiar with, and able to read, a good deal of environmental print, we can support their literacy by using that print in the classroom. Although *classroom print* includes other varieties of print, environmental print can also be displayed usefully. And print from the environment can be included in the materials for *play activities*, so that the literacy aspect of the play is encouraged. Where environmental print is used in that way, the school creates a bridge between the literacy experiences that the children bring from their homes and neighbourhood with those of the classroom. Such a link has benefits for the literacy awareness and literacy development of the children.

In the classroom

A visit to a supermarket on almost any day of the week will provide evidence of the power of environmental print. Young children, under five years of age, will be 'helping' one of their parents with the shopping. And that help will include selecting, from a wide range of similar products, the particular brand that the child, or the family, wishes to purchase. That the young children so often appear to succeed in their selection is an indication of their use of the logo, colour, shape and print of the product.

Five-year-old John was able to replicate those experiences in his classroom, because the classroom teacher had developed a collection of grocery boxes. That enabled John and his classmates to place the boxes in categories, to write shopping lists, to shop for a product, and to inform each other about the products:

John: I'm getting some cornflakes.
Steven: So am I.
John: They're not cornflakes. They're Frosties. You can see it on the box.

And, although we cannot tell what John could see on the box, we can note that he was paying attention to key features which provided the message for him.

Further reading

Hall, N. (1987) *The Emergence of Literacy*. Sevenoaks: Hodder and Stoughton.

Nigel Hall's book is about young children who, before entering school, have already begun to demonstrate that they are becoming literate. He makes the point that the text is not about those few children who reach school able to read and write, in the conventional sense of those words. Rather, it is a book about all children who are growing up in a Western, print-oriented society. These children emerge as literacy users because they construct their own knowledge about print. And an important section of the book is devoted to children's contact with environmental print. Here reference is made to a number of research articles which have demonstrated the role of environmental print as one of the foundations of children's emerging literacy.

Harste, J.C., Woodward, V.A. and Burke, C.L. (1984) *Language Stories & Literacy Lessons*. Portsmouth, NH: Heinemann Educational.

This book provides a detailed account of three- to six-year-old children learning to read and write. It does so by providing numerous observations of children's encounters with language; such evidence provides language stories from which we can begin to deduce literacy lessons. And some of these observations were of children's encounters with environmental print. The examples demonstrate for us the ways in which environmental print can support children's literacy development. Indeed, they note that children often read boxes more conventionally than they read books because the boxes are more familiar to them.

Laminack, L. (1991) *Learning with Zachary*. Richmond Hill, Ontario: Scholastic Canada.

In this short book, Lester Laminack provides an interesting insight into the pre-school literacy development of his son Zachary. There were many different activities and interactions which contributed to that development. However, an important feature was the attention that Zachary paid to environmental print and the discussions that he initiated with his father about that print. The print was in many formats, from the logos associated with products to street signs, clothing labels, print on toys and the print associated with TV programmes. Zachary's interest in environmental print was, of course, supported by his father and other significant adults who responded to his questions, his hypotheses and his more generalized statements about the print.

formula for beginning reading

It would be a misunderstanding if the reader thought that this section was going to provide a simple formula which, if followed, would ensure that all children would immediately be successful with their reading. Nevertheless, the article by Vera Southgate (1968), which presented such a formula, was interesting because it reminded us of some of the important areas that need to be considered when an approach or programme is being organized, developed and managed. The article by Southgate was published in a research journal for the purpose of alerting teachers to read and consider research reports, in the area of reading, with great caution. She argued that research which purported to demonstrate the effectiveness of a particular reading scheme, with its associated books or apparatus, should be analysed to determine whether all the factors which might influence reading development had been controlled within the research.

However, the formula can be used for purposes other than reading research reports. Each element of the formula might be considered by a teacher, when organizing for reading activities in the classroom, in order to respond to the question 'What am I doing about this aspect – and why?'

So what was the formula that Southgate put forward? She expressed the formula as:

$$\text{Reading Progress} = RD + TC + MM + MD + ML + P$$

where RD = reading drive, TC = teacher competence, MM = medium, MD = method, ML = materials and P = procedure. Furthermore, the formula was presented in this order as it accorded with Southgate's perception of the importance of the individual elements. Therefore, *reading drive* – the beliefs and attitudes of the staff about the importance of reading – was seen as the most important aspect in encouraging children's reading progress. Such a viewpoint is salutary for all of us as teachers. Do we create a reading drive in our classrooms in which our enthusiasm for reading is passed on to the children very clearly? And such a reading drive might be linked to the second part of the formula, teacher competence. As Frank Smith (1978) argues, many teachers seem to be able to help children to learn to read no matter what method they employ. In part, this might be due to reading drive, but it might also be linked to the knowledge about reading and children that the teacher brings to the task. Knowing about reading and children helps the teacher to confront the unexpected situation and to do so in an informed way. But that teacher competence also enables the teacher to plan, organize, implement and develop the reading programme to a high level in the first place. Therefore, a major part of the formula is centred on the teacher (*teacher's role*) rather than the activities of the classroom and the children.

That *medium* as an element in the formula is indicative of a major part of the debate on early reading development during the 1950s and 1960s. Now the debate so infrequently considers this topic that traditional orthography – the format in which print appears normally – is no longer a part of the vocabulary of younger teachers. Yet during the 1950s and 1960s, the question of whether to help children with early reading by changing the print (e.g. initial teaching alphabet; Pitman II 1959) or adding to the print using colour (e.g. colour story reading; Jones 1967) was a key debate. And it might have been because it was seen to be so key at that time that it was presented as the third part of the above formula.

Medium as an area of interest still remains. For example, Christopher Upward (1992a, 1992b) has debated the benefits that might accrue if the spelling system of English was changed to Cut Spelng (CS), and the word 'spelng' is indicative of the nature of what is proposed.

The next 'M' relates to *method* and typically the debate had centred upon the look-and-say/whole-word methods or *phonics teaching* (see, e.g. Chall 1967). More recently, the debate has substituted the more holistic and wider concept of the *whole-language* approach for the earlier word methods and considered that against the phonics approach. However, as can be seen in the sections devoted to these headings, the reality is more complex than the simple either/or dichotomy would suggest.

The *materials* to be used in the classroom require the teacher to consider all the books, charts, cards and other printed materials available in the classroom. This is a major task for the teacher, who will need not only to consider *reading schemes* and *real books*, but also the extent to which books are available in the classroom that are not story books or books in a narrative *genre*.

Finally, in the formula the teacher is asked to think about procedure and yet that aspect contains so many important features. For instance, the time devoted to literacy activities and the wide range of literacy activities that might be planned for the classroom, including the role of *writing* in encouraging reading development, will all be part of procedure. Procedure, if you like, covers the planning, organization and management of the reading curriculum!

The formula does perhaps provide a simple guide for considering research reports in reading because the teacher can use the formula to ask whether all the factors in the classroom were considered by the researcher. But the formula can also be used when simple solutions to the teaching of reading are proposed. Such 'solutions' can be analysed in terms of how the 'solution' meets all the factors which may be of some importance in early reading.

Further reading

Southgate, V. (1968) Formulae for beginning reading tuition. *Educational Research*, 11: 23–30.

The original article which proposed the formula for beginning reading tuition dealt essentially with research issues. However, many teachers have found that a consideration of the details of the article leads to a fundamental appraisal of the approach to reading in the early years classroom.

genres

Although genre might be thought to be more of an issue for the junior and secondary school teacher, nevertheless children in the infant classroom also require experiences that enable them to cope with the various genres that they meet in the infant classroom and the wider environment. An exploration of the different genres might demonstrate this to be the case. Alison Littlefair (1991, 1992) suggests that texts might be considered as falling into one of four major categories of genre, the first of which, the literary genre, forms a central part of young children's reading. After all, story books are for many children the texts which introduce them to books. And as teachers we might occasionally group books into subgroups of that genre when we put together collections of nursery rhymes, folk tales, poetry or animal stories, adventure stories, etc. It is very likely that children will have considerable experience of reading, and being read to, within that genre. However, young children are likely to meet other genres and need adult support, at least initially, to help them with the demands of that writing. The expository genre contains more objective writing and infant children begin to explore that genre as they write about their own science experiments, for example, or get information *by reading non-fiction* books. Then there is the procedural genre which may well be evident in the *classroom print*, as notices and lists of instructions inform children about classroom activities. Furthermore, many teachers of young children use written recipes with groups of children engaged in cooking, which brings home very forcibly the importance of following with some accuracy the procedures in such writing. Fourth, the reference genre will be brought to the children's attention in the infant classroom as they are introduced to dictionaries. But the children will need to access sequential information in other texts, and simple encyclopaedias are one example of such books.

At this point, perhaps, we need to remind ourselves that in the early years classroom it will be the literary genre that provides the bulk of the children's reading experiences. But it will also be evident that the other genres are not something waiting to be introduced in later years, but rather they will be part of the literacy experiences of the children almost as soon as they start school. That being the case, the teacher might want to demonstrate those genres from time to time. For instance, extracts from information books might be read to the class occasionally, which will help the children to begin to perceive the different register of language that is often used in such texts. So although it might be left to the older children to examine more analytically some of these differences, nevertheless younger children will at least begin to appreciate the different use and flow of language which will then help them with their own readings. Occasionally, a child might wish to read an information book with a teacher as part of a *shared reading*, where support from the teacher is provided for those more unusual texts.

Littlefair suggests that although some writers use genre and register interchangeably, it might be better to separate them. The register will be influenced by the subject being written about and the relationship with the audience for that writing. And that will determine the vocabulary to be used and the grammatical structures. We all understand that, because we write in different registers according to the task in hand, and even young children – before coming to school in many cases – soon realize that a shopping list is constructed differently from a message or story.

The main task for the teacher of young children is to ensure that there is a range of written materials that the children can experience. Therefore, in addition to the extensive number of story books in the classroom, there should also be books written in other genres. Furthermore, the teacher needs to demonstrate, share and work alongside the children in order to support them in their understanding of the various forms of writing.

In the classroom

In the early years classroom, the teacher will occasionally read from a book in a genre other than the narrative. In the brief extract below, the teacher was reading to a class of thirty six-year-olds from a text (*Famous Cities: London*) that provided some historical evidence for a project which the children were following:

Candina: It burnt a lot of the houses.
Teacher: Yes, it burnt a lot of the houses, didn't it. Shall we find out?
Fire was a frequent threat to the city of London.
Why was it a threat?
Claire: Because the fire could burn the people's houses down.
Teacher: Why could it burn the houses down?
Candina: Because they were so close together.
Teacher: So close together and they were made of?
Children: Wood.
Teacher: That's right.
Since many London houses were wooden, fires could spread rapidly.
They could spread quickly couldn't they?

Even in this short extract, we can see how the textual language could be more problematic for the children, especially if their main contact with books was through stories. The teacher was giving more explanations during the reading for that reason. The children, by hearing such texts read occasionally, would begin to appreciate the nature of the discourse patterns in such books.

Further reading

Littlefair, A.B. (1991) *Reading All Types of Writing: The Importance of Genre and Register for Reading Development*. Buckingham: Open University Press.

Littlefair, A B. (1992) *Genres in the Classroom.* Widnes: UK Reading Association.

The first of these books is the more substantial both in size and in content. The second is directed more firmly towards the classroom teacher. Nevertheless, both books extend the brief introduction to the subject given here. The 1991 title also makes links to the National Curriculum in England and Wales and demonstrates how at each Key Stage in English, there are expectations of the children's knowledge of, and ability to work with, different genres.

hearing children read

Like many other texts on the teaching of reading, the Bullock Report (DES 1975) noted the widespread use of 'hearing children read' as a classroom practice in infant classrooms in the UK. Among the teachers of six-year-old children who were surveyed for the report, a substantial number indicated that they hear their children read daily. This was especially true for those children who were regarded as poor readers. But in the majority of the 1417 classes that were surveyed, even the ablest readers in the class were heard reading three or four times a week. Such a commitment to hearing children read continued at the beginning of the 1990s (HMI 1992).

So what is the nature of the one-to-one interaction – hearing a child read? In most respects, it is similar to the fourth part of the *shared reading* sequence. So:

- the teacher and the child discuss parts of the book;
- the child reads to the teacher (and the child does so because he/she has reached that point, in his/her development as a reader, where reading in a conventional way has become possible);
- the teacher listens to the reading and supports the child where that appears to be required;
- finally, the teacher and the child discuss some aspect of the book at the end of the reading.

And all of this indicates that the role of the teacher is not a passive one. Instead, it requires an active listening to the child reading, with the teacher ready to support, guide, instruct or encourage as necessary.

However, if the teacher is listening to many children, and on a regular and frequent basis, there is a need to remain alert to the nature of the activity and ensure that it has not become ritualized (Goodacre, undated). In a ritualized interaction, the teacher might be distracted from the reader to other children or events in the classroom. Or, all interactions might begin to look alike because the teacher has become more concerned with getting through the list of readers rather than ensuring, as he or she needs to, that there is a quality to the activity, with the teacher responding according to the needs of the child and developing the interaction as is required by an analysis of the child's reading. It was for such reasons that Southgate *et al.* (1981) suggested that for older children (their

Extending Beginning Reading Project explored the reading development of seven- to nine-year-olds in classrooms) there might be less frequent but more extended sessions of the teacher and the child with a book. Such sessions, they suggested, might include a range of activities, including the child reading aloud and a discussion of the book, but also from time to time a detailed miscue analysis and/or a checking on comprehension and/or exploring the vocabulary of the book, etc.

Of course, the precise nature of the interaction will be determined by a number of factors, including the difficulty of the text being read and the miscues being produced by the reader. However, the interaction will also be influenced by the purpose that the teacher has in mind when hearing a particular child read. Overall, the teacher is likely to be concerned to help the child develop as a reader and to give the necessary support, encouragement and guidance. Besides helping children to develop as readers, the following reasons were given by teachers for hearing children read (Campbell 1988):

- to develop interest and enjoyment,
- to reinforce personal relationships,
- to give the child practice in reading,
- to develop fluency and expression,
- to check on and develop comprehension,
- to diagnose strengths and weaknesses,
- to check on progress,
- to check on accuracy,
- to provide instruction,
- to encourage the use of contextual cues,
- to teach phonics in context.

It will immediately be obvious that not all of these purposes can inform a single interaction. Some of the purposes are in conflict with each other. Therefore, the teacher will vary the purpose from child to child and also from day to day with any one child. But whatever the purpose(s), as teachers we need to ensure that our behaviour matches our purpose. As a simple example of that, if we have the purpose of developing interest and enjoyment, then the book to be read and the nature of the exchanges between the child and the teacher have to demonstrate the reality of a shared enjoyable experience. Reminding ourselves of the purpose and relating that purpose to behaviour should ensure that concerns about a ritualized activity do not become a reality.

Something that is almost inevitable when a teacher hears a child read is that the child will produce miscues. We will consider *responding to miscues* elsewhere; however, teachers will want to have in mind a number of principles to guide their actions. Because we want children to remain active learners, teachers should use the notion of minimal distraction as a guiding principle. And where support is given, then the principles will include: helping the reader with the current miscue; to do so in a way which might help with that word on another occasion; and to suggest future reading strategies.

Hearing children read can play a useful part in the primary classroom, but it requires a careful *classroom organization* for it to occur. The teacher needs to ensure that the interaction is not interrupted and that the purpose of the activity is reflected in the behaviour of the teacher and the child.

In the classroom

In order to keep each child engaged actively with the text when the teacher is hearing a reader, the principle of minimal distraction might be applied. So when six-year-old Brian was reading to his teacher, his various repetitions, self-corrections and comments received no response from the teacher during part of his reading.

Brian: Next . . . next they find a house made of . . . a house made of jelly.
Ha, ha!
'This will not do . . . This will not do, says one of the little kittens. The children will eat it all up. . .'.
And it will wobble!
'. . .all up and then there will be no house left.
And it would wobble.
Teacher: It would wobble. Go on then.

On this occasion, Brian's enjoyment of the story – in particular, the thought of a jelly (or jello) house – meant that eventually the teacher was brought into the interaction by Brian's insistent comments. Of course, on another occasion when the reader might be producing many miscues which detract from the meaning of the passage, then mediation from the teacher would be required. But, during Brian's reading, the teacher appropriately remained in the background.

Further reading

Arnold, H. (1982) *Listening to Children Reading*. Sevenoaks: Hodder and Stoughton.
In this book, listening to children reading is considered within a historical perspective and there is a consideration of what is involved in the reading process. The word listening is used to denote the active role of the teacher and that active role is demonstrated by Helen Arnold through the use of transcripts of the practice in the classroom. Miscue analysis as a means of diagnosis in a busy classroom is also debated.

Campbell, R. (1988) *Hearing Children Read*. London: Routledge.
This book is devoted entirely to the activity of hearing children read. It sets the scene by describing an infant classroom in which a child is heard reading by the teacher. As we have already noted, it details the purposes that teachers have in mind when they hear children read. However, the main part of the text is used to describe and analyse teachers hearing children read with numerous transcripts providing the basis for that description and analysis. The book concludes with some guidelines for hearing a child read based on the earlier transcript evidence.

Southgate, V., Arnold, H. and Johnson, S. (1981) *Extending Beginning Reading*. London: Heinemann Educational.
The findings from the Extending Beginning Reading Project are reported in this book, a project that explored the reading development of seven- to nine-year-olds in classrooms and considered the classroom practices to support that reading development. The report was critical of hearing children read as the authors witnessed the event with its many disruptions and overly simple teacher responses to miscues. They proposed less frequent, but longer, individual reading consultations with a variety of activities during each consultation.

home–school links

Children arrive at school with some literacy learning already having taken place. Although the literacy experiences of the children will have varied, as Shirley Brice Heath's (1983) study of two communities separated by only a few miles in Carolina, USA demonstrated so vividly, nevertheless all children will reach school with some knowledge of literacy. One problem for the school is to match that previous learning with appropriate teaching strategies which can build on those initial foundations. But this can be made home–school links are established in some links might be established with parents before ool, and particular literacy experiences might be t might involve close collaboration between the e once the children have started school, in which cas and home might together develop certain literacy activities, a *shared reading* is one of the literacy activities which is used frequently to create such a link.

The Plowden Report (DES 1967) emphasized the benefits that might accrue if home–school links are developed. In particular, it noted that when parents became involved and encouraged their children during literacy activities, then those children were likely to make good progress with reading and writing. Subsequently, studies like the Haringey Project (Hewison and Tizard 1980) demonstrated how simple home–school procedures could help in children's reading development. Parents were encouraged to become involved with their children's reading in the form of hearing them read. The children took books home to read to their parents two to three times a week. A reading card, with the book, was used to structure the reading and to allow comments to be passed between the teacher and parents. Children who had this type of support made better progress with their reading than children with other forms of school support. However, the gains made by these children were not always apparent one year after the completion of the project. This ties in with many other projects that have aimed to support children in some aspect of their learning. It serves to remind us that the development of home–school links is a long-term endeavour. Once established, the links need to be maintained and developed further to serve the needs of the children.

Since those initial attempts to establish the value of home–school links, a large number of projects have been initiated and many have been reported upon. Wendy Bloom (1987) has provided details of some of these projects. One feature common to all the successful projects was preparation for the partnership, that is, success is not guaranteed but has to be worked for. Two examples, one from pre-school support and the other related to the early years at school, demonstrate such careful attention to organizational aspects.

The Sheffield Early Literacy Development Project (Weinberger *et al.* 1990) developed as a collaborative project, which included the city's education department. Because it was recognized that knowledge of literacy on entry to school was a strong predictor of later literacy attainment, the project was based on the pre-school period. The project concentrated upon three aspects of literacy, namely: *environmental print*, looking for print in the home and local environment; *shared reading*, in a one-to-one interaction; and *writing*, introducing materials for the child. Then it suggested three key roles that parents could adopt as a model for their children: reading a paper and writing notes or shopping lists, etc.; providing opportunities, by providing the materials or drawing attention to environmental print, etc.; and providing encouragement, by praising achievement, including success in a non-conventional form (e.g. *invented spellings*). Subsequently, some of the comments made by the parents were indicative of the changed views that they developed and of the support that they gave their children for literacy as a result of this project.

In contrast, Davis and Stubbs (1988) encouraged the establishment of home–school links in a number of primary schools. They did so as part of their encouragement for shared reading to support children's development as readers. They recognized that although most early years teachers make valiant attempts to share a book with many of the children in their classes, that aspiration is fraught with difficulties. The size of classes and the need to support children in a range of literacy activities often means that a teacher will share a book with fewer children than might be appropriate and the quality of the interaction can be undermined by those other needs. A home–school shared reading programme can therefore be useful. But that does require an initial meeting to help the home and school to develop a working partnership, and it probably requires some form of booklet which indicates key features of the shared reading practice. Furthermore, the use of a reading or comment card helps teachers and parents to develop similar views of the reading process and give the children similar forms of support. So if the teacher writes on a comment card 'We looked at this book together and I've read the story to Brian', that gives the parent an indication that it is appropriate to spend time discussing a book and for the child to hear the story before being asked to contribute to the reading. However, it is not that single comment but rather a number of comments over a period of weeks and months which can contribute to a shared view of reading and support for reading.

There will be a variety of home–school link programmes that will be developed by schools. However, *shared reading* is often at the heart of those collaborative attempts to support children's literacy learning. But even though the links may focus on the natural sharing of a book between the parent and the child, nevertheless in order to make the programme successful there is a need for initial careful planning, an organization which maintains the link on a daily basis and the will to sustain the link on a long-term basis.

In the classroom

Three- and four-year-olds in a nursery classroom were encouraged to take a book home each evening to share with their parents. And their parents were encouraged to read the book to their children. Whenever possible, the nursery teacher discussed the book with each child as the book was changed:

Teacher: What was your book about?
Jamie: About Spot going to the seaside.
Teacher: Did you like the book?
Jamie: Yeah, 'cos it was lovely.
Teacher: Which part did you like best?
Jamie: The bit where Spot got splashed – I get splashed in the bath.
Teacher: Do you? Okay, so do you want to get another book for tonight?
Jamie: Yeah.
Teacher: So what have you got there?
Jamie: It's another Spot story – I like Spot.
Teacher: What do you think Spot is going to do now?
Jamie: Go to the doctor's.
Teacher: Who do you think he will see?
Jamie: His friends.

So Jamie, who was nearly four years old, had the opportunity to talk about his books, to relate the story to his own experiences, and to reflect on his choice of book. The home–school link facilitated teacher–child discussions at school and story readings at home.

Further reading

Weinberger, J., Hannon, P. and Nutbrown, C. (1990) *Ways of Working with Parents to Promote Literacy Development*. Sheffield: University of Sheffield Division of Education.

This twenty-eight page, A4-size booklet is very practical in its orientation. However, it does back the practical suggestions with theoretical views and there are references to a number of key texts. The booklet includes a jigsaw framework as a means of maintaining some form of *record-keeping* of the children's achievements. And the parents were encouraged to participate in that process by shading in the 'pieces' as the children demonstrated their literacy behaviours.

Beverton, S., Hunter-Carsch, M., Obrist, C. and Stuart, A. (1993) *Running Family Reading Groups*. Widnes: UK Reading Association.

Although Family Reading Groups link teachers and librarians with parents, they do not have as a main aim the teaching of reading, albeit that might be an indirect outcome of the meetings. Instead, the aims are 'to promote a love of books and voluntary reading' and 'to widen children's and adults' experience of children's books' (p. 9). Those aims are achieved during a series of meetings in which discussions are held and children and adults review books that they have enjoyed. The authors stress the need to consult and plan in order to achieve success with these meetings and they suggest strategies for setting up and running a Family Reading Group.

illustrations

Teachers of young children will be aware of the way in which the covers on books attract the attention of children who are beginning to emerge as readers. Many books should be displayed in *library corners* with their front covers showing, so that the illustrations can lead the children into selecting a book. Furthermore, Margaret Meek (1988) notes that a well-illustrated cover could be used to initiate a discussion about the characters and setting of the story, so that the child would be well prepared for the story and would already have anticipated some possibilities for the plot.

Therefore, as a simple, although important, starting point, the illustrations in early reading books can be seen as a lure into the book. The illustrations can attract the children's attention and encourage them to engage with books. And the bold pictures and bright colours frequently do exactly that. Jill Bennett (1991) noted that sixteen-month-old Joe would rush off to get a Spot book (*Where's Spot?* by Eric Hill) when asked 'Shall we read a book?' Although Joe was unable to read the print, he was able to engage with the pictures and, with that particular book, help to find Spot's hiding places by opening the doors, lids and flaps. Spot, as Bennett noted, is probably one of the best loved picture book characters of recent times. Yet the illustrations are very simple with little or no background, the emphasis of the pictures being on the characters –

especially Spot. Nevertheless, children from one to five years of age appear to be captivated by the representations of Spot. They are attracted to the Spot books, and others, in part because of their illustrations, but also because of the enjoyable interactions that they have with significant adults.

The illustrations in many of the excellent picture books that are now available do far more than just attract children to the book, however. In many early reading books, the illustrations are an important part of the story. For instance, in Eric Carle's *Do You Want To Be My Friend?*, the illustration of an animal's tail leads to the side of the page and takes the reader on to the next page. And in the much loved *Rosie's Walk* by Pat Hutchins, the illustrations play an even more prominent part in the story. Hearing the words of that story without any knowledge of the book, or the pictures, will only provide the listener with part of the story. The fox, a central character of the story, is never mentioned in the text, but is there on every double-page spread and plays an important part in the development of the plot.

The illustrations in many picture books are in bright colours and that appears to be part of the attraction. But the illustrations do not have to be in full colour; more importantly, they need to be there for a purpose, supporting the text, or part of the text, or creating a character, or suggesting a setting, or developing the plot.

When these purposes are met, then illustrations can provide an important contribution to the child's development as a reader, because they capture the child's involvement and engagement with the book. But the illustrations do more than that, very often because having become interwoven with the narrative, they are important in helping the child to understand and become engaged with the story. In her book *Pictures on the Page*, Judith Graham (1991) demonstrates this with great skill, and she concludes that the illustrations have the potential to create readers – a conclusion which reminds us as teachers of our important role in selecting worthwhile books for the classroom library.

Further reading

Bennett, J. (1991) *Learning to Read with Picture Books*, 4th edn. Stroud: Thimble Press.

As the title of the book suggests, it argues that children can best learn to read when presented with picture books (*real books*) rather than *reading scheme* books. And a substantial part of this text is devoted to a list of books which might be used to help young children to read and to continue reading. This list includes brief descriptions of the books in which Jill Bennett demonstrates the way in which many of the books have words and pictures that are closely connected. Indeed, she indicates, through these examples, that the illustrations add to the story that is being told.

Graham, J. (1991) *Pictures on the Page*. Sheffield: NATE.
In this text, Graham provides a very detailed account of the importance of illustrations in picture and early reading books. She argues that much of a character, setting, story and theme can be conveyed through carefully executed and detailed pictures. In that sense, she is suggesting that children can learn *story grammar* as much from pictures as from words. The debate she presents is informed by both theoretical insights as well as numerous examples of illustrations from many different books. These carefully selected pictures support the argument of the importance, in picture and early reading books, of illustrations, for they demonstrate how they support the child in his or her reading.

invented spelling

Children in the nursery classroom, although only three years old, can be encouraged to write. The use of a *writing centre*, or table, which the children can visit freely can be instrumental in that encouragement. However, more important perhaps will be the attitude of the teacher towards the children's efforts at writing. If the teacher conveys an acceptance of, and an interest in, a child's efforts, then that may contribute substantially to the child being encouraged to continue exploring written language. And that acceptance, by the teacher, may need to start with the 'scribbles' that children produce. However, what soon becomes evident is that writing scribbles can be differentiated from drawing scribbles. They can be differentiated because, as the children become more aware of the conventions of writing, so their own writing becomes more linear. Either they produce a joined-up squiggle across the page or they write separate shapes and other marks, which Judith Kalman (1991) refers to as pseudoletters – which could be letters but are not. These pseudoletters can eventually take on other attributes of writing, so that there may be no more than two of the same shapes written side-by-side, there may be gaps between groups of letters, and for some children 'bear' may require more letters than 'butterfly' because it is a bigger creature. In one sense, the writing is real writing rather than scribbles (at least as that word might be interpreted), because the children are writing according to the rules that they perceive might govern writing production. Eventually, the pseudoletters will be replaced by real letters as the children learn from the print in the environment, the *classroom print* and literacy activities, such as shared book experiences with *big books*. However, these letters may be produced as a collection which are difficult to decipher, because initially they may not be governed by the sounds of oral language.

When the children begin to use the sounds of oral language in order to construct words, or invent spellings, then we have a better chance of reading their writing. Charles Read (1971) indicated that children bring some knowledge of English phonology, learnt in the pre-school years, to their first encounters with both reading and writing. Therefore, we can follow the children's writing because it is rule-governed. Initially, we might expect that consonants will be more predominant than vowels in early invented spellings. Donald Graves (1983) suggested that five general stages of invention might be noted in the spellings of children. First, the initial consonant might be used to represent the word (e.g. 'G' for 'grass'). Second, the initial and final consonant might be used (i.e. 'GS'). Third, the initial, final and also any interior consonant might be written (e.g. 'GRS'). Fourth, to those consonants might be added a vowel place holder. That vowel may not be the correct vowel, but it might appear in the correct position (e.g. 'GRES'). Finally, the child moves to a conventional spelling of the word, 'GRASS'.

Children's progress with invented spellings may not be as tidy as the above sequence suggests, however. In part, this is because visual memory also influences each child's invented spellings. This should not surprise us, as print which surrounds children gives them support as they write. One of the first words which children might write conventionally is their own first name. Although this might be guided initially by the child's *phonemic awareness*, most children see their name in many different contexts, which will offer the opportunity of developing a visual memory for that word, as will other experiences for other words.

Although children will move gradually towards conventional spellings, nevertheless teachers should not just stand by and wait for it to happen. The many literacy activities in the classroom will give general support to the children, but additionally the teacher will also help more directly when talking with each child about the writing that has been produced. The content of the writing may be the main emphasis of that discussion or *conferencing*, but the teacher might also talk about one of the invented spellings, particularly high-frequency words, in order to guide the children towards conventional spellings. And the *classroom print* might be used to draw the children's attention to the conventional spellings of some words.

Nevertheless, although the teacher guides the children towards conventional spellings, the advantage of encouraging them to write freely, even though that means that the writing may contain many invented spellings, is that the children have to engage actively with sounds and letters in order to produce the writing. They have to think about the sounds, letters and the representation of those letters on the page. That engagement is an important part of learning to write conventionally. Furthermore, it will be obvious that such activity might be helpful when the child is reading, because the thought applied to sounds and letters in writing can be used to help the child give sounds to the letters and words when they are reading.

In the classroom

Six-year-old Sam produced a piece of writing unaided, in his infant classroom. The writing, a short story, contained numerous invented spellings as well as some conventional spellings:

one day a pig wos
rolin in sum mud and h
met one of His frens
and they Playd two
geva and they the
frma cam and tod them
to get Bac in they stiy
He wos vere cros

The writing, which can be read quite easily, demonstrates Sam's strengths as a literacy user. He is able to spell conventionally many of the words. He is also able to construct, or invent, the other words using his knowledge of letter shapes and letter sounds. These invented spellings suggest that Sam's phonemic awareness will help him to develop further as a reader and a writer.

Further reading

Graves, D. (1983) *Writing: Teachers and Children at Work*. Portsmouth, NH: Heinemann Educational.

This book includes a chapter devoted entirely to spelling in which the author indicates the five general stages of invention which he believes operate as children develop their spelling. The chapter also stresses the active role of the teacher in guiding children towards more conventional spellings.

Kalman, J. (1991) Who invented invented spelling? In K. Goodman, L.B. Bird and Y. Goodman (eds), *The Whole Language Catalog*. Santa Rosa, CA: American School Publishers.

This two-page article provides a good introduction to the notion of invented spellings. It also includes a few helpful examples. Some of these examples are in Spanish, which is indicative of the links made to the important work of Emilia Ferreiro and Ana Teberosky (1982) on invented spellings.

Temple, C., Nathan, R., Temple, F. and Burris, N.A. (1988) *The Beginnings of Writing*. London: Allyn and Bacon.

This book is divided into three main parts, one of which deals with 'The beginnings of spelling'. There are numerous examples of children's spellings within the context of their writing. The authors debate the progress that children make from pre-phonemic spelling (using letters without reference to sounds), to early phonemic, letter name and transitional spelling (which can be related to the first four stages suggested by Graves), and finally conventional spelling. They provide suggestions for the teacher to support the children's move to conventional spelling. These suggestions indicate both general support from the literacy activities of the classroom as well as more specifically bringing the children's attention to some examples of conventional spellings.

knowledge about language

As young children talk, write and read within the context of a variety of experiences, they learn to use each of those aspects of language with increased sophistication. This is important, because children learn about a wide range of subjects through language. So children learn to use language, and to learn through language, and in doing so they also demonstrate their knowledge about language. This knowledge is in the main implicit, but nevertheless it will be demonstrated during the children's talk, writing and reading. For instance, when children talk, they demonstrate their developing knowledge about the structure of sentences with each of their utterances. When they write, their *invented spellings* are indicative of a knowledge about orthography, phonology and sequences of letters. And in their reading, a *miscue analysis* will give information relating to the children's knowledge about parts of speech – they typically substitute nouns for nouns, verbs for verbs, etc. Yet, despite all their knowledge about language, the children may not be able to articulate that knowledge or indeed have the terminology of language to describe their knowledge. Recent debates and developments have considered what children might be expected to know and the extent to which that knowing might be articulated.

In the UK, the Bullock Report (DES 1975) influenced many aspects of language across the curriculum and it raised the issue of children learning about language but not in the sense of being taught formal grammar. However, it was the Kingman Committee (DES 1988a) which developed this idea more specifically. While recognizing the opposing views of the direct teaching of grammar versus no explicit teaching of language structure, the report suggested:

> We do not recommend a return to that kind of grammar teaching. It was based on a model of language derived from Latin rather than English. However, we believe that for children not to be taught anything about language is seriously to their disadvantage.
>
> (p. 12)

The report went on to describe a model of language which included: the forms of the English language; communication and comprehension; acquisition and development; and historical and geographical variation. Such a model, it was suggested, might be used to inform the training of teachers as to how the English language works and to inform professional discussion of all aspects of English teaching. Subsequently, the LINC (Language In the National Curriculum) Project was set up in order to develop materials for professional use (Carter 1990). The conflicts which arose between LINC and government ministers in the UK as those materials were developed, demonstrated the political debates relating to language education in the 1980s. But how did all of these debates and developments affect teachers and children in early years classrooms?

First, the debates suggest that teachers gain by knowing about language. As is argued in the *whole language* section, teachers need to have a knowledge about language which can inform their planning, teaching, monitoring and evaluation of children's progress in literacy. Second, the debates suggest that when talking with children about language, it is appropriate to use the terms which most adequately describe language being used. But as the Kingman Report emphasized (DES 1988a: 13), 'these terms must be acquired mainly through an exploration of the language pupils use, rather than through exercises out of context'. And the very specific example that was given in the report was that of teacher–child conferences to discuss written work. Quite simply it was suggested that terms such as word, sentence or paragraph would be used to talk about the child's writing. So the teacher should not feel restricted by avoiding the technical terms but instead should offer them as part of the discussion in an unobtrusive manner. After all, that is what many teachers of young children do already when they read a story to the class. Words such as author, illustration, character, paragraph, sentence, full-stop, etc., might all be used at various times. And, although some of these words help to describe features of a book or *story grammar*, others are more specifically related to the forms of the language. All of this helps children to acquire a language about language which subsequently will enable them to become more reflective about their own language. But it is acquired in the early years informally during the interactions within meaningful literacy events where they are supported by an informed teacher.

Further reading

DES (1988a) *Report of the Committee of Inquiry into the Teaching of English Language* (The Kingman Report). London: HMSO.

This report provided a model of the English language for use in the teaching of English. It was influential because it set the foundations for parts of the National Curriculum in England and Wales and it provided a basis for a further discussion of what might be learnt about language and how that learning might take place. Of course, the document did not concern itself in the main with the early years. But there were features, some noted above, which were of importance to the infant classroom.

Carter, R. (ed.) (1990) *Knowledge about Language and the Curriculum: The LINC Reader*. London: Hodder and Stoughton.

This book contains a collection of articles under two main headings: 'Knowledge about language – some key issues' and 'Language and the curriculum'. In the first, the Kingman model of language is developed 'in order to make it pedagogically sensitive' (p. 6). A key part of that development was, then, to ensure that teachers would recognize the relevance of the model for classroom practice. In the second part, the articles are more practical in their orientation and at least two of them, those by Yetta Goodman and Margaret Meek, are of direct interest to the early years teacher.

Bain, R., Fitzgerald, B. and Taylor, M. (eds) (1992) *Looking into Language: Classroom Approaches to Knowledge about Language.* London: Hodder and Stoughton.

This collection of articles is very much based in the classroom. The articles report on the work of teachers helping children (often young children) to learn about language. There are numerous transcripts which highlight the ways in which teachers introduce the terminology of language, and examples of the written work of children which demonstrate their knowledge about language.

language experience approach

When the Plowden Report (DES 1967), on primary schools in England, was published, it included brief accounts of practices observed in schools. It noted that 'it is quite common for writing to begin side by side with the learning of reading, for children to dictate to their teachers and gradually to copy and then to expand and write for themselves accounts of their experiences at home and at school. Often these accounts also serve as their first reading books . . . Much of the writing derives from the experiences of individual children, much from the excitement of a shared visit' (pp. 218–19). And although the report did not refer directly to a language experience approach at that point, nevertheless the description above includes many of the elements that would be a recognized part of such an approach.

In particular, the sequence of the use of the experiences of the individual children, the shared visits, the dictation to the teachers, the copying of the dictation by the child and the use of that dictation as a first reading book might all be part of a language experience approach in the classroom with young children. Nora Goddard (1974), in her book on the language experience approach, included all these elements in her discussion of this approach. In particular, she argued that the teacher of young children needs to make use of children's experiences, interests and feelings as a basis for developing literacy. Furthermore, it was suggested, the approach has the advantage of bringing together the four modalities of language (speaking, listening, writing and reading) within one activity.

The practical consequences in the classroom would be that the teacher would wish to encourage each child to talk about those experiences and interests which had been thought about. And that which had been talked about could then be expressed in drawings, paintings and in writing. For the very young child, that writing might have to be dictated to the teacher and the child could subsequently copy the writing. The writing might, then, provide the basis for a reading book for the child. The collection of writing by a child, or the writing by a number of children, can be used as part of the reading resources of the classroom. And when that reading material is organized and presented in an appropriate way it can form part of the reading collection in the *library corner*.

In the Bullock Report (DES 1975), comment was made on the purpose and meaning that was provided for the children in 'the language experience approach to reading we are advocating' (p. 103). Earlier in the report, a description was given of an infant classroom where such an approach was adopted and the benefits of the approach (which we have debated above) were noted.

Many teachers in the UK have made substantial use of language experience approaches (as well as derivatives of it, e.g. *Breakthrough to Literacy*) and aspects of the approach are still being used in many schools, especially the attempts to link children's literacy activities to that which has been experienced and is known. However, there are some issues that need to be considered. Holdaway (1979), although recognizing the many positive features of the approach, was concerned about the possibility that the writing and reading might become dull and repetitive. That is, for some children, the experiences that they dictate to their teacher might relate to common and frequent events without variation (e.g. watching television, shopping with a parent, etc.). However, such obstacles can be overcome. Goddard (1974) suggested that, although the starting point for writing and reading might be the experiences that the children bring to school, it is part of the teacher's role to provide other experiences and interests so that the children can talk about – and therefore write about – visits outside of school, about visitors to the school, collections within the school and experiences encountered second hand through the stories that are read to the class. Such class experiences can lead to individual writing but also to group or class writing where the teacher composes a description or account based on the various inputs from the children. During such a process, the teacher is able to demonstrate the ways in which spoken language is used and developed as it is presented in a written format.

The dictation of writing to the teacher is another contentious area. At the practical level, of course, this has always been a problem for teachers with even moderately large classes. Being a scribe for all the children in the class can create unproductive queues for the children and a difficult task for the teacher. Some teachers, in an attempt to overcome such problems, developed their skills as touch typists using jumbo print typewriters, so speeding up the writing of the dictations and producing 'book-like' print at the same time. However, we also need to consider whether it is in the best interests of the children for the teacher to act as the scribe (Goodman 1991).

Our insights of children as active constructors of knowledge, and the numerous examples we now have of children developing as writers (e.g. Schickedanz 1990), must lead us to question the notion of the teacher as scribe as a constant feature of a language experience approach. Many teachers now wish to see children writing on their own using *invented spellings,* rather than eventually copying the dictated writing produced by the teacher. In such circumstances, children have to consider actively the letters, sounds, words, sentences and eventually some of the other conventions of print as they write. And all of this helps them to develop their literacy.

Nevertheless, the key principle of the language experience approach is likely to underpin a good deal of the work in the early years classroom. That is, the children's experiences and interests, from both outside and within school, will be used to encourage writing, reading, play activities, drama, painting and model-making, etc., so that the children's involvement with literacy in those contexts has meaning and purpose.

Further reading

Goddard, N. (1974) *Literacy: Language Experience Approach*. London: Macmillan Educational.

Joyce Morris, in her introduction to Nora Goddard's book, states that the text is 'the best possible exposition of language-experience approaches to literacy'. Perhaps this view is based on the fact that not only does the book provide interesting classroom examples of the approach in practice, but it also includes a clear reference to the theoretical and historical underpinnings of the approach. And it does not neglect to deal with many of the important and demanding roles which confront the teacher when using the language experience approach.

Stauffer, R.G. (1970) *The Language-Experience Approach to the Teaching of Reading*. New York: Harper and Row.

This text was written by one of the key exponents of the language-experience approach in the USA. (And I used the hyphen here because Stauffer includes a section on the importance of the hyphen to denote the linking of language-experience rather than, as he notes, the less dynamic language and experience.) There are many connections between the approach as it was developed in the UK and in the USA. However, the text does demonstrate a rather stronger emphasis on the dictations to the teacher and there is a complete chapter on 'dictated experience stories'. Furthermore, there is a more formal emphasis given to word recognition. Yetta Goodman (1991: 386) argued that 'taking dictation from children and then having them read it became a way to teach children words and other subskills', thus ultimately taking the approach away from initial principles. Nevertheless, this book provides many interesting insights into the approach as it was being developed in many English-speaking countries.

left-to-right directionality

A simple feature of print in the English language is that the letters, words and sentences go from left to right. Children become aware of this principle as they develop as readers and writers. They also realize that there are other features of print, such as the usual top-to-bottom progression of lines on a page and front-to-back directionality within a book; and words are separated one from another by a space. But how do the children become aware of and understand left-to-right directionality, and the other print functions?

A starting point for that learning, and much other learning about reading as well, can be the *story readings* that parents engage in with their children at home. During such readings, the parents read from the front to the back of the book, point to some words (separated from other words by a space), and occasionally follow their reading with a finger, pointing to the words and therefore to the direction of the print. None of this is done intentionally to teach print functions, rather it is part of the close sharing of the reading between parent and child. Nevertheless, such demonstrations of reading do have the effect of helping children learn about print while enjoying stories.

Many children therefore arrive at school with an understanding of various aspects of print, including left-to-right directionality.

However, some children with less experience of literacy and few interactions with a knowledgeable adult may not have such an understanding. So, the teacher in the classroom will read stories to the children because of the benefits that are derived from that activity (Strickland and Morrow 1989b) and therefore, those children without the earlier literacy experience will begin to benefit and children with a wide range of literacy experiences at home can build upon their foundation of literacy.

However, Holdaway (1979) argued that story readings in the classroom may not be enough for some children, as they do not necessarily provide a model of the reading process. Therefore, *big book* shared book experiences are used, especially with younger children, so that the children can follow the words and directions of the print as the teacher reads to the class and points to the words during that reading. This modelling of the reading process helps the children to learn about the conventions of print.

An initial awareness and understanding of print can be more firmly established during one-to-one *shared reading* interactions. In particular, during early shared readings the teacher is likely to provide a model of the reading before inviting the child to attempt a retelling or an emergent reading of the story. And, during that modelling of the reading, children are able to confirm their developing awareness of print conventions.

During the process of learning about print children will also be *writing*. This writing, especially as it develops from earlier scribbles, will not always follow the print conventions, so that right-to-left, bottom-to-top, a lack of spaces between words and *invented spellings* may all be evident. But that 'get-it-down phase' of writing (Graves 1983) soon passes as children write, read and see others modelling the process.

Left-to-right directionality should not, therefore, be a major concern for teachers. It, and other print conventions, are developed through engagement with literacy in meaningful contexts. Of course, some children will need guidance when a discussion or conference about their writing takes place. However, children mainly learn about print incidentally as they engage with literacy during story readings, *big book* shared book experiences, shared readings and writing.

Further reading

Strickland, D.S. and Morrow, L.M. (1989b) Interactive experiences with storybook reading. *The Reading Teacher*, 42: 322–3.

This short article by Dorothy Strickland and Lesley Mandel Morrow is concerned essentially with the importance of story book reading. They stress the strategies that the teacher might employ before, during and after reading stories, so that the children will benefit from the interactive experience. And they argue that children will learn many different things during those story readings. One area of learning will be about how the book works, which includes the left-to-right directionality of English print.

library corner

The books that are made available for children to read are central to the organization for literacy in the early years classroom. And the quality of those books is of considerable importance – as we note in the section on *real books*. However, how the books are displayed, the general ambience of the area in which they are situated and the availability of a place where the children can read the books in comfort, all suggest that careful thought needs to be given to the setting up of the library corner in the classroom.

A survey of 120 primary schools and 470 classrooms by HMI in the UK, during the autumn term of 1990, indicated the widespread acceptance of the need for a library corner (HMI 1991). Almost all the classrooms had a library corner, or 'reading area' as it was called in the report. And in the classrooms through to year (or grade) 2, the corner was most usually carpeted, had bookshelves and some comfortable seating. But the value of the area for reading varied considerably, depending on how well it was organized and maintained. Therefore, the organization and day-to-day management of the library corner is very important.

The first thing the teacher must consider is the physical setting of the library corner. Most teachers want the daily use of the corner to be integrated into the literacy activities provided. Quite literally, a corner of the classroom is most often used as it provides two physical boundaries as well as two walls for displays of books, book covers, posters and the children's pictures or reviews of books that they have enjoyed. However, it may be insufficient to think only of the walls as boundaries. One further side, and perhaps part of the fourth side, needs to have bookshelves, noticeboards or small cabinets so that the corner is more clearly distinguished from the rest of the room. And these boundaries will also include some surfaces at child level for table-top displays. Carpeting the floor brings two benefits: first, there is the comfort of the soft flooring and, second, there is a reduction in noise which helps the children concentrate on their reading. Soft chairs, large bean bags and/or a sofa all add to the comfort of the library corner. If a few large soft toys of some well-known story characters can be acquired over time, so much the better. One objective will be to make the corner a very inviting place to visit, and this will be enhanced if attention is given to its physical appearance.

However, the books are the reason we want the children to visit the library corner, and therefore the selection and variety of books available is very important. Story books will make up a substantial part of the collection, but there will also be anthologies of nursery rhymes and fairy tales, picture books and poetry books, information and reference books, and each category will need to cater for children at different stages of development. Morrow (1989) suggests that five to eight books per child is a good indication of the minimum number of books required to stock a library. Not all the collection can be displayed with their covers showing, so shelving which allows for the spines of books to be displayed is important.

As part of the management of the library corner, the books that are shown front-on will need to be changed on a regular basis. Furthermore, the teacher should add to the collection as often as possible, ensuring the children are aware of recent additions. From time to time, it is useful to have a book of the week – which has been read to the class, talked about and made readily available by providing more than one copy – and occasionally to have an author of the week or month, when as many of that author's books as possible are displayed. A thematic display which utilizes a number of authors can also stimulate interest in a range of books and might include both story books and information books.

Management of the library corner need not be restricted to the teacher. Morrow (1989) suggests that children should be involved in the planning and development of the area. In particular, she suggests that they might help to develop the rules and arrange a rota for keeping it tidy. If there are notices in or around the library corner (e.g. 'Only six children in the library corner at one time please'), it will help to establish the rules, as well as adding to the *classroom print* which is used for real purposes. A lending system, whereby each child has a library card that indicates the book they have taken home, provides another functional use of literacy.

Involving children in the management of the library corner was noted by HMI as an important feature of successful reading areas.

Nevertheless, class teachers should monitor the corner constantly and ask themselves: Is the area attractive? Has it been changed for good purpose often enough? Do the children use the facility with respect? Are all the children making use of it? Are the discussions about books, and the library corner generally, demonstrating the children's interests in books? Such monitoring will enable teachers to evaluate and develop further this important part of classroom provision.

Further reading

Morrow, L.M. (1989) Designing the classroom to promote literacy development. In D.S. Strickland and L.M. Morrow (eds), *Emerging Literacy: Young Children Learn to Read and Write.* Newark, DE: International Reading Association.

The chapter by Morrow is actually about more than just the library corner. It includes a debate about the organization of the classroom as a rich literacy environment and the benefits that can accrue for the children, and there are examples from classrooms of children engaged with literacy which add to the picture presented. However, part of the chapter is about the literacy centre, which includes a library corner, writing area, oral language area, and additional language arts materials. Such an area is argued to be the focal point of the room and the library corner is a major part of the centre. Morrow considers some of the important features of the library corner and a number of her suggestions are included above.

listening area

For a number of reasons, many teachers of infant school children include in their classroom organization a listening area. First, it is provided as recognition of the power of stories in helping children to learn about reading, writing and aspects of language such as sentence patterns, words, punctuation, etc. Second, it acknowledges that although the teacher may read a story to the class once or twice a day, even that may not be enough to help children in their literacy growth. Third, teachers attempt to share a book with individual children as often as possible, but the size of the class may mean that such one-to-one interactions take place less frequently than is desired. Fourth, many children love to repeat the experience of listening to a story as it becomes familiar to them. Carol Fox

(1993) argues that children need many repetitions of their favourite stories, repetitions which give them time to explore the language and to gain greater control over the story structure, sentence patterns and words of the story and thus provide a solid foundation for their own personal reading of the story in the future. Any one of these reasons might suggest the value of a listening area; together, they present a strong case for the teacher to provide such an area.

All the listening area requires is a table, chairs, access to an electrical point and a tape-recorder. A junction box and several sets of headphones connected to that box would also permit a number of children to listen to the story at the same time. When more than one child listens to the tape, then there is a need, perhaps, for more than one copy of the book. At least one book between two children is necessary. The teacher might wish to encourage two children to listen to the story at the same time and to follow the reading with the book. In this way, there is the possibility of the children supporting each other in their linking of the storyline of the book with the tape-recording.

A number of tapes are now commercially available. However, a lack of funds should not be a deterrent. Class teachers can soon record a number of stories for the listening area, and the children are often fascinated and delighted to hear the voice of their teacher on tape.

Once a junction box has been obtained and the principle of the children working together has been established, then it might be time to isolate that area from other quieter areas. However, in most instances, the listening area can be part of the *library corner*. Morrow (1989) includes the listening area (or listening station) in her suggestions for a library corner and, given that the stories are being heard through headphones, the listening area being sited in the library corner should not be problematic as far as noise is concerned. And, of course, it would seem to be logical to store the books and tapes in the library area.

Most importantly, however, the listening area is organized and developed because it provides another opportunity for the children to listen to stories and engage purposively and enjoyably with the printed word. These listenings can further the enjoyment of books and encourage the child's literacy development.

Further reading

Hutchinson, P. (1983) *Story Chest: Teacher's Book*. Leeds: Arnold-Wheaton.

There are now a number of publishers who produce audiotapes of their books. Here, there is the suggestion of individual or group work and the reader is reminded that in these particular tapes there are two readings of the book, one at normal pace and a second, slower version, which encourages the child to read along with the story reader.

methods

Many different methods of teaching reading have been suggested over the years, each of which has emphasized the letters, sounds, words, sentences or larger units of language. Let us first look at the nature of these methods.

The English language is represented on the printed page through the use of the twenty-six letter alphabet. Therefore, teachers in early years classrooms take various steps to encourage children to look at, think about and come to know the alphabet. Indeed, for many years, children were taught to read using what was known as the 'alphabetic' method.

Using the alphabetic method, children were taught to recognize and name the letters of the alphabet in both upper and lower case. The method was particularly prevalent in the eighteenth and nineteenth centuries. Within the approach debates occurred from time to time about the order in which the letters should be taught: should the letters be taught in alphabetic order, with obvious links to the subsequent use of a dictionary, or should the letters be taught in groups? These groups of letters were established according to some criterion, for example lip movement!

The alphabetic method led to the development of reading books that at first only utilized two-letter words before moving on to three-letter words. One can imagine that these were not the most exciting of texts! (It is an interesting, and at times frustrating, task to attempt to write prose when one is so restricted.)

But learning the letter names – no matter how useful that might be – was seen to be incomplete, and the additional learning of the sounds of the letters led to various phonic methods being adopted. *Phonics teaching* is made difficult in the English language as there is not a perfect and invariable correspondence between the letters and their sounds. Nevertheless, the benefits of using phonics teaching in some form has been argued by Jeanne Chall (1967) and more recently by Marilyn Jager Adams (1990). However, *whole language* teachers counter that argument by suggesting that although it is important for children to acquire a knowledge of the letter sound rule system, that learning can take place in the context of reading and writing. However, as we shall see in the section on *phonics teaching*, a range of suggestions has been made as to how to teach the sounds of letters.

Word methods contrast with the methods which emphasized letters and sounds. And the basis for the word methods was to produce meaningful reading. However, some reading schemes which followed a word method demonstrated that meaning was not always a strong point of such texts. Indeed, because the use of word methods emphasized repetition in order to ensure that the words were met frequently, to encourage over-learning, so the strange texts of a 'look, look, look' type were developed.

Schools which followed a whole-word methodology often used flash cards, on which was printed a single word, to encourage each child to learn and practise saying the word when shown the card. The child often took the cards home in a tin to practise with his or her parents. And it was often only when the words had been learnt that the book containing the words was given to the child. The benefits of context whether provided by the sentence structure or the meaning, perhaps in the form of a story, were largely missing in this method.

In her booklet on methods, Elizabeth Goodacre (1975) distinguished between whole-word and look-and-say methods. She stated that whole-word methods concentrated upon meaningful words which could often be represented by pictures or where the card could be placed on an object. Look-and-say methods required the teacher to state what a word said so that the child could learn it. Nevertheless, both methods raise doubts as to the extent to which children were reading meaningful material.

The sentence method extends the idea of word methods by emphasizing meaning using a complete sentence. Children's interests can be used and it is possible to see the link with the *language experience approach* and *Breakthrough to Literacy*. But the logical extension is not to stay with the sentence but to expand to stories and other more complete forms of written material.

The idea of *whole language* provides such an extension. Adopting this approach, philosophy, or set of principles and beliefs, the children are encouraged to use environmental print, stories and other meaningful print material as well as to write for real purposes in order to develop as readers and writers. Kenneth Goodman's

Good

(1986) book *What's Whole in Whole Language?* provides an overview of whole language. That approach is very much based on a meaningful start to literacy and is therefore sometimes regarded as having a top-down view of literacy rather than the bottom-up view of methods which start with small parts of the whole, such as letters, sounds and words.

Further reading

Chalmers, G.S. (1976) *Reading Easy 1800–50*. London: The Broadsheet King.

The subtitle of this book, 'A study of the teaching of reading with a list of the books which were used and a selection of facsimile pages', indicates that the book provides a debate about the alphabetic method and also gives examples of the contents of those early readers. In particular, the facsimile pages provide an immediate feel for what was involved in learning to read using the alphabetic method.

Diack, H. (1965) *In Spite of the ALPHABET: A Study in the Teaching of Reading*. London: Chatto and Windus.

This book explores the various methods which have been used to teach reading. It therefore has chapters on phonic, word and sentence methods. The first chapter is devoted to alphabetic methods (alphabetic, spelling and ABC), which Diack argues were the predominant methods for the teaching of reading well into the nineteenth century. Subsequently, there are chapters which consider phonic, word and sentence methods and do so within a historical context as well as indicating their psychological and educational basis.

Goodacre, E.J. (1975) *METHODS: Including an Annotated Reading List and Glossary of Terms*. Reading: Centre for the Teaching of Reading, University of Reading.

This short booklet provides a brief introduction to the various methods of teaching reading. It debates the alphabetic, phonic, whole-word/look-and-say, whole-sentence and linguistic methods, and in addition it indicates a number of references where the methods can be explored further.

Goodman, K. (1986) *What's Whole in Whole Language?* Portsmouth, NH: Heinemann Educational.

This short text provides a very readable and succinct statement about the nature and process of a whole-language approach. It also indicates how that approach might be translated into classroom practice.

miscue analysis

Almost inevitably during any reading of a text, children (or indeed adults) will, from time to time, produce a miscue. So, instead of reading the text word as expected, the reader instead produces a miscue, or response, which is not in the text. And the word used to describe that deviation from the text is miscue, rather than mistake or error, because it indicates the strengths that the reader brings to the reading rather than negatively referring to any failure. Kenneth Goodman (1969), a key figure in the development of miscue analysis, argued for the use of the word miscue for this reason, but also to avoid the implication that good reading does not include miscues.

Teachers who share books with young children know that they produce miscues and, whether they have a knowledge of miscue analysis or not, must ask themselves: Why did the child read like that? What information was being used to produce, for instance, 'horse' for 'house'? Furthermore, because teachers ask these questions of themselves, the basis for understanding miscue analysis is already in place. As Goodman (1992: 194) suggests, 'Miscue analysis quite easily became a part of the repertoire of British teachers. For decades they'd been "hearing pupils read". Now they knew what they were listening for.'

Although most miscues by children (80 per cent) involve the substitution of one word for another, they also insert or omit words, repeat words, hesitate and self-correct. Though there are others, these six categories cover the majority of miscues produced by children. Elsewhere I describe these six types of miscue within one sentence (Campbell 1993a):

in to-to run-rub down

The dog got ^ wet [and] Tom had to // rub him dry.

In this sentence, the six miscues are:

1	Substitution	down (for the text word 'dry')
2	Insertion	in (added to the sentence after 'got')
3	Omission	and (left out during the reading)
4	Repetition	to-to (the word spoken more than once)
5	Hesitation	// (a pause longer than three seconds)
6	Self-correction	run-rub (initial attempt at the word is corrected).

Of these types of miscue, miscue self-corrections often indicate children's positive attempts to check their own reading. As Marie Clay (1972) argued, self-corrections can be indicative of reading progress. Repetitions and hesitations are often used to give the reader more time to consider the next word and in that sense are positive; they might be viewed more negatively if they occur too frequently. An analysis of insertions and omissions often leads to the view that the readers are editing the text into their own dialect or level of understanding, and as such they demonstrate a real involvement with the text. Occasionally, the omissions might, more negatively, be made to avoid a difficult word or phrase.

However, it is substitutions which are the most frequent and helpful miscues for teachers. They are helpful because teachers can analyse a substitution to consider the use that a child is making of the language cue systems. In other words, teachers can compare the observed response/spoken word with the expected response/text word for syntactic and semantic acceptability and graphophonic appropriateness.

In our earlier example, the reader had substituted 'down' for the text word 'dry'. We could ask of that substitution:

1 *Syntactically*, is the miscue acceptable structurally within the sentence – that is, does it still make a sentence?
2 *Semantically*, is the miscue acceptable meaningfully within the sentence – that is, does it make sense?
3 *Graphophonically*, is there a degree of similarity between the spoken word and the text word – that is, is there first letter similarity?

And by analysing this example it suggests that all three language cue systems were being used. However, on other occasions, such an analysis will be made more difficult because of the need to look graphophonically at word endings, or word middles, rather than just first letters. Also, where the substitution is in the middle of a sentence, rather than the last word of the sentence, a judgement will have to be made as to whether syntactically and semantically the sentence was acceptable up to and including the miscue even if the complete sentence is not. Such complexities become less problematic the more frequently the teacher attempts a miscue analysis and therefore becomes more knowledgeable about it and more familiar with its use.

Of course, miscue analysis is not something that is attempted for its own sake. Miscue analysis might be conducted rather formally and very specifically to determine the reading strengths and weaknesses of the reader, or more informally while the teacher is sharing a book with a child. Indeed, it could be argued that once a teacher is familiar with miscue analysis, it is inevitable that every shared reading or hearing a child read involves a miscue analysis because the teacher's knowledge now prompts him or her to ask: Why did the reader produce that miscue? Miscue analysis encourages teachers to become more diagnostic as listeners. But this diagnosis is not in itself sufficient, it is there because it enables us to move forward to consider literacy planning. We can use the information from the miscue analysis to assist us in determining what sort of literacy experiences the child now needs in order to develop further as a reader.

Many teachers of young children become familiar with miscue analysis not only through sharing books with children but in a variety of other guises. So the *running records* that are a part of *reading recovery* involve the use of miscue analysis (or many of the principles of miscue analysis). Additionally, part of the Standard Assessment Task testing procedure for reading at Key Stage 1 (seven years of age) in England and Wales used, at least in the initial years of operation, running records. All of this points to miscue analysis as a means of finding out about young children's reading.

In the classroom

While sharing a book with a child, teachers have the opportunity to consider the miscues produced by the reader and, therefore, build a picture of the child as a reader. So when five-year-old Richard read to his teacher, the miscues on the first few lines provided interesting insights into Richard's strengths:

Richard: In the light of the moon
the(a) little egg lay on a leaf.
One Summers(Sunday) day(morning) the warm sun
came out(up) and – pop – out of the egg
a very(came-t) a tiny and very hungry caterpillar.
He looked(started-t) to look for some food.

(See Campbell, 1992, for the complete transcript.)

Although he needed some support from his teacher (indicated by '-t'), nevertheless Richard maintained the sentence structure and, especially initially, the meaning of the text during the first six substitutions that he produced. And although there might have been less attention to the graphophonic features, nevertheless his 'Summers' for 'Sunday', and 'out' for 'up', plus the verb ending -ed, suggested that that area was not neglected as he read. Richard was just five when this interaction took place, which serves to remind us of the strengths which he demonstrated as he read.

Further reading

Campbell, R. (1993a) *Miscue Analysis in the Classroom*. Widnes: UK Reading Association.
Miscue analysis is widely recognized as a useful means of assessing children's development as readers and diagnosing current strengths and weaknesses. However, the procedures used may appear to be oriented more towards the researcher than the classroom teacher. This book attempts to provide a simple but concise description of miscue analysis for use by the classroom teacher. It includes, additionally, sections on more recent developments such as retrospective miscue analysis.

Goodman, Y., Watson, D. and Burke, C. (1987) *Reading Miscue Inventory: Alternative Procedures*. New York: Richard C. Owen.
For teachers who require very detailed procedures for making a full miscue analysis of an oral reading, this book will suffice. The theory of miscue analysis is debated and practical procedures for collecting miscue data are provided. Then the procedures for miscue analysis are considered; alternative procedures with varying degrees of intensity are also noted. In all, a very thorough text for reference purposes.

National Curriculum

A National Curriculum has now been established in England and Wales, which indicates the areas to be covered and the levels of attainment to be expected at certain stages within schools. Furthermore, as one might expect from a centrally directed curriculum, there has been an avalanche of documents which have sought to explain the curriculum, levels of attainment, suggested programmes of study and some notes of 'non-statutory' guidance on the implementation of the curriculum into the classroom. With such a wealth of information, it might be thought that it would be relatively easy to describe the English element (speaking, listening, reading and writing) of the curriculum. However, that is not the case, as aspects of the curriculum, and of the testing, have been changed on a regular basis and it is difficult to predict what the next changes might be. Nevertheless, English along with mathematics and science are regarded as being the core curriculum subjects for the early years up to seven years of age (Key Stage 1). And English, at least, will surely remain central in the classroom activities for infant school children. (Our discussion will concentrate on the reading and writing components of the English curriculum.)

It might have been expected that the Bullock Report (DES 1975) would have set the scene for English teaching in primary and secondary schools for a longer period of time than events subsequently demonstrated. However, just as it was a concern about standards of reading which led to the setting up of the Bullock Committee, so too it was similar concerns about standards which led to further explorations of the curriculum in general and English in particular. The Kingman Committee was asked 'to recommend a model of the English language as a basis for teacher training and professional discussion, and to consider how far and in what ways that model should be made explicit to pupils at various stages of education' (DES 1988a: 1). Following this report on *knowledge about language*, a working group was immediately set up under the chairmanship of Brian Cox to produce a blueprint for the National Curriculum in English (DES 1988b). This report included the attainment targets that were to be set, separately for reading and writing, in the area of literacy. Subsequently, the *English in the National Curriculum* document (DES 1989) provided the fine details and statutory requirements for the teaching of English at Key Stage 1 for children in infant schools aged five to seven. In particular, the attainment targets for the testing at the end of Key Stage 1 at seven years of age were indicated. The following year the *English in the National Curriculum (No. 2)* document (DES 1990) detailed the curriculum and attainment targets for the other three key stages at eleven, fourteen and sixteen. These four key stages contained ten levels of attainment, the first three of which were, at the time, designated for the early years up to seven years of age.

Because there have been changes to the attainment targets, and it would appear that further changes might occur, it is difficult to provide precise details of the expectations for each child. However, if we consider some attainments that were contained in the first draft order (DES 1989), then in reading (Attainment Target 2, AT2) the sequence was: at Level 1 the child should be able to 'show signs of a developing interest in reading' and an ability 'to recognize individual words or letters in familiar contexts'; at Level 2 the child should be able to 'read accurately and understand straightforward signs, labels and notices' and 'demonstrate a knowledge of the alphabet' but also 'read a range of material with some independence, fluency, accuracy and understanding'; at Level 3 that reading should be fluent 'and with appropriate expression' and the children should be expected in discussions to demonstrate an 'understanding of the way stories are structured'. Within Key Stage 1, it was Level 2 that was to be regarded as the norm for the majority of the children. The testing of the children using *Standard Assessment Tasks* (*SATs*) was, as we shall note in that section, to create a number of problems.

Progress within writing (Attainment Target 3 or AT3) suggested a similar expectation of the child from letters, to writing and subsequently more sophisticated writing. So at Level 1 'isolated letters, words or phrases to communicate meaning' were expected, whereas at Level 2 the child would have to 'produce, independently, pieces of writing using complete sentences, some of them demarcated with capital letters and full stops or question marks', and for story writing there had to be 'an opening, characters, and one or more events'. At Level 3 the demand upon punctuation became more pronounced as the independent writing now needed 'complete sentences, mainly demarcated with capital letters and full stops or question marks', and there needed to be 'a wider range of sentence connectives than "and" and "then"'.

The attainment targets for reading and writing appeared to create, among early years teachers, two slightly conflicting responses. First, that the expectations were no more than those they might expect from the majority of the children at seven years of age. Therefore, there would be no need to adjust in any major way the teaching and learning of literacy within the classroom. But, second, there was some concern about a utilitarian approach to literacy, that literacy was to be more concerned with functional uses rather than with personal growth. Allied to this concern was the sense that there was to be more attention to the parts (i.e. knowledge of letters and use of punctuation rather than reading and writing for meaning). This concern was deepened as the draft revised version of *English in the National Curriculum* (SCAA 1994) was made available, with extensive sections on phonics, punctuation, spelling and handwriting.

These worries were alleviated somewhat, in the early versions of the National Curriculum, by the programme of study for reading, which included recognition of the *home–school link* ('reading activities should build on the oral language and experiences which pupils bring from home') and which suggested a wide range of reading to 'include picture books, nursery rhymes, poems, folk tales, myths, legends and other literature' as well as the 'pupil's own writing ... [as] part of the resources for reading'. And *story reading, shared reading, play activities, reading non-fiction* and *environmental print* were all part of the recommendations. And for writing there were suggestions of 'frequent opportunities to write in different contexts and for a variety of purposes and audiences', and that the children should see the teachers demonstrating writing and there should be both chronological and non-chronological writing.

There were, however, suggestions in the programme of study which were to prove to be more contentious. The suggestion that the teacher 'should introduce pupils to terms such as punctuation, letter, capital letter, full stop, question mark' might have been seen initially as a gentle introduction to some aspects of a *knowledge about language*. However, in subsequent years, with changes in the assessment tasks, such an emphasis upon *punctuation* in the early years changed quite dramatically the writing demands, with an emphasis upon capital letters and full stops becoming as important as the writing content.

Just as the programmes of study contained much that the early years teacher might have expected, so too the non-statutory guidance contained a good deal of supportive suggestions. Those notes contained suggestions for planning, organization, resources, schemes of work and the role of the teacher. The *teacher's role* included acting as a 'responsive and interested listener ... an organizer ... a partner/guide ... a reader of books and children's own stories in order to provide an example ... a support ... a praiser ... a monitor ... a recorder'. All of this indicated the importance of the teacher and suggested a complex and facilitating role in the early years classroom. The guidance also included an example of a visit and the ways in which such a visit might enable a range of worthwhile reading and writing to take place. This example suggests that the use of themes or topics was still to be valued.

But, of course, the National Curriculum has created a great deal of heated debate. Many teachers saw the development as a vindication of the principles, beliefs and methods which they had been carrying through for some years. Others saw it as a means of restricting teachers, with its imposition of content and activities upon the early years curriculum. As the debate continues, I must leave it to the reader to remain in contact with the current and future developments and outcomes.

Further reading

DES (1988a) *Report of the Committee of Inquiry into the Teaching of English Language* (The Kingman Report). London: HMSO.

DES (1988b) *English for Ages 5 to 11* (The Cox Report). London: HMSO.
DES (1989) *English in the National Curriculum*. London: HMSO.
DES (1990) *English in the National Curriculum (No. 2)*. London: HMSO.

You may wish to consult one or more of these documents, which were instrumental in putting into place the English component of the National Curriculum in England and Wales. What these documents contain is the enormous detail of the developments of the National Curriculum for English which the above section has merely outlined.

Fisher, R. (1992) *Early Literacy and the Teacher*. Sevenoaks: Hodder and Stoughton.

Ros Fisher has written about the important and various roles of the teacher of literacy in the early years. This is important because comment has been made, incorrectly, about the non-teaching demands of a real books approach or invented spellings. This book demonstrates instead the complex and demanding role of the teacher as facilitator, model, manager and assessor. Furthermore, the book is permeated with references to the National Curriculum as it might influence the teaching of literacy in England and Wales. There is also a chapter devoted entirely to the development of English in the National Curriculum, which provides an extended summary of such developments.

nursery rhymes

Traditionally, a part of children's early language development has been associated with the learning of nursery rhymes. Such learning often takes place as part of the rich exchange of language that occurs at home and at school as adults and children play with language. Some of this handing down of language culture also occurs between children, as one generation of children pass on to the next generation the rhymes and stories associated with certain games and activities (Opie and Opie 1959).

So already it is apparent that although this section is entitled nursery rhymes, and nursery rhymes are a very important part of the language learnt by young children, nevertheless the rhymes that children enjoy will take us into other areas as well. At the very least it is useful to think about finger plays, nursery songs and poems in addition to traditional nursery rhymes. Bernice Cullinan (1989) provides a comprehensive listing of the various kinds of literature that young children enjoy and benefit from. As well as story books in various forms, and the value of *story readings* with those books, she also lists finger plays, nursery rhymes, songs and poems as important early experiences for young children.

During the first year of a child's life, parents share events such as 'Round and round the garden, went the Teddy Bear. One step. Two steps. Tickly under there', as well as numerous other finger plays. Such games bring the adult and the child together in a shared enjoyment of language. And even at one year of age, one notes the child's awareness of sequence, memory and recall of the event, as well as anticipation of the final outcome, after just a few experiences of a particular game. Adults can also share nursery rhymes with children, at the same time engaging them in physical movements, as when Humpty Dumpty 'fell off the wall'.

So nursery rhymes are important because they are enjoyable and they provide a rich opportunity for sharing language. Dorothy White (1954/1984), in her detailed diary account of her daughter's involvement with books before school age, made frequent comment about Carol's love of rhyme and rhythm. There was even the suggestion that Carol might have been offered poetry in a foreign language without destroying that enjoyment, because what intrigued Carol was the rhyme and the rhythm of the language.

However, nursery rhymes are not only enjoyable, they also enable children to develop an understanding of language which contributes to their subsequent reading development (Meek 1990). Meek argues that if we teach children nursery rhymes, then their awareness of phonology should follow naturally. We can see why if we look at part of the 'Hickory, dickory, dock' nursery rhyme. In this the first two lines end with 'dock' and 'clock'; a rhyming is created by the -ock endings. Children will recognize this link without being taught about it directly. Such recognition, or phonological awareness, of -ock and numerous other rhymes is an important part of children's subsequent reading development.

The link between early experiences with nursery rhymes and later reading development appears to be well established. Peter Bryant and his colleagues (e.g. Bryant and Bradley 1985; Goswami and Bryant 1990) have indicated that children with a knowledge of nursery rhymes at three years of age appear well disposed for acquiring *phonemic awareness* within the next year and success at reading and spelling at six years of age. And we need to remind ourselves that such success appears to be derived from the natural shared enjoyment of the language and laughter in nursery rhymes.

At play groups and nursery schools and in reception or kindergarten classes, teachers will want to replicate these experiences by making copious use of finger plays, nursery rhymes, songs and poems. Children can be encouraged to learn the rhymes, to present them in unison, to act them out and to represent them on paper. The latter is most likely to be in the form of drawings initially, but will soon include the children's writing as well, even if not presented conventionally.

As part of the learning of these various rhymes, the teacher will develop some of them as big books, or big sheets, so that the children not only hear the words but also see them regularly in print. Holdaway (1979), in his description of the development of *big books*, indicated that nursery rhymes, songs and poems were used for many of the big sheets that were produced for the children in his classroom.

In classrooms where time is spent on nursery rhymes, the laughter and enjoyment initiated at home can be replicated in school. And the learning that is derived from such experiences is of real benefit to the children both immediately and as a foundation for the future.

Further reading

Bryant, P. and Bradley, L. (1985) *Children's Reading Problems: Psychology and Education*. Oxford: Oxford University Press.

In part of this book the authors describe the various studies that they have conducted which suggest a link between children's knowledge of nursery rhymes at three and four years of age and their subsequent sensitivity to rhyme. This sensitivity to rhyme, and therefore phonological and phonemic awareness, supports the children in their development as readers. Such studies should give further encouragement to parents, play group leaders and teachers to devote time to the enjoyable activities of finger plays, poems, songs and nursery rhymes.

Matterson, E. (1969) *This Little Puffin . . . Finger Plays and Nursery Games*. London: Puffin.

There are, of course, many books which provide numerous nursery rhymes. This is but one example of that genre. However, it does also include many interesting finger plays, which the youngest children at home as well as those in the play group or nursery classroom will enjoy.

organic vocabulary

What is an organic vocabulary? It is that vocabulary that comes from children individually and means something to them, indeed has an intense meaning for them. As Sylvia Ashton-Warner (1963) indicated in her work with Maori children, these include fear words (e.g. ghost, tiger, skeleton, bulldog, frightened and police), sex words (e.g. kiss, love and touch), words of locomotion for the boys (e.g. aeroplane, jet and tractor), words of domesticity for the girls (e.g. house, mummy and doll) and others (e.g. school, socks, frog, porridge and beer). (Would the same words appear in lists from young children today, in your classroom and in your culture?) Bettleheim and Zelan (1981) suggested that words which have emotional significance for children are readily learnt. Such a view was based on their teaching of 'non-readers of long standing' (p. 30). So the words which come from children and which are intensely felt might provide a springboard to literacy development.

Ashton-Warner (1963) wrote on a card, for each child, the key organic word that he or she had stated each day. They were what she called 'one look' words; that is, they were intensely felt and therefore would be remembered after only one look. These words were always provided without pictures because the pictures were in the child's mind with individual and emotional representations. Interestingly, the words that could not be remembered by the children, Ashton-Warner concluded, were probably ones that she, as the teacher, had inappropriately written. These were words that were not intensely felt and therefore of little importance to the children, so the cards were disposed of by the children. The children shared their words with each other, and these words came to be recognized and spoken because they were felt and known.

The children's words could be used, Ashton-Warner argued, to develop dynamic material that could then be utilized to form the first reading material for each child. So each child would be asked to write a word, two words, a sentence or more (with a general vocabulary including 'then', 'I', 'and', 'the', 'to', 'me', etc., which provided the reading material for that child and for others as the writing was shared. With the group of children that Ashton-Warner was working with, it was vital, she suggested, that the first reading books were drawn from their own words and culture before they encountered books from European culture. But then if the first reading was drawn from 'Daddy', 'Mummy', 'ghost', 'bomb', 'kiss', etc., wouldn't that be preferable she argued to 'Come John come. Look John look'. The argument that Ashton-Warner was making against *reading schemes* can be extended, for isn't it vital that the books that children first meet are *real books* that have a relevance and meaning for the children? And, of course, it was important that the Maori children moved from their own organic reading, 'reaching further and further out to the inorganic and standard reading, [so that] there is a comfortable movement from the inner man outward, from the known to the unknown' (p. 62), from their own self-constructed books, to those constructed by the teacher which reflected the children's words and writing, and finally to books available from publishers.

The sharing of the organic texts was an important part of Ashton-Warner's approach. Part of that sharing included the children working in pairs reading their writing to each other. And although she did not use the terms 'purpose' and 'audience', she was demonstrating to the children that there was a purpose to their writing and a real audience to appreciate their efforts. Subsequently, that sharing led to group discussions about the writing which she suggested were 'the climax of the whole organic purpose' (p. 65).

In the infant classroom today, many teachers encourage children to write about events which are of importance to them. In this sense, the notion of using each child's organic vocabulary has developed, albeit in somewhat different ways, in many classrooms.

Further reading

Ashton-Warner, S. (1963) *Teacher*. London: Secker and Warburg.
This book details the author's use of a key or organic vocabulary with Maori infant school children aged four to six years in New Zealand. Inevitably, literacy was just a part of her teaching, and therefore the book is about more than just organic vocabulary. It tells about her teaching in various classrooms as she attempted to help build a bridge from one culture to another, from Maori to European. It was a process she described as 'creative teaching' and the extension of her teaching outside of the classroom where nature and number were learnt is vividly portrayed.

The principles that Ashton-Warner put forward are regarded as being part of a *language experience approach* and, as Veatch (1991) argues, one of the antecedents to *whole language*. In particular, the respect for the children's own ideas, the children's choice of words and the flexibility required of the teacher in support of the learner would appear to accord with whole language views.

paired reading

The term 'paired reading' is used to describe a reader, most often an adult, and a beginning reader, usually a child, reading together from a book chosen by the child. In this sense, it would appear to be similar to *shared reading* or *hearing children read*. And perhaps in some cases, in the early years classroom, the term might be used to describe such teacher–child interactions with a book. However, there are differences between paired reading and those other classroom interactions. First, as originally put forward by Roger Morgan (1976) in the USA, paired reading is a relatively structured reading of a book which follows clear guidelines, and we shall explore that structure in a moment. However, as often applied with young children in early years classrooms, paired reading is used to describe two children reading together from a book where the more competent reader supports the reading of the less advanced reader.

Paired reading as originally conceived in the USA has been popularized in the UK by Keith Topping (e.g. Topping and Lindsay 1992) and was a central feature of the very large Kirklees Project, another example of a *home–school link*. The structure of a paired reading, as described for that project, includes the following:

- the children choose their own books;
- paired reading should last between five and fifteen minutes each day;
- paired reading should take place five days a week;
- a quiet and comfortable base should be provided where both child and adult have a clear view of the book;
- before the reading, the book should be discussed;
- at natural pauses during the reading discussions can take place;
- such discussions can check on comprehension and prediction;
- when the child makes an error (miscue), the adult reads the word;
- the child repeats the word spoken by the adult;
- the child should not be asked to break up or sound out the word;
- praise should be given for the correct reading of difficult words, self-corrections, and longer pieces of reading;
- with more difficult texts, both adult and child read all the words out aloud;
- finger pointing by the child, if required, is encouraged;
- when the child feels confident to read alone, a non-verbal signal is used by the child to silence the adult;

- the adult stops reading and praises the child for signalling;
- when reading alone, if the child struggles on a word for more than five seconds, or struggles and gets the word wrong, the word is read by the adult and the pair revert to reading together.

Typically, such a set of instructions can be presented as a flow chart, which indicates the sequences of reading, instruction and support. It will be apparent that there are links with shared reading: the child and adult work together with a book; at times they read together; the adult supports the reader when miscues are produced and provides encouragement at appropriate moments;and the child takes over the reading when confident to do so. However, there are also differences. For example, in a shared reading, the child and the adult read together and the child is encouraged to read alone when it seems appropriate to do so; meaningful miscues might be ignored; because telling a child what a word is does not help him or her to develop his or her own strategies for reading and often does not help him or her when he or she next meets that word and other responses can be adopted (Campbell 1994). Furthermore, in a shared reading, the flow from the adult reading to the child reading is dictated by an awareness of what the child can do by both child and adult. For many teachers of young children, the strict interpretation of the 'rules' of paired reading might not tie in with the wish to develop a collaborative reading and enjoyment of a book. Nevertheless, a number of the aspects of paired reading can be debated by teachers and with parents in order that the important role of the adult when sharing a book can be considered and developed.

Although paired reading is written about most frequently in the way that we have just considered, it may be that it operates somewhat differently in many early years classrooms. There, the term is used often to describe a sharing of a book between two children. In such a situation, a competent reader provides support to a less advanced reader during the reading of a book. Although the competent reader might be told by the teacher to read a word when necessary, nevertheless it is likely that a number of different kinds of support will be given, drawn probably from that child's perception of what adults do when they share a book with a child. Teachers argue that both children benefit from these peer-tutored paired readings and that the competent reader learns as much as does the less advanced reader. Teachers should, of course, monitor such child–child interactions in order to assure themselves that it is proving worthwhile. And paired reading in this form is only one of many different literacy activities that take place in the classroom.

In the classroom

In one year-2 classroom, the children were regularly engaged in peer-tutoring paired reading. For instance, Andrew acted as a tutor for Joanna, the reader:

Joanna: The cat, the bird and the tree.
The cat. The bird. The bird is up in the tree.
The cat runs to the tree.
The cat// (// = hesitation)
Andrew: ... looks
Joanna: ... looks up. He sees the bird in a tree.
The little bird is singing, up in the tree.
The cat is near the tree.
The (He)// – He jumps up into the tree.
He climbs up//
Andrew and Joanna: ... and
Joanna: ... up and up.
As the cat climbs up the little bird looks down.
She – He (She)//
Andrew and Joanna: ... looks
Joanna: ... at the cat. The cat
Andrew: ... sits
Joanna: ... sits firmly (very)
Andrew and Joanna: ... still.
Joanna: He is on a branch.
The little bird is//
Andrew: ... afraid
Joanna: ... afraid of the cat.
The big cat jumps//
Andrew and Joanna: ... from
Joanna: ... the branch.

(For a complete transcript, see Campbell and Stott, 1994.)

Even in this short extract, it is evident that Andrew did not interrupt the flow of the text although he did support Joanna by providing the word when Joanna hesitated. He also read in unison with Joanna to guide her reading. Furthermore, he did provide time for Joanna to lead the reading. Both children seemed to enjoy the reading session and both may have benefited from this experience of reading.

Further reading

Topping, K.J. and Lindsay, G.A. (1992) The structure and development of the paired reading technique. *Journal of Research in Reading*, 15: 120–36.

This short article describes paired reading both as initiated by Roger Morgan and as developed by Keith Topping for the Kirklees Project. The summary flow chart presents at a glance the structure of the interaction. A brief review of research studies indicates the strengths of adult–child interactions centring on a book. Finally, there is a debate regarding the theoretical framework of this procedure. In this section the authors claim that although the procedure may have been developed from behavioural psychology, it can be seen to meet the needs of both real book approaches and more direct teaching methods.

Topping, K.J. and Wolfendale, S. (eds) (1985) *Parental Involvement in Children's Reading*. London: Croom Helm.

As the title suggests, this edited collection of papers provides a detailed account of parental involvement in the reading development of their children. One section of the book is devoted to home–school programmes which used paired reading between parent and child to encourage the children's reading (pp. 109–59). Among the contributions in this section is a paper by Roger Morgan, who developed this particular form of adult–child interaction with books.

phonemic awareness

When children read they use cues from a number of different sources, including the contextual cues of syntax (how the words are strung together into sentences), semantics (the meaning element of the writing) and pragmatics (the recognition that particular words are normally expected to appear in particular kinds of writing).

Then there are those cues which are linked more to the word itself, in particular the letters and associated sounds of those letters. And most writers would acknowledge that children make use of all these sources at various times. For instance, Kenneth Goodman, who might be regarded as emphasizing contextual cues, nevertheless recognizes the importance of the graphophonic cue system when children read. So if children are making use of the graphophonic or letter–sound cue system, then what knowledge do they need in order to succeed?

Goswami and Bryant (1990) use 'phonological awareness' as a blanket term to cover the general awareness of sounds that children might require for reading. And one specific aspect of that generality is phonemic awareness. The phoneme is the smallest unit of sound and typically each alphabetic letter (grapheme) has an associated phoneme. So in the word 'mat' we can recognize that there are three phonemes: m, a and t. A number of writers, including Adams (1990), stress the importance of phonemic awareness for children to progress with reading. However, Adams also recognizes the catch-22, that children who have acquired phonemic awareness have also learned to read. Such a view led Goswami and Bryant (1990: 26) to conclude that 'it is most unlikely that the progress that children make in reading is determined by their sensitivity to phonemes. On the contrary their progress in learning to read (or to read in an alphabetic script at any rate) is probably the most important cause of awareness of phonemes.'

Such conclusions might leave teachers in a quandary as to what learning experiences to provide in the classroom. They need not do so, however. First, because the range of reading experiences such as *story reading, big books, shared reading* and *sustained silent reading,* all provide opportunities for children to learn about reading, to learn to read and to develop an awareness of phonemes. Furthermore, the alphabetic friezes, opportunities for writing and enjoyment of *nursery rhymes* will more specifically encourage children to think about and develop an awareness of phonemes. Nursery rhymes are particularly helpful because they encourage children to think about other aspects of phonological awareness, namely onset and rime.

The terms 'onset' and 'rime' are debated in Goswami and Bryant (1990). However, put simply, the terms recognize the opening unit (onset) and end unit (rime) of a word. So in the word 'mat', the onset is provided by the 'm' and the rime by the 'at'. It is the rime element which is used so extensively in nursery rhymes, while alliteration is developed by manipulating the onset unit of words. Children's awareness of onset and rime and their ability to manipulate them may be especially helpful for their developing literacy. And it can be developed naturally with nursery rhymes and using books which place an emphasis upon rhyme and alliteration. Colin Harrison (1992) reminds us of the way in which a number of books can help with that process (e.g. *The Cat in the Hat* by Dr Seuss).

Such experiences will also encourage children towards another advance in their reading, namely being able to read a word by analogy. As Harrison indicates, the use of analogies might be crude in the first instance, being no more, he suggests, than perhaps 'the word cat begins with a c, so perhaps this new word which begins with c is going to begin with the same sound' (p. 22). However, these readings by analogy can become more sophisticated as children read new words and do so by utilizing their recognition of onset and rime units. Therefore, words such as 'sight' and 'fight' can be determined because of a knowledge of 'light' and a recognition of the rime unit 'ight'.

The use of analogies is aided when the word is met in the context of meaningful reading. Then, reading the new word by analogy is supported by the confirmation that the word will fit in the sentence and will construct meaning. It is important, therefore, that children are able to select their reading from a wide range of interesting books, many of which have been selected by the teacher for the classroom because they contain rhymes, rhythms, alliterations and playful use of language.

Further reading

Goswami, U.C. and Bryant, P. (1990) *Phonological Skills and Learning to Read*. Hove: Lawrence Erlbaum Associates Ltd.

In this quite technical book, Usha Goswami and Peter Bryant debate the importance of phonological awareness, phonemic awareness, onset and rime, and analogies in children's early reading development. In order to support that debate, they use evidence from a number of experimental research studies in psychology, including many of their own or allied studies from Oxford. Among the features which emerge from those studies are the importance of nursery rhymes in children's earliest language experiences and the constructive way in which children infer some of the rules of language during the process of reading.

Harrison, C. and Coles, M. (eds) (1992) *The Reading for Real Handbook*. London: Routledge.

The first chapter in this book, 'The reading process and learning to read', is written by Harrison himself. In it, the importance of phonemic awareness and learning by analogy is made clear. Although the writing draws attention to some of the theoretical insights from Peter Bryant's work, it nevertheless makes clear and helpful links to classroom practice.

phonics teaching

There is little disagreement with the view that children's reading development is supported by their knowledge of letters and sounds. What is more contentious is how children acquire that knowledge – that is, is it learnt during the process of learning to read or does it need to be taught in order to read? We note in the section on *phonemic awareness* that Goswami and Bryant (1990) conclude that progress in learning to read is probably the most important factor in becoming aware of phonemes. Therefore, a range of reading and writing activities becomes vital in order that children are involved with language and can actively construct their knowledge of letters and sounds.

A second area of contention concerns how teaching should take place if it is considered necessary to teach phonics; or at least ensure that knowledge of letters and sounds is being acquired. Three areas in particular are of concern: emphasis, timing and teaching (Campbell 1990b). First, a phonics teaching approach to early reading development would, of course, place great emphasis upon the direct teaching of phonics in some form. However, where a *whole language* or *real books approach* is adopted, then the emphasis is upon authentic reading and writing, with some attention being given to letters and sounds. Second, if a phonics approach is being adopted, then phonics are taught almost immediately upon entering school; however, a whole language approach emphasizes the development of reading and monitoring that development for knowledge of letters and sounds. Inevitably, the teaching style would differ also, from the direct and systematic teaching of phonics in a phonics approach, to the incidental teaching which arises from the children's reading and writing within a whole language approach.

In addition to the major questions of emphasis, timing and teaching, teachers have to address the question of the nature of any teaching which takes place. Do we know what should be taught? A number of suggestions have been made, but there is no agreement on the approach to be adopted.

A starting point, as we note in the section on *methods*, is teaching the alphabet. Indeed, such an approach would be to follow a methodology used in the nineteenth century. Knowledge of the alphabet is often seen to be important because children who know the alphabet can usually be expected to succeed with reading. However, can the children read because they know the alphabet, or do they know the alphabet because they have engaged in many literacy activities which have enabled them to read and learn the alphabet? Furthermore, there are problems if it is the letter names of the alphabet that are learnt, as it might not be especially helpful to children when deciphering words; for example, the letters see-ae-tee are joined together only with some difficulty to produce the word cat.

Because of such difficulties, it has been argued that children need to learn the letter names and their usual sounds. Such an approach which emphasizes the consonants and short vowels, it is argued, might be most helpful to children. However, the letters cannot be learnt easily in isolation from a word. In most circumstances, a neutral vowel (uh) is added when a single letter sound is uttered (e.g. ruh rather than (r)), and that has consequences when the letters are combined to form a word: ruh-uh-nuh (run or runner?).

Reducing the amount of single letter learning and drawing the children's attention to such combinations as consonant blends (br) and consonant digraphs (ch), is a partial recognition of the single letter problem. And another approach might be to teach consonant vowel combinations rather than single letters. So the word cat could be taught as ca-t or c-at, if the teacher wished to persist with this form of phonics teaching. As to which might be the preferred combination, perhaps the notions of onset and rime might help us. However, before that we should first look at another aspect of phonics teaching, namely phonic rules or generalizations.

Although phonic rules are more truly expressed as phonic generalizations, in classrooms they are often stated as rules. Examples of such generalizations include the so-called magic 'e', which indicates that when a word ends with a silent 'e' the preceding vowel is long. However, when Clymer (1963) conducted a study of such generalizations, he found that the magic 'e' rule only applied in some 60 per cent of cases. In another example – when there are two vowels side by side, the long sound of the first is heard and the second is usually silent – Clymer noted that in only 45% of cases did the generalization apply. Lefevre (1964) summed it up when he suggested of the rule, when two vowels go walking, the first one does the talking, 'There is no place here (or anywhere else) for that nonsensical "rule" of phonics' (p. 179). Perhaps it is easier to teach reading than it is to teach phonics.

However, returning for the moment to the question of letter combinations, they might remind us of notions of onset and rime discussed in the section on *phonemic awareness*. So if a teacher were considering ca-t or c-at, then onset and rime (Goswami and Bryant 1990) would indicate that c-at would be preferred because it links to children's knowledge of rime. But we also need to remind ourselves that that knowledge is probably derived from *nursery rhymes* and other language games, finger plays, songs and poems. Children 'develop phonological awareness through language play' (Goswami 1994: 36). In other words, children do learn about letters and sounds through engaging with language in many different contexts.

However, even though children might be expected to learn about letters and sounds through many language and literacy activities, nevertheless teachers will want to take the opportunity to draw the children's attention explicitly to aspects of letters and sounds. Schonell (1951) suggested that phonics teaching should only occur incidentally and arise naturally out of the materials being read to the child. Some teachers take the opportunity to extend such incidental teaching into displays which might emphasize objects that all begin with the same letter. Or, as Schonell suggested, from time to time playing language games such as I-Spy.

Whole language teachers are likely to operate in a manner similar to this. As Kenneth Goodman (1986: 38) stated: 'Whole language programs and whole language teachers do not ignore phonics. Rather they keep it in the perspective of real reading and real writing.' So just because whole language teachers preach meaningful reading and writing, with an emphasis upon the whole rather than the parts, it does not, or should not, mean that they are unwilling to talk about letters and sounds with the children. As Goodman (1993) indicated in a later text, whole language teachers assess their pupils' development as they read and write and then support and help as needed. More directly, Mills *et al.* (1992) demonstrated how within a whole language classroom attention is given to letter–sound relationships as a natural part of language and literacy learning; nursery rhymes, songs, talking about reading and writing and classroom print, which includes alphabetic friezes, all help children to construct their knowledge of letters and sounds. Furthermore, teachers in such classrooms will monitor the children's development in those areas through the use of *miscue analysis* and a careful reading of the children's *invented spellings*.

The teachers will do so because they will want to ensure that the children are making good progress with an important aspect of the reading process.

Further reading

Adams, M.J. (1990) *Beginning to Read: Thinking and Learning about Print*. Cambridge, MA: MIT Press.

This book created quite a stir when it was published. It was suggested by those who wished to argue for phonics teaching that here was the case that indicated the need for explicit and substantial phonics teaching in classrooms. Yet, in reality, Adams was somewhat more circumspect with her conclusions. For instance, she indicated that 'to be most productive it [phonics instruction] may best be conceived as a support activity, carefully covered but largely subordinated to the reading and writing of connected text' (p. 416).

Among the concerns which were registered by those who might follow a whole language approach were: that the book was largely based upon a psychological perspective with an emphasis upon studies of word recognition, and that many of the references used by ethnographic studies of linguistics and pedagogy were ignored. Indeed, two advisers to the Centre for the Study of the Teaching of Reading, Dorothy Strickland and Bernice Cullinan, felt it necessary to write an afterword to the book which presented some of those emergent literacy perspectives.

An issue of *The Reading Teacher* (Vol. 44, No. 6, February 1991) devoted a large section to the debate about the book. The contributors, and the response from Adams, demonstrated the political dimension to the debate and that there were strongly held views on the subject of phonics teaching.

play activities

Most nursery and infant classrooms are likely to have a play area or home corner conveniently situated so that the children can engage in play activities during the course of the school day. The emphasis upon play is apparent because there are well-established views on the benefits that can accrue from such activity. The social and emotional benefits might appear to be obvious, but there is also recognition of the foundation that is provided for cognitive learning through play; 'discovery, reasoning and thought grow out of children's spontaneous activity' (Manning and Sharp 1977: 12).

And teachers recognize that it is insufficient just to designate an area for play. So materials and equipment are made available so that the structured play enhances learning. More recently, perhaps, there has been wider recognition of the ways in which the play area can be developed in order to encourage literacy learning.

The inclusion in the play area of literacy materials is a starting point for the encouragement of literacy learning. Such materials include various books, magazines, brochures, telephone directories, notices and instructions for reading, and alongside these paper, notepads, envelopes, letter pads and blank forms with a variety of pencils, crayons, coloured pencils and felt-tip pens for writing. These materials will encourage children to become involved in literacy behaviours during play. Not only can the teacher extend this involvement by reminding the children about the materials and suggesting possible uses for them, but also by providing demonstrations of these suggestions during brief visits to the play area.

In order to promote literacy learning, the teacher can also, in discussion with the children, develop the play area setting so that it becomes more specific (e.g. a restaurant, a dentist's waiting room, etc.). The designation of the area will have to be changed from time to time as the role-playing becomes static and the children's enthusiasm begins to wane. A number of authors have written about the ways in which the play area can be developed and we shall look at some of these in a moment.

Inevitably, in making the area more specific, it becomes clearer what reading and writing materials to provide. The clear designation of the area can also help the children in providing a purpose for their writing. In her account of developing the play area in her classroom into a hairdresser's, then an optician's and finally a restaurant, Helen Dutton (1991) noted that there were six main categories of writing produced by her six-year-olds: letters, messages, personal notes, instructions, factual descriptions and stories. This list is indicative of the literacy learning and purposeful writing that can be generated by structured play where the opportunities for literacy are organized and encouraged.

So what are some of the play area adaptations that might be used in order to encourage literacy? The list is almost never-ending. However, a number of authors have made suggestions, and very often descriptions of these suggestions as they were put into practice. For instance, Morrow and Rand (1991) suggest a number of possibilities, the first of which they describe in detail.

Veterinarians' offices: A number of rooms, or areas, might be developed, including a waiting room which could include magazines, books and pamphlets about pet care. Notices, similar in kind to those found in waiting rooms, including examples of *environmental print*, and posters could be provided. There would be a link to the nurse's desk which would have a telephone, address book, appointment cards and patient forms. Then there would be the office itself with prescription pads and patient files. And Morrow and Rand suggest the children could be reminded to read to their pets while waiting their turn. All of this provides opportunities for literacy behaviours. Wray and Medwell (1991) describe a similar arrangement in a classroom with four- and five-year-old children. There, they noted, a dentist's surgery had been developed and a wide range of literacy-like behaviours were evident.

Restaurant: Menus could be developed by the children according to the type of restaurant or fast-food establishment. Order pads and cash registers would encourage child–child interactions. And the children could model fish, chips, muffins, etc., with dough, which when baked hard and painted could be used as part of the activity. (Fiona MacLeod described such craft work in her description of the fish and chip shop in 'Down at the chippy' in Hall and Abbott, 1991.)

Newspaper office: The very nature of this adaptation demands literacy. There would be a telephone for the reporters plus writing pads and typewriters or a computer. There would need to be reference texts of various kinds to help with the general news, sports, weather, travel, fashion, etc. And the children could make a newspaper for the class or, according to the children's age, perhaps for other classes in the school.

Supermarket or grocery shop: One of the advantages of this play area is that the cartons, packets, plastic bottles, and adverts from magazines and newspapers, can all be used to provide a wide range of literacy messages that can be read by even the youngest children because they will recognize these examples of *environmental print*. Labels and prices on the shelves can add to the literacy learning and mathematics.

Post office: The immediately obvious links to literacy are with letters, envelopes and stamps. But there are also forms to be filled, pensions(!) to be obtained and the various posters on the walls to be considered. A development of this is to set up a letter service in the classroom or the school so that the children write to each other.

Petrol station and garage: Such a play area would bring into the activity maps of the immediate local area as well as more widely. There would be the usual magazines associated with cars, repairs to be arranged for the toy cars and bills to be paid.

Travel agency: The numerous holiday brochures provide a colourful source of literacy and the children will be able to relate some of the destinations to their own holidays. Passports, visas and travellers' cheques might all have to be produced by the children. Catherine Coleman (1991) notes that in her classroom this adaptation led to planning and problem-solving as well as to literacy.

This list could be expanded to include a wide range of shops and services that exist in the community. In most cases, teachers will know what is the most appropriate based on their knowledge of the locality. The creation of something familiar to the children might be most appropriate for the youngest children in particular. In many instances, members of the local community are willing to help with supplying posters, old forms, etc., and perhaps to visit the school briefly to speak and answer questions about their work.

It will have become obvious that teachers have a very important role in this activity: first, in discussing with the children the area and finding materials to stimulate literacy; second, in moving in and out of the activity to suggest and demonstrate literacy behaviours. Furthermore, some of the literacy produced by the children can be collected, which will be useful as a means of making *assessments* of the children's growth as literacy users.

In the classroom

The three- and four-year-old children in one nursery classroom used many props, clothes and furniture to develop their imaginative play when they visited the home corner. One of the props, the old telephone, was used frequently by them to have 'conversations'. However, when the teacher added a telephone messages pad, it encouraged the young children to write as well as to speak.

Of course, at such a young age much of the writing was presented unconventionally. Nevertheless, the scribbles often contained the vertical and horizontal lines as well as circles that are used to construct letters; the shapes were increasingly presented in a line; letters began to appear (A R I Y L 4 P B); and later *invented spellings* (e.g. mmy) and names (e.g. SAM) were occasionally written. So the introduction of a very simple pad and pencil into the play area had positive literacy outcomes. This is especially likely to be the case where the teacher models the literacy for the children initially.

Further reading

Hall, N. and Abbott, L. (eds) (1991) *Play in the Primary Curriculum*. London: Hodder and Stoughton.

There are nine chapters by different contributors in this book on play in the primary curriculum, which are divided into two sections. The two chapters in the first section provide the theoretical background for socio-dramatic or structured play in the classroom. And part of the argument here is that play remains important and need not be constrained by the National Curriculum in the UK. The second section contains reports, from seven classroom teachers, on the development of the play area, or home corner, as a travel agency, hairdresser's, restaurant, etc. These case studies provide evidence of the ways in which literacy can be developed from structured play.

Morrow, L.M. and Rand, M.K. (1991) Promoting literacy during play by designing early childhood classroom environments. *The Reading Teacher*, 44: 396–402.

In this short article, the authors argue that play in the early childhood classroom can be organized and developed in order to promote literacy learning. The authors set the scene by providing a brief theoretical statement about the value of play in young children's learning. Then there is a review of a study carried out by one of the authors, Lesley Mandel Morrow, which indicates the benefits which accrue when teachers introduce literacy-related materials into the play area and when they suggest and model literacy behaviours for the children. A number of different adaptations to the play area are suggested and some of these were noted above.

punctuation

As children develop as writers, their scribbles become linear as first pseudoletters and eventually letters are written. Subsequently, as we note in the section on *invented spellings*, the children's writing, if constructed freely, will be governed by the sounds of oral language and we then find it easier to decipher their writing. Eventually, the children will write with many of the words written conventionally. However, that writing is unlikely to be marked with punctuation, at least initially. Most frequently, the children will use 'and' to connect the meaning units that are written rather than making use of commas and full stops. Indeed, when children read, it is likely to be speech marks, question marks and exclamation marks, rather than commas and full stops, that are noted first. In Lester Laminack's (1991) record of Zachary's literacy learning, the exclamation mark was noted to be the first punctuation which Zachary commented upon when he was four years and ten months old. Teachers can support such learning, for instance when reading a big book, by commenting upon the punctuation marks.

Nevertheless, for teachers of young children, it may be the demarcation of the sentence, with the use of capital letters and full stops, which is encouraged when the children are writing. The development of the National Curriculum in England and Wales has placed emphasis on this aspect of punctuation because the assessment of the children's writing at seven years of age, Key Stage 1, places great importance upon the use of capital letters and full stops to signal a sentence. This emphasis on the punctuation of sentences has increased as the National Curriculum has been refined. However, the expectation of the 1994 *Standard Assessment Tasks* that children need to demarcate 50 per cent of their sentences in order to achieve Level 2, and 90 per cent in order to achieve Level 3, has caused concern that this will lead to more attention being paid to conventions rather than to content and flow of writing (Anderson 1993). In particular, such emphasis might encourage teachers to teach the demarcation of sentences directly. However, there is no evidence to suggest that such a strategy would be effective. So what might teachers do in order to encourage the use of punctuation marks?

As with much of literacy learning, a good starting point in the promotion of an understanding of punctuation is to ensure that children have many opportunities for reading and writing. And during this reading and writing the teacher will support the child's efforts, respond to the child's questions and draw the child's attention to aspects of the print. And when it is appropriate, the teacher will comment upon aspects of punctuation; importantly, this is done in the context of the child's current experiences with print. When the teacher or child is reading from a book, the teacher might comment on the use of speech marks by indicating: 'Those speech marks tell us when the boy is talking, don't they?' In the same way, when a child is editing a piece of writing, for inclusion in a book or for a display, the teacher might guide the child's attention to aspects of punctuation by suggesting, 'Should we put a full stop here at the end of your sentence?' Such comments during reading and writing, just like parental support when oral language is being developed, will guide the child towards an understanding of punctuation. But it need not only be during one-to-one interactions that children are helped towards an awareness and understanding of punctuation.

Teacher demonstrations of reading and writing provide useful opportunities to talk about, or refer to, punctuation in a meaningful context. The shared book experience with *big books* enables teachers to demonstrate *left-to-right directionality* and other conventions of print as they model the reading of the book. And during or after a reading of a big book, teachers can comment on the use of capital letters and full stops as well as other aspects of punctuation so that the children are made aware of those conventions. Similarly, during teacher demonstrations of *writing* in front of a group or the whole class, teachers can comment upon that writing, supported and guided now by the children. And while writing in front of the children, teachers can think aloud, 'Now, what's that first sentence again?', as Brian Cambourne (1988) suggested. Such think-aloud comments bring concepts and aspects of punctuation to the children's attention. Demonstrations of literacy used in this way help the children to an understanding of the use of punctuation.

Further reading

Ferreiro, E. and Teberosky, A. (1982) *Literacy before Schooling*. Portsmouth, NH: Heinemann Educational.

Emilia Ferreiro and Ana Teberosky present some evidence of children's progress, between the ages of four and six, in their understanding of punctuation marks. As we might expect initially, children assume that there is no distinction between punctuation marks and letters. When children begin to differentiate between them, it is the dots (e.g. full stops and colons) which are noted to be different, whereas question marks and commas continue to be confused with similar letters or numbers (e.g. ? and 2 or S; or the comma ',' and 9). By six years of age, many children recognize that punctuation marks serve a different purpose to letters, although they may not yet be able to use the marks themselves in their writing.

reading drive

When introducing the idea of reading drive, as part of the *formula for beginning reading*, Vera Southgate (1968) suggested that among all of the factors which she had explored this was, in her view, the one which she felt to be most important: 'I think that the most decisive factor influencing children's reading progress is the beliefs and attitudes of the staff about the importance of reading' (p. 26). So reading drive was considered to be important and the rest of the quotation indicated that reading drive was concerned with the attitudes and beliefs of the staff. She further indicated that it was in schools where reading was given prime importance, that a reading drive was likely to be in place and most children would learn to read 'early and well' (p. 26). Furthermore, in a statement which would be reflected upon subsequently by Frank Smith (1992; see the section on the *teacher's role*), Southgate suggested that the progress made by children in learning to read would be 'almost regardless of the media, methods, materials or procedures adopted' (p. 26).

So reading drive would appear to be linked very closely to two other areas which are explored in this handbook, namely *school policy* and the *teacher's role*. The views of the teachers in the school about reading and writing will be reflected in the school policy, which will indicate the ways in which practices derived from those views might be implemented in the classroom. And provided that the policy suggests the prime importance of literacy, and the teachers are committed to an implementation of that policy in a dynamic manner, then there is every likelihood of a reading drive permeating the school. From such a starting point, the role of the teacher in the classroom will take over and the beliefs, actions and enthusiasm for literacy can then be conveyed to the children. Where the children are immersed in a sub-culture of an emphasis on, and enthusiasm for, literacy, then there is every chance that they will be facilitated in their literacy learning. Similar sentiments were recorded by HMI (1991) in their evaluation of the teaching and learning of reading in primary schools in England. They suggested that 'a major determinant of that [reading] success is what the teacher and the school bring to the situation' (p. 15).

In part, the reading drive will be derived from the positive perceptions that the teachers have about the children's ability as active learners to be competent literacy learners and to become literacy users. A number of reports have stressed the need for teachers to have positive expectations about what the children can achieve (e.g. Alexander 1992). These high but realistic expectations, which lead to a range of literacy activities being provided in the classroom by teachers enthusiastic about literacy, will create a reading drive which seems to have benefits for the children.

None of this means that teachers do not have to think about planning, organization, literacy learning and worthwhile interactions. But the knowledge that teachers need about reading, writing and children has to be matched by a drive to make it happen in the school and the classroom. In many respects, this dual requirement can be seen in books which provide insights into particular ideas or methods. For instance, in Sylvia Ashton-Warner's book, *Teacher* (1963), there are a number of interesting insights regarding *organic vocabulary* and a *language experience approach*, and yet the book also tells us about an enthusiastic and knowledgeable teacher who demonstrated great concern and empathy for the children she taught. We are left with a feeling that, despite any constraints that might have been imposed upon her, here was a teacher who would have overcome the odds and provided a drive and enthusiasm in the classroom which would have helped the children as literacy learners. And there are other books and articles which describe classrooms and schools in which a similar picture is presented. From such writing we are left with an awareness that teachers and schools should create a drive for literacy and that a reading drive has to remain in place throughout each school day.

Further reading

Southgate, V. (1968) Formulae for beginning reading tuition. *Educational Research*, 11: 23–30.

This short article, you may recall from the section on *formula for beginning reading*, explores the areas needing consideration when research reports are read. However, it also emphasizes reading drive as a vital part of any consideration. And although only a few lines are devoted to the exploration of reading drive, nevertheless the suggestion that it is the most important factor leading to children's reading progress ensured that it received considerable attention.

Goodman, K., Bird, L.B. and Goodman, Y. (1991) *The Whole Language Catalog*. Santa Rosa, CA: American School Publishers.

Although a substantial part of this text is written by Kenneth and Yetta Goodman, there are also hundreds of other contributors. There are many reports throughout the book of 'great teachers'. These contributions are made by colleagues who have witnessed particular teachers at work and have then described these teachers and the children in the classroom. These teachers, of course, work in a variety of contexts and in different styles. But each of the reports is suggestive of teachers who have created a reading (or literacy) drive in their classrooms. The children are left in little doubt about the importance and enjoyment of reading and writing, because everything that these teachers do seems to emphasize literacy. And in such circumstances the children appear likely to develop as literacy users.

reading non-fiction

Both at home and at school, young children have many opportunities to engage with story books. The initial story readings that the children hear not only enable them to learn about books, they also inform them about the structure of the narrative or literary *genre*. Such knowledge provides a good basis for children when they read story books either in the form of a *shared reading* or on their own. Eventually, however, children also read other books and these books may be structured somewhat differently, and use a vocabulary that is not typically found in story books. The teacher might then be concerned with how to help young children when reading non-fiction. We will explore specific strategies below, but first it is important to remind ourselves of the important learning that occurs when engaging with stories. Margaret Meek, in her Foreword to Carol Fox's (1993) book, indicates 'that children use storying to sort out their own knowledge and ideas until they learn the contexts, as well as the forms, of non-narrative genres' (p. viii). So the primacy of story in children's learning to read and reading to learn remains. Therefore, in helping children to read non-fiction, we need first to provide numerous opportunities for story reading and story writing. However, in addition, the teacher will also use opportunities to support children's reading of non-fiction, especially older infants. At the very least, such opportunities will include reading aloud, shared readings, thematic work and writing.

In the majority of readings aloud by the teacher, it will be *story readings* that are used. However, occasionally the teacher might read a short extract from an information book – not as a replacement for the daily story reading, but additional to it. These short readings from information books might occur, for instance, at the end of a period of *sustained silent reading*. Such readings are not designed specifically to teach about the structure of non-fiction books, they are there because the class may have been exploring a particular topic and the teacher, having found an interesting item, reads it out to the class. Of course, the outcome of such readings is that the children will be informed not only about the subject matter but also indirectly about the organization, grammatical structure and flow of some information books. Furthermore, it should not surprise us if some young children bring an information book to a *shared reading* with their teacher. During these one-to-one interactions, the teacher is able to support the child's reading of the text and also to make comments about the nature of information books.

Involvement with information books occurs during other literacy activities. For example, when children are engaged in thematic or topic work, they often need to consult a variety of books to find out more about their interests. The reading of this variety of materials written in different registers needs to be supported by the teacher so as to avoid simple copying of sections from the books. Demonstrations and guidance from the teacher are required, so that the children can make the best use of their reading skills in the context of reading differently arranged texts. This variety of reading by young children is now included as part of the National Curriculum in England and Wales (DES 1990).

The reading of non-narrative texts can also be facilitated by arranging for opportunities for the children to write in non-narrative forms. Although Valerie Cherrington's (1990) example of children working together to write an information book is of eight- and nine-year-olds, it does demonstrate some of the activities that are required to accomplish the task. The children had to locate information, use a variety of reading strategies including *scanning and skimming*, understand and extract information from the texts, record and store the information that was collected, and compose their own text collaboratively. All of this required substantial support from the teacher. The obvious outcome of the writing was that the children added to the information books available in their class library. Furthermore, the writing that had taken place was concerned with 'realistic tasks: with real reasons for inquiry, real reasons for writing and real audiences in mind' (p. 153). However, not only were the children learning to write in a non-narrative form, they were also able to take that learning to their subsequent reading of non-fiction.

Further reading

Neate, B. (1992) *Finding Out About Finding Out: A Practical Guide to Children's Information Books*. Sevenoaks: Hodder and Stoughton.

Bobbie Neate suggests initially that her book is aimed especially at those who work with primary children. However, the subsequent emphasis in the text is on junior school children aged seven to eleven rather than younger children. Nevertheless, there are many aspects of the book that will have applications for the teacher of younger children. The list comparing narrative and expository texts (pp. 49–51) has a general relevance for all teachers, which will raise questions about the provision of literacy activities in the classroom to support children's reading of information books.

reading recovery

Most teachers of young children recognize literacy to be the main area for emphasis within their classrooms. This being the case, a wide range of literacy activities should be provided by the teacher within a well-organized classroom so as to encourage each child's growth as a literacy user. Yet in every infant class there are some children who do not progress as well as the teacher would like. In such circumstances, teachers normally consider ways in which the classroom, or the teacher's time, might be reorganized to provide more support for these children. Developing a firm foundation for children as literacy users is crucial for subsequent learning through literacy. Reading recovery is a programme which bears these concerns in mind, but which has developed towards a system of support for these children beyond, and additional to, that which could be provided in the classroom.

Reading recovery was developed in New Zealand (Clay 1985), but has subsequently been used widely in the USA as well as other English-speaking countries. It is regarded as an early intervention programme rather than a remedial programme. In New Zealand, the programme is adopted with those children who, after a range of diagnostic tests, are regarded as being in need of support after their first year in school, usually when they are close to their sixth birthday. A key part of the diagnosis is the *running records* of the children reading from what Marie Clay (1985: 17) refers to as 'an easy text, an instructional text and a hard text'. From such records, the teacher is able to determine the 'error rate' and the strategies adopted by the children. But Clay suggests that no one mode of assessment is sufficient on its own to provide a detailed picture of the child as a reader, and therefore other procedures need to be used as well. These include letter identification (both upper- and lower-case letters); the Concepts about Print test, which indicates children's knowledge of the use of print in books (i.e. it suggests whether the children know about how a book works); and word tests and writing tasks (either writing down all the words that the children know or writing a story). With all this information the teacher is able to compile a detailed picture of the children's literacy development. This is important, because the reading recovery programme attempts to build on that which is known.

The children selected for reading recovery are given thirty minutes extra intensive individual teaching each day. And because reading and writing are seen to be interwoven and supportive of each other, both are part of that extra teaching. The programme starts with 'roaming around the known', where the teacher and child get to know each other, working with the literacy that the child has demonstrated to be confident with in the diagnostic assessment. When the teaching programme commences, it typically includes reading and writing each day. This teaching usually has a format as follows (Clay 1985: 56):

- re-reading of two or more familiar books,
- re-reading yesterday's new book and taking a running record,
- letter identification (plastic letters on a magnetic board),
- writing a story (including hearing sounds in words),
- cut-up story to be rearranged,
- new book introduced,
- new book attempted.

Most of these activities, especially the emphasis upon reading short story books and writing stories or a sentence, are likely to be part of the infant teacher's normal provision within the classroom. However, very detailed instructions are given for each of these activities and this is why an extensive training programme is suggested for reading recovery teachers.

Reading recovery is discontinued when it appears, from the reading and writing on the programme, that the child is able to cope with the normal activities of the rest of the class without regular individual guidance. As a guide, this is usually after fifteen to twenty weeks of reading recovery. Marie Clay (1985) provides evidence to suggest that children make considerable gains during their period of intensive individual instruction. Ted Glynn and his colleagues (1989), in their independent evaluation of reading recovery for the New Zealand Department of Education, also found that children who had attended reading recovery programmes made substantially more progress than comparable children who did not attend such sessions. However, as with a number of other support programmes, there was some indication that these children failed to progress further once reading recovery was discontinued. This serves to remind us of the need to monitor each child's literacy development and to ensure that progress is continued through the provision of appropriate literacy activities.

Although in the normal classroom intensive individual attention is difficult to provide without support from other adults, nevertheless there are likely to be elements of reading recovery that teachers of young children will wish to employ. Furthermore, such provision is likely to be for the whole year, rather than for the short but intensive period suggested by reading recovery. Even without the resources required by reading recovery, some of its principles are likely to be utilized, including diagnosing the children's strengths and weaknesses, ensuring that the children read and write each day, and giving individual support as often as possible – which implies careful organization of the classroom.

Further reading

Clay, M. (1985) *The Early Detection of Reading Difficulties*. Auckland: Heinemann Educational.

Clay, M. (1993) *Reading Recovery: A Guidebook for Teachers in Training*. London: Heinemann Educational.

For any teacher wishing to consider reading recovery in greater detail, one of these texts is essential. For instance, the diagnostic procedures noted above are provided in great detail and they therefore allow the teacher to carry out the assessments in an appropriate manner. These texts also demonstrate what information can be gained from the assessments. From such knowledge of the child as a reader and writer, Marie Clay then proceeds to describe the details of the programme.

reading schemes

A reading scheme might simply be described as a collection of books written with the express purpose of helping children to learn to read. In the USA, they are referred to as basal readers and comprise workbooks and ancillary materials, which suggest a tighter control of the teaching. In the UK, reading schemes more typically contain the central collection of books focused on a small group of characters. Given that teachers of young children have a similar goal to that of reading schemes (i.e. helping children to learn to read), many schools use such materials. The HMI (1991) survey of 470 primary classes in 120 schools indicated that more than 95 per cent of the classes used reading schemes to some extent, albeit 'usually supplemented by other fiction or non-fiction books' (p. 7). Teachers who use reading schemes can point to the perceived advantages of such materials, and in particular that they provide a structure to the teaching of reading. (In 1988, Kenneth Goodman and colleagues suggested that the tight organization and sequence of basal readers was the main strength of graded reading materials. However, they also suggested that such a structure was a major weakness, as it did not allow for easy modification and adaptation by the teacher.) The provision of such a structure might nevertheless be important, especially when large classes are to be taught. Furthermore, the children's reading progress can be monitored by teachers and parents (and perhaps the children themselves) using the books of the scheme.

Features of reading schemes include: a controlled increase in vocabulary, which may lessen the demands placed upon the child; frequent repetition of vocabulary, once introduced, in order to reinforce the learning process; the use of simplified short sentences to match the child's own repertoire of relatively short sentences; and perhaps if the reading scheme is phonic-based, then the systematic inclusion of particular letters and letter combinations.

Yet the use of reading schemes has been a contentious issue for many years (Burt 1893), and more recently the arguments in support of *real books* have emphasized that debate. In part, the concern about graded reading schemes can be linked to the two different philosophies underpinning the production of texts. Some reading schemes are based on look-and-say principles, where a controlled vocabulary and a high repetition rate are evident. On the negative side, this has led with some schemes to the 'look, look, look' type of writing which seems to be divorced from the world of natural language. Other schemes are based on phonics teaching and in some texts that has led to the pedestrian 'cat sat on the mat' type of material for the children to read. And in neither of these types of reading schemes is there a flow of language with a forward-moving narrative and cohesive links between the sentences. However, in recent years, publishers have attempted to meet these criticisms and have produced schemes with a greater reliance upon stories and the use of natural language. And schools in the UK, having considered the structure that is provided by the reading schemes and the adequacy of the books in such schemes, have moved towards a policy with a number of different possibilities.

First, some schools use just one major reading scheme in order to teach their children to read. Often the school will develop themes based upon the characters or events from the scheme in order to consolidate or extend the learning. Of course, where there is a reliance upon one scheme, then it will need to be selected carefully by considering in detail the stories, illustrations and teacher's manual, which will indicate the philosophy behind the scheme, as well as determining whether the books will meet the interests of the children. Second, because it will be difficult to find a scheme that meets all the needs of the school, more than one reading scheme can be used, and a new structure can be created based on the texts from the different schemes. Third, although the intention is to encourage the children on to story books after using a reading scheme, some schools make it their policy to use a scheme for a short period of time only and then use story or real books to facilitate the children's reading growth. Fourth, because of the concerns about the language in some reading schemes, schools might use the natural language books in some of the more recent reading schemes. These schemes have small story books, often of just eight or twelve pages, written in a natural language and with different characters in each book. Nevertheless, these schemes attempt to provide a sequential development of difficulty through the large collection of stories. Fifth, some schools use *real books* throughout the school in order to encourage reading development. In such circumstances the careful selection of each book is important for ensuring that there is a good storyline written in a natural language and which will be both interesting and meaningful to the children.

Although as we noted earlier 95 per cent of classes in the UK use a reading scheme, the number using a single reading scheme is much smaller. Nevertheless, whatever use is made of carefully selected reading schemes, decisions will need to be made about the organization of the classroom and the provision of the various literacy activities that are discussed in this handbook.

Further reading

Donaldson, M. (1989) *Sense and Sensibility*. Reading: Reading and Language Information Centre, University of Reading School of Education.

Recently, reading schemes have been criticized for their lack of meaningful stories written in a natural language in a forward-moving narrative. Margaret Donaldson explores the real books/reading scheme issue, along with a number of other debates, and suggests that a general condemnation of reading schemes is inappropriate. In conclusion, she argues for 'the reading of text which is very simple, but which is not stilted in its sentence forms and is linked to familiar and interesting themes' (p. 33). Such a conclusion reminds us that what is required is a careful consideration of the quality of all the texts that we provide for children as they develop as readers and beyond.

real books

Real books, not unlike big books, is a term used to describe two different notions. First, as we shall deal with it here, 'real books' describes the materials that might be used in a classroom to encourage children's early reading development. It is used in this way to indicate those books which are written for the purpose of telling a story. This can be contrasted with those books which are written for the purpose of teaching children to read and which might be referred to as *reading scheme* books (or 'basals' in the USA). Second, as we will see in the following section, the *real books approach* refers not only to the books to be read but also to a philosophy about the teaching and learning of reading.

The impetus towards the use of real books, as the materials by which young children's reading development is encouraged, emanates from a concern about many reading schemes. After all, a reading scheme is likely to be based on short sentences, a simple vocabulary and the repetition of words, which often leads to uninteresting texts that restrain children's learning (albeit that a number of key words are likely to be learnt and mastered). Barrie Wade (1990) is very critical of reading schemes and demonstrates that concern by presenting a text back to front, as well as in the appropriate order, where the ordering does not appear to influence the meaning of the text. We would normally expect stories to have a forward-moving plot and children would share that expectation. Indeed, children's implicit understanding of story structure may mean that they are well placed to use real books from the earliest moments in their contact with print.

Although the emphasis upon real books, and the benefits which they can bring, may appear to be a recent innovation, teachers have expressed concern for many years about books written especially for teaching reading (i.e. reading schemes, basals or reading books). As an example of this concern, let us consider Mary Burt's strong words from 1893:

> At the end of the year we had proved that the reading-book was of no earthly use – unless to make good materials for bonfires. We had satisfied ourselves that reading-books made children timid towards real books, and thwarted the intention of the schools to teach 'the essentials' – or at least one of the essentials, namely 'readin''.
>
> (p. 172)

So what are the qualities which one would expect to find in real books? In part, we touched briefly upon the qualities of real books when mention was made of predictable books in the *big books* section. Real books are written with natural language, and they are predictable and meaningful, which means as Liz Waterland (1988: 46) indicates that 'the story, however simple, [can] be read aloud by an adult in a natural, interested manner and without sounding lunatic'. Most frequently, these books are written about people, animals and events, which are a reflection of the real world and therefore the children are able to contextualize many of the stories and to learn from them. Jill Bennett (1991: 7) develops this view and suggests that it might be the 'intrinsic humour of nearly all the books [which] seems to be what attracts children to them'. The *illustrations* in real books are there to support the text and, as Graham (1991) has argued, illustrations can extend the meanings of the story and also help the children to understand the story. In addition, real books are often written in a way that produces a rhythm or flow to the words, so in Eric Carle's *The Very Hungry Caterpillar* there was 'On Monday he ate through ... On Tuesday he ate through ...', etc., which produces a predictability but also a rhythm to that part of the story. And then there is repetition. Real books often contain aspects of repetition, but the repetition is based on units of language rather than single words (which might be evident in a reading scheme). So if we stay with *The Very Hungry Caterpillar*, then despite the variety of eating 'he was still hungry' at the end of each day, and children appear to enjoy the repetition of that sentence with its predictability and rhythm.

Overall, as Barrie Wade (1990) argues, real books with their forward-moving narrative and logical connections and consequences give emotional and intellectual sustenance to a child. Of course, just because a book is not part of a reading scheme and has been written by an author (rather than a publisher) does not necessarily make it a worthwhile real book. Nevertheless, there are now hundreds of books which children find interesting and which provide sustenance in the sense noted above. And a number of the texts have lists to help us make a start with our own selections. Both Wade (1990) and Slaughter (1992) include a list of books for children, each with a brief description or comment; Bennett (1991) does the same but in greater detail. Our reading of some of these stories to children and the children's responses to them will help us to determine the quality of these real books.

Further reading

Bennett, J. (1991) *Learning to Read with Picture Books*, 4th edn. Stroud: Thimble Press.

Jill Bennett's book was first published in 1979 and its popularity is indicated by the fact that it is now in its fourth revised edition. In addition to arguing the case for real books, and demonstrating how she has used those books in her classroom, she notes the qualities she would expect to find in them. However, for many teachers it is the very detailed list of real books and Jill Bennett's sensitive comments on them which are the great attraction of this booklet.

Meek, M. (1988) *How Texts Teach What Readers Learn*. Stroud: Thimble Press.

The title of this short booklet clearly conveys its message. Through a detailed consideration of some children's books, Margaret Meek shows us how the quality of real books not only helps children to learn to read but also how those stories teach about language, discourse and writing. And reading these multi-layered texts, as a reflective reader, assists in learning about life.

Wade, B. (ed.) (1990) *Reading for Real*. Buckingham: Open University Press.

The ten chapters in this book are written by teachers and educators. Much of the book is devoted to real books as materials. So a consideration of reading schemes, the power of stories, the attributes of real books and lists of real books are available for the reader. These sections provide a useful and detailed extension to the comments made above on real books. The text goes beyond real books as the reading matter to be used and also considers teaching and learning within classrooms when a real books approach is adopted.

real books approach

A starting point for the real books approach is indeed the books to be read. And as we noted in the previous section, such books are real books in the sense that they are story books, most frequently, which are written to tell a story rather than to teach a child to read, at least directly. However, some of the key features of story books – natural language, predictability, repetition and rhythm, illustrations, characters and humour, forward-moving narrative with logical connections and consequences – do facilitate children in their development as readers. Furthermore, teachers give extra support by working alongside the children in one-to-one *shared readings* of the books. Such shared readings are an important feature of a real books approach, where the quality of the book, the efforts of the child as an active learner, and the sophisticated and changing role of the teacher all contribute to the making of a successful interaction.

Margaret Meek (1982) and Frank Smith (1978) have both argued the importance of the book, the child and the teacher to encourage reading development. Shared reading within a real books approach provides those elements. However, the approach extends far beyond just real books and shared readings and includes many other literacy activities within a carefully organized and managed classroom. Furthermore, the approach implies working with a view of teaching and learning which emphasizes the whole rather than the parts, and learning experiences rather than frequent direct teaching. So a real books approach refutes any suggestion of it being one of minimalist teaching, as suggested by Phillips (1990). Indeed, those teachers who attempt to follow a real books approach would argue that it involves a complex teaching role requiring a sound knowledge both of children and of reading.

In practical terms, teachers working with a real books approach make a careful selection of books for the children and organize the classroom so that uninterrupted shared readings can occur. However, the organization of the classroom encompasses more than this, because teachers will want to ensure that there are areas for literacy activities to occur. So the room will usually contain a *library corner*, *listening area* and *writing centre*. And these areas will be developed to attract the children to them. The furniture will be arranged so as to support carefully managed movement and interaction in the classroom. Part of classroom management will be to ensure that there is sufficient *time* being devoted to literacy. In some respects it could be argued that the *classroom print* should be so great that the children are always engaged in literacy. However, it is important for teachers to ensure that not only is print available in the classroom, but that that print is used with the children either as a class, a group or as individuals.

A real books approach also recognizes the importance of the home in supporting literacy development and therefore *home–school links* should be a feature of a school adopting this approach. And the wider environment should be used to form a foundation for some of the *language experience approach* activities in the classroom, which enable links to be made between reading and writing as one supports the other. The above indicates that a real books approach is not a non-teaching approach. The teacher is constantly engaged in the *assessment* of the children so as to ensure that needs can be ascertained and subsequently met.

The real books approach does involve far more than just the books to be read and shared readings. Nevertheless, the books are important as are the interactions between the teacher and the child or children. Therefore, teachers using a real books approach will use other opportunities to share books in order to encourage reading development. *Story readings*, shared book experiences with *big books*, *hearing children read* and *sustained silent reading* are all fundamental aspects of a real books approach, as they provide the opportunity for teachers and children to interact with worthwhile and meaningful books when learning to read and the enjoyment of reading can be brought together.

Further reading

Campbell, R. (1992) *Reading Real Books*. Buckingham: Open University Press.

This book describes the principles and practices of a real books approach. It was written at a time when critics of real books were describing the approach as a simplistic non-teaching movement involving just real books and repeated readings of them. Although the text does note the importance of the books to be read and the use of shared readings, it suggests that the real books approach involves far more. The book debates classroom organization and management together with literacy activities. Classroom examples are provided in many of the chapters.

Harrison, C. and Coles, M. (eds) (1992) *The Reading for Real Handbook*. London: Routledge.

Colin Harrison and Martin Coles have gathered together a number of articles which emphasize literature-based approaches to early reading. The articles are arranged into three broad sections concerned with theories about learning to read, the books to be used and, finally, the organization and practices required to encourage children to be readers. The text argues that teachers need to have a sound understanding of the theory and principles which provide the rationale for the practice, so that at times of debate a strong defence can be made for the real books approach. The authors outline these theories and principles and in each chapter provide the reader with some questions to reflect upon.

record-keeping

Teachers of young children will want to keep a record of the literacy developments of each child in the class. This is because having a systematic and detailed account of each child's literacy growth enables the teacher to reflect upon the activities that might be provided in order to build upon that child's current strengths and support the child's needs. Of course, the records serve other purposes as well, as they can form the basis for discussions with parents about a child's progress and can be passed on to other teachers who teach the child subsequently. The records can also be used to form the basis for any teacher assessments that might be required as part of a National Curriculum. However, what the teacher in the busy classroom will want to compile are records on each child which are informative yet do not take up too much of his or her time.

The records that are kept will be based upon the observations, interactions and analyses that will be part of the *assessment* procedures in the classroom. These occur throughout the school day, although there are particular times when information can be collected in greater detail. *Shared readings* provide a good opportunity for the teacher to learn about the child as a reader. During such interactions, a *miscue analysis* or *running record* can take place and a discussion with the child can add to the information. *The Primary Language Record* (CLPE 1988) includes a pro forma, 'Reading Sample Form', for providing a description of the reading by the child during such an interaction. Used on occasions as an informal observation of the child's reading, it can add other details to the miscue analysis or running record. The form includes:

- the title of the book;
- whether it is a known or unknown text;
- overall impression of the child's reading;
- strategies used by the child when reading aloud (which implies some reference by the teacher to miscue analysis);
- the child's response to the book; and

- a reflection by the teacher about the child's development as a reader and the support now needed for further development.

This sample of the child's reading could be added to the regular record that is kept of the shared readings with each child. Such reading diaries might include:

- the date;
- the book read;
- the teacher's comments on what are perceived to be significant features of the child's reading;
- responses to the reading; and
- the extent of any teacher support.

Such a diary would, over a period of time, provide some interesting insights into the child's progress as a reader. All of this information provides an extended narrative or description of each child as a reader. From that description, particular aspects can be extracted as necessary. In some schools, a record sheet is used in an attempt to provide an immediate visual impression of what a child has achieved. Liz Waterland (1988) provides a reading wheel on which certain reading behaviours can be noted. The use of the wheel to record the information is indicative of the non-linear development of literacy growth. The Sheffield Early Literacy Development Project used a jigsaw, for similar reasons, to enable parents to see their children's development with *environmental print*, *writing* and *shared reading* (Weinberger *et al.* 1990).

The obvious way to maintain a record of a child's writing is to retain samples of that writing, often chosen in collaboration with the child. These samples can be kept in a scrapbook or portfolio, and over a year they build up to a very complete record of the child's progress. And over a three-year period, these samples provide not only a detailed picture of the child as a writer but also provide a wealth of information to help teachers evaluate the literacy policy of the school. The sample of writing requires some additional comment by the teacher in order to contextualize the writing product, so that any support the child might have received can be recognized. Typically, the teacher needs to date the work, and provide information about the stimulus for the writing, the extent of teacher support, whether the work was independent or collaborative, whether *invented spellings* were used, whether a word book/dictionary was used, etc. All of this information is important so that the writing can be analysed in the most informative way. The sample of writing should be sufficient to demonstrate the child's growing knowledge of story structure, ability to organize and structure the writing according to purpose and audience, as well as indicating knowledge of conventions, such as spelling and punctuation.

Although each school is likely to develop somewhat different record-keeping practices, nevertheless certain principles will underpin that practice. Myra Barrs and Gillian Johnson (1993) suggest that observation-based records should be based upon:

- regular, frequent and systematic recording (some recording takes place daily);
- the recording of normal behaviour in favourable contexts (the children are assessed in normal classroom situations rather than in special and artificial contexts);
- an emphasis on positive recording (focusing on the child's strengths);
- recording that includes evidence from home (thus emphasizing the *home–school link*);
- records which stress the links between different aspects of language (so that reading and writing growth can be looked at together);
- records which view non-conventional reading and writing as information (miscues and invented spellings are good examples of such information);
- records which include contributions from children (which might develop from small beginnings where the child helps with the selection of writing for the portfolio);
- helpful structures for recording (an open structure which suggests areas for information but which encourages observations and comment rather than checklists);
- recording in different contexts and in different formats (so that we are not reliant upon just one type of record to judge a child's literacy progress).

This extensive list of principles can be used to judge the earlier suggestions for record-keeping in this section. The list might also be used by teachers to evaluate their own record-keeping practice.

Further reading

Barrs, M. and Johnson, G. (1993) *Record-keeping in the Primary School.* London: Hodder and Stoughton.

This short book provides a very readable and practical introduction to record-keeping. The examples are drawn from primary schools but they are of particular relevance to infant school teachers. As Myra Barrs was associated with the development and use of the Primary Language Record, the discussion of that language record is well informed. For teachers in England and Wales, who need to consider record-keeping in the context of the National Curriculum, there are numerous helpful links.

responding to miscues

During the literacy interaction of *hearing children read*, children spend part of the time reading out aloud to their teacher. This is also the case in some of the later instances of *shared reading*. During such oral readings, some miscues are inevitably produced by the reader. And the teacher will have to consider how to respond to these miscues using a variety of strategies.

A starting point for many teachers and parents is to consider the pause–prompt–praise continuum (Glynn 1980). These three 'p's' remind us to wait before mediating in a child's reading, thus giving the child time to think about his or her own reading, to provide some response or prompt if it is required, and subsequently to praise the child's efforts.

But what should be the format of the teacher's response or prompt? Elsewhere I have suggested that teachers working in the normal classroom environment use a number of different responses to support a child's reading (Campbell 1992). And using the example of five-year-old Richard reading from Eric Carle's *The Very Hungry Caterpillar* I was able to demonstrate the five main strategies that teachers adopt and suggest the reasons for the use of those responses.

First, teachers may use the strategy of non-response:

Richard: In the light of the moon
the (a) little egg lay on a leaf
Teacher: —

In this example, Richard miscued the text word 'a' and read 'the', although later on the same line he read the word 'a' accurately. This miscue did not alter substantially the meaning of the book and the teacher, working to the notion that meaning is the essential feature of reading, decided not to mediate.

Second, teachers may use a word-cueing strategy, which involves the teacher in reading the part of the sentence that leads up to the miscued word and to do so with a rising intonation which draws the child back into the interaction as the reader:

Richard: one cupcake and
one slice of salami (watermelon)
Teacher: one slice
Richard: one slice of watermelon

Importantly, this strategy seems to work very frequently (Campbell 1994), and perhaps it does so because it does not draw the child's attention away from the text, it informs the reader of the need to reconsider a word and it does so by reminding the reader of some of the semantic and syntactic cues. Additionally, as Marie Clay (1972) has shown, children who can read well often use the strategy of restarting a sentence to help themselves with a word which is creating a problem. Therefore, by using this response, teachers help children to develop strategies which they will be able to use themselves later.

Third, teachers may use a soft, non-punitive 'no' as a means of informing the reader that a miscue has been produced:

Richard: He looked (started)
Teacher: No.
Richard: He starts (started)
Teacher: Yes.
Richard: He started

So without a great deal of disruption of Richard's reading, the teacher was able to help him read the verb correctly, if not completely accurately. And it would appear that many teachers use this response especially where the miscued word is at the beginning of the sentence and, therefore, where the word-cueing strategy cannot be used by the teacher.

Fourth, the teacher might very simply provide the word for the reader:

Richard: out of the egg
a very (came)
Teacher: came
Richard: came a tiny and very hungry caterpillar

This response by the teacher is predictably successful. The child hears the word and can echo the word in the reading. However, although it may provide for immediate success, this teacher response may not help the child in the long term. The child has not been involved with the word and therefore teachers often find that after telling a child a word the same word can be miscued two or three lines later. The response does not encourage the child to be an active learner or encourage the child towards independent reading. For these reasons, teachers will wish to use this response sparingly.

It was, in part, because Southgate *et al.* (1981) found this response being used so frequently that they were critical of teachers spending substantial periods of time in hearing children read. But many teachers will, of course, use a range of responses. Nevertheless, they will provide the word on occasion in order to maintain the flow of reading, or because they are working with a very young beginning reader and they wish to give extra support in the early stages.

Fifth, the teacher will occasionally use a response that draws attention to the letters and associated sounds in words:

Richard: he ate through
two peppers (pears) //
Teacher: They do look a bit like peppers.
And they do begin with a 'p'.
But they might be something else do you think?
Richard: pineapples – eh –

So, following Richard's miscue of the word 'pear', the teacher responds with a number of comments which include an emphasis upon the initial letter 'p' in the text word and Richard's miscue. Although this strategy did not help in this instance, it did remind Richard of the graphophonic cue system. This might be another response that the teacher would wish to use sparingly because it takes the reader away from a meaningful reading of a book. However, its occasional use will draw attention to the importance of letters and sounds in reading.

The teacher needs to respond to the reader's miscues with care. In particular, the teacher will want to keep the child involved with the book as an active reader, to provide responses which create minimal disruption to the reading, and to help the reader not only with the immediate reading but also to use responses which help the child to develop strategies for the future.

In the classroom

In the section above, we looked at the various responses that a teacher made when sharing a book with five-year-old Richard.

However, these responses were drawn from various parts of the book and it might create more coherence if we look briefly at the beginning of that reading – with the various comments and discussion removed and just the reading by Richard and the response by the teacher left in place. Your familiarity with this piece of reading by Richard might also support you in your consideration of the teacher's responses:

Richard: In the light of the moon
the – the (a) little egg lay on a leaf
One summer's(Sunday) day(morning) the warm sun
came out(up) and – pop! – //
Teacher: out
Richard: of the egg
a very(came)
Teacher: came
Richard: came a tiny and very hungry caterpillar

An interesting feature of this opening is that the teacher did not respond to the first four substitutions. This non-response seems appropriate for this five-year-old reader. After all, each of the miscues did not alter substantially the nature or meaning of the story which Richard read. Later, the teacher did provide two words when it seemed necessary to keep Richard on track with his reading. We know that the teacher in this example continued to use a variety of responses. But even this short example from the beginning of the reading serves to demonstrate how, in the context of a busy classroom, the teacher can support a reader in a shared reading of a book and respond to the miscues in a way which helps the reader rather than distracting him or her from the book.

Further reading

Arnold, H. (1982) *Listening to Children Reading*. Sevenoaks: Hodder and Stoughton.
Eleven pages in this book are used to consider the ways in which a number of researchers have described and analysed the various teacher responses to miscues within the normal classroom.

Campbell, R. (1988) *Hearing Children Read*. London: Routledge.
This book is devoted entirely to the literacy activity of hearing children read. However, within that analysis, fourteen pages are used to consider the teacher response to children's miscues and excerpts from more than twenty different interactions are used to illustrate the various teacher responses and their influence upon a child's reading.

Campbell, R. (1992) *Reading Real Books*. Buckingham: Open University Press.
The examples of Richard's miscues are debated more extensively in this book. Furthermore, the complete shared reading between the teacher and Richard is provided, so that it is possible to contextualize the miscues within a total reading.

Campbell, R. (1994) The teacher response to children's miscues of substitution. *Journal of Research in Reading*, 17: 147–54.
This article considers the various teacher responses that are used following children's miscues of substitution. Using data from a research study, it explores the teacher responses to almost 3000 cases of substitutions. The analysis indicates the particular usefulness of the word-cueing strategy to help readers immediately and to support them in subsequent readings.

running records

In early years classrooms in England and Wales, especially among teachers who have taught a year-2 class recently, there will be some knowledge of running records. This knowledge might derive from the experiences with that mode of assessment as part of the testing arrangements for Key Stage 1 of the National Curriculum. However, an awareness of running records will also have come from other sources. First, where teachers have used miscue analysis at some stage, then the concept and practice of running records is readily understood, because of the similarities between these two modes of diagnosis and assessment. Second, even where miscue analysis is unknown, most infant teachers during shared readings will have kept some form of record of the child's progress and that record-keeping may well have included some reference to words that the child was unable to read. So normal classroom literacy activities provide a basis for an acceptance of a process that is already implicit in the teacher's everyday working.

The running record is a simple means of recording the oral reading of a child. It is simple because it does not require a duplicate of the pages being read and the reading is not tape-recorded. Because the teacher codes the oral reading of the child on to a plain sheet of paper, a running record can therefore be taken at any time. Indeed, the development of the running record was to meet these very needs of the teacher for the day-to-day activities of the classroom with young children (Clay 1985), although it was based on the more detailed *miscue analysis* developed in the USA (see Goodman *et al.* 1987, for a consideration of this mode of diagnosis). So how is a running record coded?

Each child reads aloud from the book he or she has selected. This reading to the teacher is recorded on to a plain sheet of paper, and each word read accurately is recorded with a tick and miscues (or errors as Marie Clay, 1985, refers to them) are noted using a number of conventional marks:

/	word read correctly
T	word told by the teacher
the	substituted word
it–the	substitution sequence
O	omission of word
SC	self-correction of word by the child

For example

The boy saw a dog. ///it–the/

It can be seen at a glance that the reader read four of the five words accurately and substituted the word 'a' first with 'it' and then 'the'. Marie Clay (1985) suggests that the text word might be written under the miscue so that the nature of the substitution, etc., can be seen at a glance. However, many teachers of young children are able to record the reading and recognize the coding in relation to the text (providing the title of the short book is noted at the top of the sheet) because of their familiarity with the books in the classroom. There are other miscues that are produced by children, so the teacher might have to represent repetitions using an 'R' for example. However, as a starting point, the short list of conventions above will account for much of the child's reading of a book.

Once the reading is completed, then, as with a miscue analysis, the teacher may ask, 'Why that miscue?' And this raises the issue of which language *cue system*, or systems, the child was using in order to produce the miscue. Marie Clay suggests that the letters M, S and V might be inserted on to the coding, these letters representing meaning, structure and visual cues being used. Such an analysis is not dissimilar to a miscue analysis, because meaning (M) will be indicative of the child using the semantic language cues, structure (S) will suggest the use of the syntactic cues and visual (V) will indicate some use of the graphophonic cue system. When an analysis is undertaken, it will be noted that one, two or all three of the cue systems may apparently have been used by the child; it is seldom the case that children only use one of the cues throughout a reading. But we also need to recognize that when we undertake such an analysis, we are making our best judgement of what the child might have done. We can never be totally sure because we cannot get into the mind of the reader, although the miscue analysis or running record enables us to get close to achieving that goal. Such analyses can be used to help to determine the literacy activities that might be provided to support the child in the classroom.

Although the running record is a development from miscue analysis, it is important to remember that it is a simplification of that mode of diagnosis and that some information might be lost in that simplification. As an example, it is well known that when a child's oral reading is audio-recorded for subsequent miscue analysis, there are many points where the listener has to listen two, three or more times in order to be sure that the coding of the miscues is accurate. Coding straight on to a plain sheet of paper will include some errors by the teacher, or there will be some codings which on reflection after further hearings of the reading might be interpreted differently. Therefore, it might be the more complete miscue analysis which teachers will use, especially with children who may require extra attention. Nevertheless, the use of a running record may be helpful in a busy classroom for gaining some insight into the reading strategies being adopted by the children, and the teacher can use that information to evaluate the range of literacy activities provided in the classroom.

Further reading

Clay, M. (1985) *The Early Detection of Reading Difficulties*. Auckland: Heinemann Educational.

Part of this text, which very largely is about reading recovery, describes running records. This description of running records is nevertheless comprehensive and provides sufficient information to enable us to understand this process. For those teachers in the UK who have been involved with SATs and therefore have carried out a running record in a more limited way, this text will provide greater insights into this mode of assessment.

Campbell, R. (1993a) *Miscue Analysis in the Classroom*. Widnes: UK Reading Association.

This short book attempts to provide a simple but concise description of miscue analysis for use by the busy classroom teacher. Inevitably, given that the emphasis is upon the classroom, there is also a section on the use of running records in which the coding used is described. The link to miscue analysis is more firmly established by using the same short passage and the oral reading of a child for both a miscue analysis and a running record.

scanning and skimming

Scanning and skimming are two reading techniques, or styles, which are often regarded as part of the repertoire of older readers. For instance, in their study of secondary school reading, Lunzer and Gardner (1979) referred to four styles of reading – scanning, skimming, receptive reading and reflective reading – and indicated the need for children in the ten to fifteen age range to be able make flexible use of each, according to the demands of the text and the purposes of the child. They defined scanning and skimming as follows:

> Skim reading is a rapid style used mainly to establish what the text is about before deciding whether and where to read… Scanning is a kind of skimming to see if a particular point is present in the text – or to locate it.
>
> (pp. 26–7)

Many teachers of young children might react initially to these definitions by suggesting that such skills can be left until later. Their priority will be to get children to read, most usually with story books, so that there is a good foundation for a subsequent variety of reading and reading to learn. However, a closer analysis might suggest that although teachers of young children might not necessarily introduce the terminology, or teach scanning and skimming directly, nevertheless they will appear as part of the interactions between the teacher and child centred on a book.

When teachers use *big books*, in a shared book experience with the children, that literacy activity teaches the children about how to use story books. Simple messages such as front-to-back and *left-to-right directionality*, and the reading of the complete text, will be demonstrated by the teacher and learnt by the children. These messages are useful because they will help the children to use the books in an appropriate manner. But we know that not all the books that are used are likely to be read in that most normal of ways.

There are occasions when the youngest of readers need to use scanning. A simple example is when children start to consult a dictionary to find the spelling of a word. At that point, the normal strategy of front-to-back reading will not be very helpful. So young children will have to be encouraged to scan the text in order to find the initial letter and then subsequently the actual word that is required.

In order to facilitate such learning, some guidance from the teacher will be required. Such guidance will also be required when children begin to consult information books while engaged on thematic or topic work. Of course, much of this work might be based on the experiences of the children, but the teacher should attempt to extend those experiences and knowledge. This extension could be developed by the teacher arranging visits and bringing artefacts into the classroom. Nevertheless, it should also include using information and reference books. And the teacher will want to avoid this degenerating into low-level learning (Alexander 1992) where the children might, for instance, copy large chunks of the book. Instead, the teacher will want to encourage the children to use the books in order to locate, and extract, specific information that will be useful to them. This suggests that the teacher will talk with the children individually, in groups and as a class, about the process of scanning.

A similar argument can be put forward in relation to skimming. Take, for instance, the task of selecting a book to read. The child will use a number of strategies to help him or her in that endeavour. So the *illustrations* might be used as a guide to selection, and a growing knowledge of authors can also be helpful. However, at some stage, the child will want to glance through the book and get a feel for what the story is about and to decide on the basis of that skim read whether to select the book or not. Children can be helped to develop such a strategy by the demonstrations that the teacher might give in the *library corner* or when introducing a book prior to a *story reading*.

It has not been the aim of this section to suggest that scanning and skimming are major areas for teachers of young children to consider. However, they are reading styles which the teacher is bound to introduce and demonstrate as the children begin to approach books for a variety of purposes. And it is important that the teacher provides these introductions and demonstrations because it enables the children to gain flexibility in their reading.

Further reading

Southgate, V., Arnold, H. and Johnson, S. (1981) *Extending Beginning Reading*. London: Heinemann Educational.

This book is the report of the Extending Beginning Reading Project, which studied in depth the literacy practices in numerous schools and which concentrated upon eight- and nine-year-old children in their year three and four classes. The extensive study had looked at the wide range of literacy practices in classrooms for those age groups. And it came up with a substantial number of recommendations, including that there should be support for 'a gradual transition to the realization that skimming and scanning are as legitimate for certain purposes as reading every word' (p. 291). There is no particular section on these reading strategies, but throughout the book there are ideas to encourage children to become sophisticated and reflective readers. Part of that sophistication is that children should have flexible strategies for dealing with print.

school policy

Throughout this book, there are suggestions about literacy activities and practices for use in the primary classroom. In the main, these activities are contextualized within the classroom where the teacher works together with a number of children. But, of course, the majority of teachers work in schools alongside colleagues. And it would seem strange if each teacher worked in isolation from the other teachers in the school. Indeed, there is evidence to suggest that schools which are successful in helping children with literacy learning often have a school policy on language.

The members of the Bullock Committee (DES 1975) argued the case for a school policy very emphatically when they suggested that 'a coherent strategy, understood and agreed by the staff, is the best instrument for improving standards of reading and language' (p. 212). Such a view was substantiated by HMI (1991) when the teaching of reading was evaluated during visits to numerous schools in England in 1989 and 1990: 'clear well-formulated policies for reading were strongly associated with good standards' (p. 13).

Why should the existence of a clearly written and comprehensive school policy on language and literacy be helpful in encouraging standards of literacy in the school? At the simplest level, of course, it will mean that there are plans for the organization, management and monitoring of reading and writing in order to meet the literacy aims of the school. All teachers will recognize that need, namely to have planned for the literacy teaching and learning which will take place in the classroom (and that includes *whole language* teachers (Goodman 1986), even though occasionally they are accused, falsely, of just allowing learning to happen).

However, it is not just the existence of the school policy that is important. The means by which the policy is established is also important. In particular, where the staff have taken time to debate the development of the school policy, then there is a better chance of that policy being offered in each classroom. Robin Alexander (1992), in reporting upon the evaluation of the Primary Needs Programme in Leeds, indicated the value of such a debate:

> equally important was dialogue on matters of purpose and policy within each school, especially between head and staff. Without such dialogue, and the associated openness in management and decision making, there could be a substantial gap between a school's espoused philosophy and its classroom practice.
>
> (p. 149)

So debate reduces the likelihood of a gap between the policy and the practice. However, it does more than that; debate encourages collaboration between staff and becomes part of the continuous learning process for all the teachers in the school. The roles of the headteacher and the language coordinator in providing leadership and guidance for other colleagues during such a debate and subsequently in supporting the teachers in the classroom, whenever possible, can also be helpful.

The policy then sets the framework for the literacy teaching and learning in the school. But it is useful to think of it as a framework within which teachers can work flexibly. That does not mean that each teacher is at liberty to ignore the policy, but it does allow each teacher to develop his or her particular strengths in the classroom, consistent with the policy agreed in collaboration with colleagues. No two teachers are exactly alike and therefore it would be unreasonable to expect all classrooms to be exactly alike. So there is flexibility, but it is a flexibility within the framework of the school policy.

Of course, the policy is always being developed so that in one sense it is never finalized. HMI (1992) made the point that many of the school policies which they had come across needed to be revised in the light of the requirements of the newly developed National Curriculum in England and Wales. But the school policy on literacy has to be revised constantly for other reasons. Teachers new to a particular school can only acquire a real feel for the policy if they are able to take part in debates with colleagues about that literacy policy. The policy has to be revised regularly for that reason but also all teachers should be developing their knowledge of literacy, and regular debates about aspects of school policy will help in that development. Such regular debates should also ensure that the policy remains appropriate.

Although the school policy may have to be a relatively short and succinct statement of plans and practices, nevertheless the debates which take place will have to address very minute details of classroom practice. For instance, during a staff discussion on the school policy, the practice of shared book experience using *big books* might be debated. Is that best practised as a group or class activity? How is it best fitted in during the school day? What might the children be expected to learn during that activity? What variety of strategies might the teacher employ in order to encourage that learning? Not all of the responses to such questions might be written up as part of the school policy document, but having been a part of a debate about such issues can be helpful to the teacher in the daily task of teaching literacy in the classroom. And that can have a beneficial effect upon the literacy learning experiences of the children.

Further reading

HMI (1991) *The Teaching and Learning of Reading in Primary Schools.* London: DES.

This short document provides details and findings from a survey of 120 primary schools, which took place in 1990, during which some 470 classes were visited by HMI. That evidence built upon other data collected during more general visits to 3000 primary schools from 1989. The specific visits were arranged as part of an analysis of reading standards and the effectiveness of literacy teaching in primary schools. And, as noted above, this report, like the Bullock Report (DES 1975) and the subsequent HMI (1992) paper, stresses the importance of a school policy for literacy planning and teaching. Such a policy, developed collectively, implemented carefully and monitored effectively, was an important feature of schools with high reading standards.

shared reading

Shared reading involves a child and a teacher (or other adult) reading together, in a one-to-one interaction, from a book. It is a practice used frequently in early years classrooms (reception, years 1 and 2 in the UK, or K-2 in the USA). It is also a practice commonly used by many parents at home. Often the *home–school link* is emphasized by the schools producing small booklets for the parents which describe the main features of the interaction.

Shared reading is a practice which places importance upon each of the three elements of the interaction – the child, the book and the adult – as well as the interaction itself. Frank Smith (1978) and Margaret Meek (1982) are among a number of writers who have argued that the interaction between child, book and adult is an important basis for reading success. The principle underpinning this literacy event is that in order to learn to read the child needs to read, just as there is a need to cycle in order to ride a bicycle. This interaction enables the child to learn to read naturally. Reading with the support, guidance and encouragement of the teacher, or other adult, is an important requirement. Nevertheless, the child is perceived to be an active learner attempting to make sense, in this instance, of the print. And the book most usually will be one selected for its natural language (*real books*), which is meaningful and of interest to the child and in which the flow of language and predictability facilitates the child's reading.

Although the active role of the child and the quality of the book are important, the *teacher's role* is very important. The teacher will model the reading as well as supporting, guiding and encouraging the child during the reading of the text. The teacher will also attempt to develop a discussion of the book and encourage the child to initiate questions about the book.

Of course, shared readings will cover a variety of interactions. They do so because as the child develops as a reader, he or she will take greater control over the reading of the book and the adult's role will therefore be reduced as a reader, although increased as a guide and supporter. There is some indication of a sequence in shared reading.

First, the teacher might read the book to the child. During such a reading, the teacher or child might make comments about the story, the characters, the illustrations or make connections from the text to life experiences. Just occasionally, the child might be drawn into the reading of the story where the flow of words allows the child to predict the language with some ease. In Eric Carle's *The Very Hungry Caterpillar*, the repetition of the sentence 'But he was still hungry' very quickly enables young children to contribute to the sharing. At the conclusion of the reading by the teacher, the child might retell the story in his or her own words. Such retellings may be a useful growth point for the child as well as giving insights to the teacher about the child's understanding of the specific book and reading more generally.

Second, the teacher might once again lead with a reading of the story during which a similar sort of discussion to that noted above might take place. However, following this reading, the child is encouraged to provide an emergent reading of the story. It will be an emergent reading because, although the child might convey the general structure and meaning of the story, the precise wording of the story will not be maintained. There will be places where the child reads a word, phrase or sentence from the text but it will not be a fully conventional reading. Such emergent readings with some limited attention to the conventional print requires careful listening by the teacher. We need to look at the strengths that the child displays as the story is recalled and as he or she begins to insert some of the text words into the reading.

Third, the reading of the book starts to resemble the teacher and child reading alongside each other, but not always in unison. At times, therefore, the adult will read and the child will be fractionally behind and echo the words. At other points, the teacher will recognize the growing confidence and ability of the reader and so will encourage the child to lead the reading, the teacher now echoing the child's reading. This drawing back by the teacher will, on occasions, mean that the teacher drops out of the reading altogether. The child therefore reads alone, although the adult is always listening to the reading and ready to support as necessary. During this form of shared reading, the teacher encourages the child to read or leads the child in the reading not in any mechanical way, but because the teacher is in tune with the child's intentions and ability with the particular book being read.

Fourth, the child will have reached a level of attainment which allows him or her to produce a more conventional reading of the book. However, although the child may be more confident and independent as a reader, the teacher will still need to provide support by listening to the child (*hearing children read*). Also, the teacher will note the miscues (*miscue analysis*) that are produced and consider how to respond to them in order to provide support and encouragement for the reader.

During each of these forms of shared reading, the teacher will discuss (*discussions*) with the child aspects of the story, the characters, plot, setting and illustrations. And as Margaret Meek (1988) demonstrates in her book *How Texts Teach What Readers Learn*, that discussion will on occasions include a discussion of the cover, author and publisher.

Shared reading as described in this section is a one-to-one interaction. However, Don Holdaway (1979) debates the use of shared readings with *big books* in the context of a group of children working together. Such a strategy is important for teachers to consider, particularly with younger children. However, many teachers find it useful to progress from group readings with a big book to one-to-one interactions of shared reading.

Teachers place an emphasis upon shared reading because it provides an opportunity to support each child's reading in order to help them develop as readers. Furthermore, it enables the teacher to analyse the reader's developing strategies, strengths and needs.

In the classroom

When five-year-old Kirsty shared her book *Dizzy Dog* with the teacher in a reception class, there was first a reading of the book by the teacher to Kirsty. Furthermore, during the reading by the teacher, there was a discussion about the story, often using the illustrations, and at appropriate moments during the reading Kirsty was brought into the reading in a natural way:

Teacher: It's fallen all the way down the stairs – bump, bump, bump.
Now.
The dog gets out of the box
And what does he try to do?
Kirsty: Stand up.
Teacher: Yes.
The dog falls...
Kirsty: ...over.
Teacher: ...over.
Yes.

Such readings by the teacher with discussions about the text provide the support that enables young children like Kirsty to provide an emergent reading, and later a conventional reading, of the book. The use of a rising intonation as the teacher read 'The dog falls' led Kirsty to provide the completion of the sentence, 'over'. So although it was the teacher who was reading, Kirsty was being helped to read by being given an opportunity to take part.

Further reading

Campbell, R. (1990a) *Reading Together*. Buckingham: Open University Press.

A complete chapter in this book is devoted to a discussion of shared reading, in which two complete transcripts of children reading to their teacher are provided. The miscues produced by the children and the support given by the teacher are discussed. The important role of the teacher in this and a number of other teacher–child interactions is emphasized.

Campbell, R. (1992) *Reading Real Books*. Buckingham: Open University Press.

As part of a consideration of the real books approach to reading, there is a chapter on shared reading. Here, too, there is a transcript of a child reading to his teacher, but interestingly the example indicates that although a sequence of development may be the case with shared readings, each shared reading may be more complex than that sequence suggests.

Davis, C. and Stubbs, R. (1988) *Shared Reading in Practice*. Milton Keynes: Open University Press.

A substantial part of this book is devoted to the practical problems of setting up shared reading as a school practice and of encouraging parental involvement. It provides a useful description of strategies and practices to aid those school and home–school processes.

Standard Assessment Tasks

Standard Assessment Tasks (SATs) are national tests that were devised in conjunction with the National Curriculum in England and Wales. Therefore, this section, like that devoted to the *National Curriculum*, is difficult to write because of the changes that have occurred during their operation and future developments are unknown.

The first national testing using SATs at Key Stage 1, for seven-year-olds, took place in the summer of 1991, although pilot tests had been carried out in some schools prior to that first year of testing. The first year of testing demonstrated that there were problems with the tests and the equal application of them in all schools (even with monitoring processes in place). Furthermore, the publication of the results and their interpretation created something of a public furore, and this was especially the case with reading and writing in the core subject of English. For the SATs of 1992, a number of changes were made to the tests and the testing procedures with the effect of reducing somewhat the time commitment of teachers. Subsequently, further changes were made for the 1993 SATs. But by this time classroom teachers had become disenchanted with this mode of testing, in part because it did not appear to add greatly to their knowledge of the children. Therefore, in many schools the tests were boycotted, and even where the tests had taken place the results were not forwarded to the authorities for publication. Such disquiet led to a major review of the assessment procedures for the National Curriculum (Dearing 1993). That review proposed a substantial slimming down of the testing, although it was proposed to retain SATs for reading and writing at Key Stage 1 in the 1994 national tests.

The considerable amount of time that had to be devoted to SATs was a major concern for teachers working with young children, especially as it seemed to reduce dramatically the time that was available for teaching each summer term. There were perceived to be other problems as well, which were linked to the purposes of the assessment. The tests were expected to provide a diagnosis of children's needs, yet teachers believed that the tests told them little which they did not already know. The tests were also expected to provide a summative picture for parents about their own children and collectively a picture of the performance of the school for interested parties. Meeting the needs of diagnosis and summative information with one set of tests was not unproblematic. But perhaps we should look briefly at the nature of the SATs, at least as they were first utilized in 1991 (SEAC 1991), in order to consider these other issues.

For the Key Stage 1 testing in 1991, all children were tested for competence at Levels 1 and 2 and some children at Level 3. That meant when the results were released, the children were placed in one of four categories, including those who were 'working towards level 1'. For Level 1 in reading, the children had to be able to tell about a story book, to indicate that they recognized that print conveyed the message and to name three letters correctly. At Level 2, each child had to read three of the labels in the classroom (incidentally encouraging the development of *classroom print* in the early years classrooms in England and Wales). Next a story book, designated a Level 2 book, had to be read by the child, with the teacher keeping a *running record* of that reading once the child had reached the passage of approximately one hundred words which constituted the test. If the teacher had to tell the child a word, this was recorded, because after eight words the child was deemed to have failed at Level 2. However, if successful, the child proceeded to tell about the story and, with another book, had to indicate some knowledge of story structure. For Level 3, a more difficult book had to be read silently and retold to the teacher, who would then ask some questions about the text; the children also had to demonstrate an ability to use information books.

At first sight these tests might be welcomed because they replicate a number of literacy events that teachers use regularly in the classroom with six- and seven year olds. However, that being the case, it might be asked whether anything was being added to the teacher's diagnosis of the child as a reader. But the allocation of a child to a particular level and the reporting of the results was to prove to be even more problematic. The boundary of Levels 1 and 2 demonstrated one of the problems. If a child was told nine words, then they would be regarded as being at Level 1. Yet the running record of such a child demonstrated his considerable strengths as a reader (Campbell 1991). Nevertheless, being told nine words rather than eight meant being at Level 1 – and inappropriately being regarded as a non-reader in the national media. In part, this example demonstrates the substantial difference that existed between Level 1 attainments and those of Level 2.

The reporting of assessment results to the parents of children was problematic because no account was taken of the age of the children. Although in theory the Key Stage 1 was testing attainment at seven years of age, in fact many six-year-olds were tested. And there was inevitably a range of eleven months in the ages of the children tested. As might be expected, the results of the test in any one class reflected the ages of the children as much as it reflected the attainments of the children – 86 per cent of the children on Level 1 were born in the summer, i.e. the youngest in the class (NUT 1991). Furthermore, comparison between achievements of schools were frequently reflections of the social backgrounds of the schools. And, inevitably, given the importance that began to be attached to the levels achieved, then the tests began to become the curriculum. Level 2 books were stocked by local shops and became the most sought-after books by parents and many schools.

A similar description could be provided for the SATs in writing.

However, let us simply consider one aspect of the writing tasks at Key Stage 1, namely *punctuation*. As the SATs were refined each year, punctuation began to figure more prominently in the assessment. In particular, the ability to demarcate a sentence with a capital letter and full stop became an important criterion for achieving Levels 2 and 3. And as a result, some teachers and children restricted the writing in terms of content in order to concentrate on that aspect (Anderson 1993). This may not have been in the best interests of the children.

Although the SATs have been too time-consuming and interpreting the results has been fraught with difficulties, this does not mean that an *assessment* of children's development as literacy users is not required. We need to know about children's progress so that an analysis of their strengths and weaknesses can be determined and literacy activities be provided to help them further. And as part of the *home–school link*, parents should be kept informed of their children's progress. Assessment is an integral part of the teacher's monitoring of the classroom. Time may determine whether SATs will become a useful part of that assessment.

Further reading

SEAC (1991) *Standard Assessment Task: Teacher's Pack Key Stage 1. 1991*. London: HMSO.

This pack includes a range of materials giving instructions for carrying out the standard assessment tasks at Key Stage 1. Additionally, there is a collection of forms for recording the results. However, most importantly for our purposes, there is a 'Handbook of Guidance for the SAT' and a 'Teacher's Book'. These two booklets provide the details of the SATs procedures. Similar packs have been produced for each of the years of testing and together they provide an indication of the changes and developments in this area.

NUT (1991) *Miss, the Rabbit Ate the 'Floating Apple'! The Case Against SATs*. London: National Union of Teachers.

The NUT conducted a survey of 2550 year 2 teachers in 1750 schools in order to determine the usefulness of the 1991 SATs. The results demonstrate the considerable amount of time being devoted to the activity and the concerns about appropriateness of levels and unfairness to younger children. The report contains many comments from teachers which highlight the influence of the SATs on normal classroom activities.

story grammar

Many children have the advantage of having stories read to them at home. Additionally, they may have heard *nursery rhymes*, played finger games and perhaps witnessed or played games which have involved language stories. And they may have heard events described by adults as well as beginning to tell their own stories about things which have happened to them. All of this enables the children to develop their language. One aspect of this development is that the children will begin to acquire, intuitively, a knowledge about story grammar or story structure. They will not have been taught this grammar directly, but their own telling of stories will indicate that a knowledge of story grammar is being acquired. Indeed, evidence of such knowledge, albeit limited, is apparent among some two-year-olds as they tell stories (Applebee 1978).

So what is the story grammar that is being learnt? There are a number of ways of describing it, although most descriptions include some key elements, including the characters, setting (indicating time and/or place) and a plot with a problem or wish leading to some resolution (the plot might contain a number of events or episodes). Stories are also expected to have a beginning, middle and end with the use of a consistent past tense. Applebee debates the way in which children from two to five years of age gradually demonstrate greater control over the use of a formal opening phrase ('Once upon a time'), a formal closing ('happily ever after') and the use of a consistent past tense when asked to tell a story. In more sophisticated story structures, there might also be description and dialogue.

In most circumstances in the classroom, the structures suggested above would be more than adequate for the teacher in order to analyse the children's development as story writers. However, Applebee extends his analysis to consider how complexities in children's stories are accommodated. Using ideas from Vygotsky (1962), he suggests a series of stages in story development from heaps with unconnected sentences, to sequences and primitive narratives in which events are linked to a central core of the story, to chains in which there are links between incidents, and finally to narrative in which there are complex links between events.

Most teachers of young children will not be familiar with such sophisticated analyses of children's story writing. However, teachers will be aware that as children develop as story writers, so they are able to distance themselves from the story; the stories, that are told or written, are less likely to be about home and family. The stories will also be decreasingly concerned with reality and will be noticeably more complex. And this complexity can be detected in the use of characters, setting and plot.

Some knowledge of story grammar will therefore help the teacher to analyse the children's development as story writers and to give support, if required, to extend the children's knowledge. Furthermore, the developing knowledge of story grammar among children, even though that knowledge may be implicit, is important because not only does it help children in their own writing, but it also enables them to understand more thoroughly the stories they hear read to them and which they read themselves. And that is important because stories have a role in the socialization of children. Stories can pass on the cultural heritage of society, inform about ways of behaving and moral values, and help children to come to terms with fears. More succinctly, Trelease (1989: 13) suggests that the purpose of literature is 'to provide meaning in our lives'.

So if the development of a story grammar is important for each child, how can it be encouraged? In part, this question has already been answered, because we noted in the introduction to this section that hearing stories read aloud can be instrumental in enabling children to acquire a story grammar. The work of Carol Fox (1993) indicates the extent of that knowledge among pre-school children where they had enjoyed many story readings at home.

Therefore, *story reading* in the classroom by the teacher and opportunities for the children to read stories will be used to support their learning of story structure. And the provision of a wide variety of story books in the classroom will underpin these readings. Writing stories frequently, with encouragement and feedback from the teacher and a real *audience* for the output, will also help children to develop a story grammar knowledge. The use of direct instruction is more problematic. However, Temple *et al.* (1988) suggested that mini lessons might have a part to play. Such mini lessons might simply involve the use of appropriate language when, for instance, discussing the cover of a book. So the teacher might ask, 'Who do you think are going to be the main characters in this story?' while showing the book cover. This introduces to the young children the term 'characters' and requires the children to make explicit their partial understanding of story grammar. Similar discussions while looking at stories written by a child also make explicit the child's knowledge. The concern about the more direct teaching of a story grammar is that children might then begin to check off the use of characters, setting and plot in their stories rather than concentrating on the story to be written. Anyway, as two-year-olds demonstrate, story grammar can be learnt incidentally through engagement with stories. And it is that provision of stories which should be emphasized in the classroom.

Further reading

Applebee, A.N. (1978) *The Child's Concept of Story*. Chicago, IL: Chicago University Press.

This book has been very influential in the many debates on story grammar. It is derived from the author's PhD thesis, although modified by 'reflection and reformulation' and is therefore quite technical and contains a substantial amount of theory. Nevertheless, there are detailed and informative chapters devoted to young children's developing awareness of story grammar. This analysis is extended subsequently to a chapter on the response of the adolescent to literature.

Fox, C. (1993) *At the Very Edge of the Forest: The Influence of Literature on Storytelling by Children*. London: Cassell.

Carol Fox carries through a detailed study of the stories of five children who each provided numerous storytellings into a tape-recorder at approximately four to five years of age. These storytellings indicated that the children had acquired an understanding of story grammar, as well as many other complex aspects of language. This knowledge appeared to have been acquired because the children had heard many hundreds of stories read to them at home during their pre-school years.

Her analysis of the children's story structure in part utilizes ideas from the work of Labov. Such an analysis considers: *abstract*, the opening remark; *orientation*, character, setting, time; *complicating action*, what happened; *resolution/result*, the outcome of events; and *coda*, the closing of the story. But, Fox argues, such an analysis also includes *evaluation*, the narrator's stance to what happened.

Temple, C., Nathan, R., Temple, F. and Burris, N.A. (1988) *The Beginnings of Writing*. London: Allyn and Bacon.

This text presents story grammar as part of a more general book on writing in the early years. Chapter nine, entitled 'Writing in the poetic mode', explores children's story writing and utilizes story grammar as a means of doing so. There are many examples of children's stories in this practical book and Applebee's ideas are acknowledged by the authors. Part of chapter nine considers suggestions for classroom practice; space is also given over to debate the dilemma of how far the direct teaching of story grammar, if at all, should be utilized.

story readings

The reading of a story by the teacher to the children is a very important part of the school day. In nursery classrooms before five years of age and in infant classrooms between five and seven years of age, teachers will want to ensure that there is time available each day for stories to be read to the children. This attention to story reading in school will, in many instances, be a reflection of the time spent on this literacy activity at home, where parents will have read to their children on a regular and frequent basis. But it is not enough to say that this is a very important literacy activity. We need to consider why it is thought to be so important, and what the benefits are to the children and what is the nature of the activity.

The results of the longitudinal Children Learning to Read Project in Bristol, directed by Gordon Wells, suggested that story readings by parents had a positive influence upon the literacy development of their children (Wells 1986). Listening to the stories, watching the parent handle the book and being involved in discussions about the stories were all regarded as being important for the child. But we are not just reliant upon the data from that study to inform us of the importance of story readings. Teale (1984), in his survey of numerous studies into home and school story readings, demonstrated the considerable evidence that exists to indicate the positive effects of this literacy activity. Furthermore, many articles and books by Margaret Meek (1982, 1988) have provided us with a detailed analysis and argument to sustain the view that these story readings are fundamental in helping children to learn about reading and to learn to read.

An important first part of the benefits to be gained from story reading relates to the enjoyment that children get from this activity. This enjoyment comes from at least two sources. First, there is enjoyment of the stories that are read, which indicates the need for the adult to think carefully about the books that are selected for reading. Second, there is enjoyment of the sharing of the book with the parent at home and the teacher at school. And this enjoyment is important because it can motivate children to learn to read. Furthermore, we do not just want to teach children to read, but hope that they will find the contact with books so interesting, worthwhile and enjoyable that they will want to continue reading once their independence as readers has been established.

There are many other benefits to be gained from story reading. For instance, very specific concepts about books and print can be learnt. How do you know how to hold and use a book unless you have seen books used by others? And children can be made aware of front-to-back and *left-to-right directionality*, which are fundamental to reading books written in English, while listening to story readings (Strickland and Morrow 1989b). If the reading allows the child to see the book, then the orthographic features, including the separation of one word from another by a space and the fact that each word is spoken, can be noted.

During story readings, children will also learn about authorship, especially where the adult reading the story takes time to comment about the writer. And in most circumstances, at least initially, it will be stories that are read rather than other book genres. This has the advantage for children that they will come to the story with some notion of story structure. They will do so because they will have heard stories relayed, made up stories themselves and heard stories as part of the rhymes associated with some of the games that they will have played. This background places the children in a good position for developing an implicit knowledge of *story grammar*. By listening to many story readings, their awareness of character, setting and plot, beginning, middle and end, episodes, problem and resolution with consistent use of past tense will all develop. As Carol Fox (1993) demonstrates, children who have heard many story readings develop an awareness of story structure as well as other aspects of language. Such an awareness helps young emerging readers not only to understand the stories that are heard, but it also helps them with their own attempts to write, often in story format. Story readings, then, help children to learn patterns of discourse as well as new words, new syntactic forms and new meanings (Dombey 1988).

If all of this learning is to take place, then story reading becomes a very important part of the school day. And teachers who recognize its importance will want to avoid it becoming the last thing on the agenda of each school day. Indeed, many teachers find that so much can be developed from, as well as learnt during, story readings, that the beginning of the day seems like a more appropriate time for many of the readings. (Teachers of very young children may not wish to restrict themselves to just one reading per day.)

The selection of the book to be read is an obvious first step for the teacher. Will the story read well? Do the *illustrations* add to the telling? Will the children enjoy it? Does the story relate to others that have been read? Have a number of books by the same author been read? Will the children be able to make connections from the stories to their own lives? Is the story more complex than some others that have been read? ('Occasionally read above the children's intellectual level and challenge their minds' suggests Trelease, 1989, p. 80.) Of course, not all these questions apply for each book, but they are among the questions that the teacher might ask as books are selected for reading. And because the book selected will have been read by the teacher before reading it to the class, it will enable the teacher to read the book with enthusiasm, pacing and emphasis, and often with eye contact with the class.

Prior to the reading of the book, the teacher might discuss the cover with the class and note the author; Meek (1988) provides an example of such an introduction with one child. Beyond the cover and the author, part of the discussion might be to make *text-to-life connections* derived from the characters and setting of the story to the world that is known by the children. All of this gives the children some prior knowledge before the reading begins and helps them with their understanding of the story. The background knowledge also helps the children to make predictions as to the events and the outcomes of the story.

During the reading itself, teachers will likely have differing goals. In the nursery classroom and the reception or kindergarten class, teachers will expect interruptions as the children predict events, ask questions, relate the text to their own experiences and make comments. As a means of facilitating the children's involvement with, and learning from, the story, the teacher might encourage such interruptions. The teacher could do so by breaking off the reading to respond to the children, then gradually moving the discussion back to the actual reading. Later, with older children, it might be that the teacher will want to concentrate on the reading of the story and emphasize the discussion at the end of the read. In any discussion after the story has been read, the teacher will not only ask 'what' questions, but also 'why' questions and queries about the children's feelings towards the story.

All of these possibilities indicate not only the importance of the story readings for the children but also the subtlety of the *teacher's role* during the literacy activity. In particular, teachers recognize that achieving a worthwhile interaction during the story reading, while maintaining the storyline for the listeners, requires considerable skill.

It will have become obvious when reading this section that there is some discrepancy between the one-to-one interaction of parent and child story reading at home and the teacher and class at school.

Can the children all benefit at school? How will they be able to detect left-to-right directionality if the teacher has the book? One answer is provided by *big books*, which can be used to demonstrate print features with younger children while the story is being read. The more general question of whether the children will benefit or not, may lie in the hands of the teacher. The careful selection of books, the timing and setting of the story reading, and the skilful reading of the story are demonstrated daily by many teachers in schools. And the evidence is that children learn about reading, and in part to read, from such organized and well-managed story readings.

In the classroom

When a reception class teacher read the story of *Bertie at the Dentist's* to a class of five-year-olds, there was inevitably a considerable amount of discourse around the story; inevitable because very young children always want to comment about the story, ask questions, make predictions and link the story to their own experiences. This can be demonstrated by a brief extract:

Teacher: Bertie nearly fell off.
Katrina: He didn't though.
Teacher: No, he didn't.
Why do you think he nearly fell off?
Katrina: Because he's on the edge of the arm.
Teacher: He nearly fell over the edge of the arm, yes.
'You sit here, Bertie', said the dentist.
He began to wash his hands.
Why do you think he washes his hands?
Why does he?
Helen: So you don't get germs.
Teacher: So you don't get germs, that's right. He has to be all lovely and clean. And as Claire said he washes with the soap.
Bertie was fascinated. He had never seen soap in a bottle before.
Robert: I have.

Interestingly, the teacher appears to be able to both encourage the children to be involved in the story by asking questions and accepting and using comments from them, and to maintain the storyline by returning to a reading of the book wherever the discussion allows for it to occur naturally.

Further reading

Campbell, R. (1990a) *Reading Together*. Milton Keynes: Open University Press.

In this book, I provide two examples of story readings from an infant classroom. The first of these, of *Bertie at the Dentist's* (Bourma 1987), included a substantial amount of dialogue between the children and the teacher as the story was read. The second, a reading of *Whistle for Willie* (Keats 1964), contained more of an immediate reading of the story followed by an extended discussion. These transcripts, like others that have been reported (e.g. Dombey 1988), provide opportunities for the reader to gain insights into the way teachers read stories to children and to glean some of the principles behind the practice.

Teale, W. (1984) Reading to young children: Its significance for literacy development. In H. Goelman, A. Oberg and F. Smith (eds), *Awakening to Literacy*. London: Heinemann Educational.

In the chapter by Bill Teale, he explores the evidence for the use of story reading, the benefits to the children and the nature of the interaction. There are numerous references to the research which had been conducted on this literacy activity at the time of writing. This review of the literature led Teale to conclude that the 'results from research consistently indicate that being read to is one type of experience that delightfully and effectively ushers a child into the world of literacy' (p. 120).

Trelease, J. (1989) *The New Read-Aloud Handbook*, 2nd revised edn. London: Penguin.

This is a very practical book. After the initial chapter on why reading aloud is so important, there are chapters entitled 'When to begin to read-aloud', 'The stages of read-aloud' and 'The do's and don'ts of read-aloud'. The seven pages of do's and don'ts will appear very simple to experienced and successful teachers (e.g. 'the most common mistake in reading aloud is reading too fast', p. 81), but as a starting point they provide important messages that have to be learnt by the adult. A large part of the book is devoted to a list of books that might be used for story readings, and in the description of these books Trelease makes links with other similar texts, or books by the same author.

sustained silent reading

The idea of a period of time set aside for the whole class to read silently to themselves appears to be derived from suggestions put forward by Hunt (1970), although the practice would probably have already been in place. Initially, the abbreviation USSR (Uninterrupted Sustained Silent Reading) was used. However, perhaps for historical and cultural reasons, that soon became SSR (Sustained Silent Reading), and McCracken (1971) was using the abbreviation a year after Hunt's article appeared. So what is SSR and why is it considered to be an important school practice.

Stated in its simplest form, SSR is a period of time set aside each day in the classroom (or even throughout the school) for the children to engage in personal reading. In many classrooms, this personal reading time is associated with the rule that there is silence, so that no one is disturbed by talking or movement around the room. If there is to be no movement, then it is a prerequisite that the teacher has organized the classroom to ensure that each child has a personally selected book to read and perhaps another book to hand if the current book is nearly finished. Typically, the teacher should also spend the same time reading as this provides a model for the children. The children should be informed as to how much time they have for their reading; this is usually about ten minutes, although it can be extended for older children to as much as twenty-five minutes. Teachers of very young children might initially devote less time to this activity, say five minutes, with the intention of increasing it in due course. We shall note later some other variations that might be required for teachers with the very youngest of children in school.

The time devoted to SSR is important because as teachers we wish not only to teach children to read but, having done so, also encourage them to read. Despite the wish of teachers to encourage children to read for enjoyment, as well as to read for information, there is evidence (e.g. Southgate *et al.*, 1981, in their study of eight- and nine-year-olds) that in primary classrooms children do not often get the opportunity to read for any sustained period of time. It was such evidence that led Southgate *et al.* to argue that more opportunities for personal reading should be given to children in the classroom. It would be strange if teachers, who devote so much time to the teaching of reading, then deny the children any opportunity to engage in that activity.

In terms of organization within the classroom, many teachers find that placing the SSR period alongside a natural break in the day (e.g. lunch time) can be useful. After all, the whole class is usually brought together before and after such natural breaks in the day and it is relatively easy to link that with a quiet time spent reading. At the conclusion of the reading, it is useful to spend a short time sharing some of the reading experiences. The teacher can demonstrate this sharing by reading a short part of the book that he or she has been reading or telling the children about an interesting phrase or word that was in the story. Children will begin to recognize that teachers have been reflecting on their reading and will want to make a similar contribution to the sharing. However, as McCracken (1971) indicated, there is no formal writing of reports or records kept about the books read; it is a time to enjoy books and to share some of that enjoyment with others in the class.

In many classrooms, the silent reading period might be referred to using a different term. Two of these, which are used quite frequently, are DEAR (Drop Everything And Read) and ERIC (Everyone or Enjoy Reading In Class). Either of these may be preferable with younger children, as the word silent no longer appears. This could be important, because although it might be reasonable to have a quiet class engaged with books, it may be difficult to have a silent class. Some young children may mouth the words of a book – even when they believe they are reading silently. So in such circumstances, it might be sensible for the teacher to encourage quietness rather than attempting to insist on silence. Furthermore, these two acronyms indicate a variation on the theme. In classrooms operating DEAR or ERIC, the teacher could encourage reading in pairs, groups sharing and talking about a book, or other arrangements ensuring a sustained involvement with a book. All of these strategies can be used as a means of moving the children gradually to the point where they can each read silently on their own with a book of their own choosing.

When working with very young children, many of whom will not be able to read, at least in the conventional sense, it might be asked whether sustained silent reading is possible, at least in some recognizable form. The answer would appear to be 'yes', although adaptations might need to be considered. For instance, rather than thinking of the children reading, it might be necessary to ask instead whether the children are demonstrating reading-like behaviours – looking through a book, turning the pages, building up the story from the pictures, etc. And, rather than engaging the whole class on the activity, it might be appropriate to work with a group from the class initially, so that the teacher can demonstrate the activity on a more individual basis. Later, it might be possible to combine the groups so that the whole class is engaged on sustained silent reading.

Many children do appear to get a good deal of enjoyment from this activity, in part because it gives them time to read a book undisturbed by other events. Eleven-year-old Stephen reflected on his experience with this reading time and commented:

> I enjoy ERIC very much and I look forward to it every day. ERIC was a brilliant idea and I wish someone could have thought of it earlier, then I could of had 10 minutes silent reading for 4 years if it had been thought of when I was in the first year. ERIC has encouraged me to read more at home because it shows how much fun reading can bring.
>
> (Campbell 1990a: 66)

Not all children are as positive, but if it does encourage children like Stephen to read at home and at school, then sustained silent reading will have served its purpose.

In my description of this literacy activity at the beginning of the section, I suggested that it might include the teacher reading at the same time as the children in order to serve as a role model. The importance of the teacher as a model for reading has often been stressed and there is some research evidence to substantiate it (Wheldall and Entwistle 1988). However, what may be more important is the overall ethos towards literacy, the *reading drive* in the classroom perhaps (Campbell and Scrivens, 1995). And what this seems to suggest is that where reading is not given a high priority, then the teacher as a reading model may be vital, but even that might not be successful. However, if there is a strong reading drive and the teacher conveys a real interest in, and an enthusiasm for, reading, then acting as a role model may not be essential. In such circumstances, sustained silent reading becomes one of many important literacy activities which can contribute to the children's reading development.

Further reading

Campbell, R. (1990a) *Reading Together*. Milton Keynes: Open University Press.

One of the main chapters in this book is devoted to sustained silent reading. There is a discussion of the origins of the activity and guidelines for it in practice are debated. The chapter also includes case studies of two schools in which ERIC and SQUIRT (Sustained Quiet UnInterrupted Reading Time) were part of the daily school routine. The role of the teacher is also considered in a final section on sustained silent reading.

Edelsky, C., Altwerger, B. and Flores, B. (1991) *Whole Language: What's the Difference?* Portsmouth, NH: Heinemann Educational.

This book is about the philosophy and practice of whole language. One part of the book considers 'What whole language looks like in the classroom'. A series of scenes are depicted and, of these, scene four (pp. 92–5), explores a classroom where DEAR is in operation. The authors have conveyed the sense of involvement of the children with their books, and teachers will find the description of a classroom in action very useful.

teacher's role

Whenever a debate takes place on the teaching of reading in the early years of primary education, it often focuses on the methods of teaching – or a linked issue of standards of reading. In the early 1990s, the methodology debate focused upon *phonics teaching* and *real book approaches*. This is an important debate because we do need to think carefully about the ways in which the literacy learning experiences of the children are structured in the classroom. Unfortunately, such is the intensity of the debate, that on occasions it appears that 'debate' is not the appropriate word to use; Nicholson (1992) goes so far as to suggest that a 'reading war' might more correctly indicate the intensity of the beliefs and arguments. However, in one important sense, such involvement in the debate could mean that a crucial issue risks becoming minimized. This issue concerns the role of the teachers and the importance of their role in enabling children to develop as readers and writers. This importance, especially in relation to the methodology debate, was expressed very succinctly in a quotation by Frank Smith (1992), which was published in *Reading Today*: 'Methods can never ensure that children learn to read. Children must learn from people' (p. 34).

This emphasis upon children learning from people, which recognizes parents at home and teachers at school as the main contributors to children's reading development, is indicative of current thinking and theory. For instance, Teale and Sulzby (1989) refer to literacy as a complex sociopsycholinguistic activity. The use of this term emphasizes literacy not only as a cognitive and language skill, but one with a social learning dimension. Children need to learn from people and the role of teachers is, therefore, vitally important.

Throughout much of this handbook, the importance of teachers is recognized. During the prior planning and leading on to the organization and management of the classroom, it is teachers who are responsible for ensuring that the arrangements are satisfactory. And the time that is devoted to literacy and the progress of the children is monitored and recorded by the teachers. Furthermore, within most literacy activities, it is the teachers who facilitate the children's learning by guiding, supporting, instructing and encouraging. In such circumstances, the knowledge, skills and enthusiasm of teachers are vital.

Teachers need to have a knowledge of reading, children and pedagogy. This knowledge is required so that when an unusual circumstance is met, the teacher is able to think the problem through based on information that will help in the analysis and evaluation of the situation. Although it is useful to know the various activities and strategies that might be used to encourage literacy development, teachers also need to have the background knowledge 'about reading in general and about [those] children in particular' (Smith 1978: 3). That knowledge will provide the basis for the teachers to become more skilful in their practice. And the roles of the teacher as an organizer, manager and teacher are important, because these skills set the scene and provide the background to the children's learning. Finally, teachers need to be enthusiastic about books, reading, writing, learning and teaching, and be able to convey that enthusiasm and vitality to the children.

The need for teachers with knowledge, skills and enthusiasm can be demonstrated more clearly if we briefly consider one of the literacy activities of the classroom. Story reading provides a good example, because whichever methodology is argued for, *story reading* is likely to be part of the literacy activities provided (Campbell 1993b). For the story readings to be successful, the teacher needs to know about the story books that are available. In part, this knowledge will be gleaned from colleagues and from the experience of story readings over a number of years. The teacher will also know why story readings are important and that knowledge will influence the nature of the story reading. Because the teacher knows about books, and will have read a particular book before presenting it to the children, the actual story reading will demonstrate the skill of the teacher as the book is read. Therefore, the story reading will be delivered in a positive, enthusiastic and skilful manner – the pace of the reading, the intonation and emphasis, the involvement of the children, the eye contact with the class, etc. All of this will capture the children's attention, interest, thoughts and feelings. In contrast, story readings in the hands of an adult or teacher without such knowledge, skill and enthusiasm are unlikely to be successful and the learning opportunities for the children will consequently be reduced.

Therefore, although there have been a few reports of children who appear to have discovered how to read without adult support, in the main it is the quality of the teaching that will determine the success of children's literacy learning. And this teaching quality, although it must be concerned with literacy activities which are appropriate for the child, will be dependent upon the knowledge, skills and enthusiasm of the teacher. The teacher's role is very important.

Further reading

Campbell, R. (1992) *Reading Real Books*. Buckingham: Open University Press.

In this book, I consider the various aspects of a real books approach to reading. An exploration of the various activities which make up the approach was necessary because critics were suggesting, incorrectly, either that the approach consisted merely of real books and shared readings or that it was a non-teaching approach. Neither of these views is correct; first, the approach is about far more than real books and shared readings (although they are important) and, far from being a non-teaching approach, 'it requires subtle and sophisticated teaching' (p. 81). Throughout the book, the requirement for skilful teaching is emphasized and the final short chapter is devoted to the importance of the teacher.

text-to-life connections

It is a feature of the *language experience approach* that the teacher attempts to base the child's early literacy learning on those experiences that the child is able to communicate to the teacher. Making such connections between that which is known and has been experienced with the initial reading and writing activities in the classroom would appear to be a sensible practice, as it reduces the abstract nature of the written language. In the section on *organic vocabulary*, we noted that Sylvia Ashton-Warner was of the view that the first books that children read should be drawn from the children's deeply felt experiences in their own culture. Furthermore, it was suggested that such texts should include those words of emotional significance to the child which were linked to those experiences. Making text-to-life and life-to-text connections is not uncommon in the classroom, and we will explore below some particular interactions where that is especially the case. However, it is not just in the classroom that such links are made; parent–child interactions also appear to make substantial use of such connections.

Tizard and Hughes (1984), in their study of four-year-olds talking and thinking at home, and in the nursery classroom, included some information on parent–child story readings. As one might expect during such story readings, the children asked many questions, which often linked the story with their own experiences. The parents reflected upon these attempts to make sense of the stories and they, too, often made connections between the story content, characters or setting and the known experiences of the child. Of course, the parent is advantaged in knowing about the child's interests and fears, so that such connections can be made very specifically and linked to known current interests. In one of the examples that Tizard and Hughes provide (pp. 62–5), it is shown how a mother was able to allay her child's fears about separation from her parents and the dangers of travel by making connections between those elements in the book being read and the child's past experiences and, in the case of travelling, future plans.

In the classroom, teachers do not have the advantage of dealing with just one child. Even on those occasions when the teacher is engaged in a one-to-one interaction, such as *shared reading* or *hearing children read*, it is still necessary to manage the activities of the rest of the children in the class. Nevertheless, despite this there is evidence to indicate that in a number of literacy activities teachers do use the opportunity of the interactions, centred on a book, in order to contextualize the learning within the experiences of the child or children. *Story reading* with the whole class is a first and obvious example where teachers attempt to make links between the experiences of the children and the story being read.

During story readings in the nursery or early infant classroom, the teacher will not expect to read the story straight through without comment or interruption from the children. Indeed, many teachers encourage such interruptions to the story in order to begin a discussion of the book. During such breaks, the teacher will talk with the children about various aspects of the story and frequently attempt to make connections from the text to the life experiences of the children. And the children will make connections from their lives to the text as they comment or interrupt the reading by the teacher. The extent of the discussions about a book can be gauged by exploring transcripts of teachers and children involved in a story reading, for example the five-year-olds listening to the reading of *Bertie at the Dentist's* (Bourma 1987) in Campbell (1990a). Such evidence indicates that teachers of young children make text-to-life connections before, during and after the reading of a story. These connections help the children to understand the story, to predict parts of it and to place it within a framework of their own experiences. (The discussion about dental floss during that particular story reading was helped by one of the children explaining how it is used to keep teeth clean.) Furthermore, there are occasions when making connections between experiences and the text may help a child to come to terms with concerns that he or she may have about a particular experience or fear.

Meeting the particular concerns of a child might be more easily accommodated during one-to-one interactions. Shared reading and hearing a child read are such literacy activities, and here too the teacher can use the experiences of the child to help him or her understand aspects of the book. Teachers often use a discussion before the book is read in order to think about the characters, setting, plot and illustrations so that when the story is read the child has some knowledge with which to help him or her with the reading. When a teacher is able to make a connection between the child's experience and these various aspects of the book, then the understanding is likely to be more securely fixed. It is for this reason that teachers make text-to-life connections not only before a reading, but also during the reading and after the reading has been completed.

In the classroom

During the reading of *Bertie at the Dentist's* (see p. 145), the teacher had reached the point of reading about the soap in the bottle which Bertie 'had never seen . . . before':

Robert: I have.
Teacher: You have.
Children: I have.
Robert: I've seen hair washes.
Teacher: You've seen what?
Robert: Hair washes.
Teacher: What do we call hair washes? Don't call out. Hair – what do we call it? In a bottle, Hair?
Sarah: Hair shampoo.
Teacher: Hair shampoo.

John:	I've seen it coming out of taps.
Teacher:	You've seen soap coming out of taps, yes that's right. What do you have to do John?
John:	Wash your hands.
Teacher:	Yes, but what do you do to the tap? Do you know?
John:	You press the thing in.
Teacher:	You usually have to press it, that's right.
John:	And it comes down on to your hands.
Teacher:	That's right, yes.

So it was Robert's comment in response to the teacher's reading which led to a short discussion about 'soap in a bottle'. This discussion, which linked the text to the life experiences of the children, was helpful in enabling the children to contextualize the story within their own view of the world.

Further reading

Mason, J.M., Peterman, C.L. and Kerr, B.M. (1989) Reading to kindergarten children. In D.S. Strickland and L.M. Morrow (eds), *Emerging Literacy: Young Children Learn to Read and Write*. Newark, DE: International Reading Association.

This chapter in the edited book on emerging literacy does not deal exclusively with text-to-life connections. Indeed, it is a relatively small part of the debate presented about the various aspects of the interactions which take place during story book readings. Nevertheless, the linking of life experiences to the text being read is noted and it is useful to consider that link alongside the other suggestions that are made by the editors.

thematic work/topic work

Many teachers of young children find that a *language experience approach* helps children to express their thoughts and feelings about objects and events related to their personal experiences. These thoughts and feelings can be expressed orally and then written down for themselves and others to read. Almost inevitably the children and the teacher together gradually move from that interest, on the immediate and personal, to a wider range of interests and questions. And arising out of these interests and questions are likely to be themes or topics which become important for the child, a group of children or the whole class. Topic studies are useful for a number of reasons. Holdaway (1979: 145) suggested that they are a 'source of strong motivation to produce various forms of writing'. This is one of the main reasons for the popularity of this approach with teachers of young children. Reading and writing for authentic reasons and which serve a variety of purposes are almost guaranteed when topic work is used in the classroom.

How should the topics for study be selected? Many teachers are concerned that if the topics are always selected by the children, they could be rather restrictive and limiting in the way that they incorporate other subject areas naturally. Conversely, if the topics are always selected by the teacher, then are they really derived from the children's interests? There might be advantages if the teacher and children can together discuss and agree the subject of the topic and the path along which that topic might be developed. Alternatively, in some classes there may be class themes which the teacher and children develop together, while at other times the children might be engaged on individual topics where the impetus comes from each child with the teacher acting more as a guide and support in order to help the children in their endeavours.

What is important about this work is that it is sustained over a period of time. Judith Slaughter (1992) demonstrates how some teachers achieve sustained involvement in themes derived from the story books read to the class. Very often the use of the story book to develop a theme will be apparent in the early years classroom, and we noted in the section on *story reading* how that can lead teachers to use story reading at the beginning of the day because the stories can be used to support learning based on a real interest in the topic. Don Holdaway (1979) also provides a case study of a class in which the reading of Eric Carle's *The Very Hungry Caterpillar* was used as the interest and stimulus for the development of a theme on caterpillars and other insects. The sustaining of interest over a period of time is important because it allows for a deep exploration of the topic. Holdaway suggests that worthwhile written expression arises from a topic when the children have a depth of experience and adequate time for reflection. Teachers do have an important role to play in providing the opportunities for that sustained involvement with a topic, rather than allowing superficial attention to be given to a topic before the children move on to another area of interest.

So themes encourage children to read and write for authentic purposes, especially where adequate time is allowed for the children to become intensely involved with the theme. Often, the theme will also require the children to begin to explore other areas of the curriculum as a natural outcome of pursuing the questions generated by the theme. This extension into other areas of the curriculum is a welcome by-product of thematic work. The Plowden Report (DES 1967) welcomed such flexibility in the curriculum and debated the value of topics, projects or centres of interest as means of integrating the curriculum and stimulating the reading and writing experiences of children. Furthermore, the advent of the National Curriculum in England and Wales (DES 1990) did not halt the use of thematic work, especially with younger children, although initially there were fears that that would be one outcome of the changes. Perhaps of greater concern is the recognition that not all topic work facilitates children's literacy development. Robin Alexander (1992) notes that topic work could result in low-level learning, and this is a timely reminder of the *teacher's role* in monitoring the activities of the children in order to ensure that worthwhile learning takes place. This issue was debated by the Bullock Report (DES 1975), where it was recognized that when the children were following their own interests, it was important for the teacher to monitor the literacy experiences that were being generated by the topic and to keep a check on the direction of the work. However, here as with most aspects of classroom life, the careful and skilful organization and management of the classroom by the teacher facilitates the learning opportunities of the children.

Using themes or topics with young children means a range of interests can be covered. This is because children have so many questions to ask based on their curiosity about the wider environment. Teachers need to support such interests by helping with the planning, supporting the inquiry when it is under way, and providing many opportunities for reading and writing (as well as other forms of expression) as the children seek explanations and answers to their questions.

Further reading

Pluckrose, H. (1988) *School: A Place for Children?* London: Franklin Watts.

Only a small section in this book deals directly with thematic work, at least to the extent that an example is detailed. However, the whole of the book is about children, learning, the classroom, the learning experience and the role of the teacher, all of which provides the foundation for themes to be developed. Interestingly, Pluckrose refers to tightly constructed themes in order to emphasize the key role of the teacher, not to control the elements of the theme but to encourage and support the planning of the theme with a learning web, and two very detailed learning webs are given as examples. This book is directed at general issues rather than dealing specifically with literacy.

time for literacy

It might be regarded as self-evident that in order for children to develop their understanding and use of literacy, they need to spend time engaged with reading and writing. Frank Smith (1978: 5) stated that 'to learn to read children need to read', and he made a somewhat similar statement about writing: 'writing is learned by writing' (Smith 1982: 199). These statements emphasize that children need to spend time reading and writing in order to become proficient readers and writers. An analogy is often made to learning to ride a bicycle or play a piano; in order to become proficient at riding a bicycle or playing the piano, many hours have to be devoted specifically to those tasks. The same could be said for literacy. But as Smith (1978: 5) recognized, 'the issue is as simple and as difficult as that'. And the difficult part is that it still requires the teacher to organize and manage the time for the many literacy activities that enable children to develop as literacy users.

In the classroom, there are perhaps three elements that the teacher needs to consider. First, how will the classroom be organized and managed in order to ensure that literacy activities are predominant? Second, how much time should the teacher devote to supporting the children with literacy? Third, how much time should each child devote to literacy activities? These questions are important because although we all recognize the need to devote time to literacy in order to help children to develop as literacy users, nevertheless, as teachers with pressures from many sources, we need constantly to remind ourselves of that fact in the classroom. Harris (1979) indicated that the research evidence suggests that the single most important characteristic of successful reading teaching was the amount of time spent on reading.

Therefore, there is a need to think about, and plan for, time for literacy.

The beginning of such thinking and planning has to be devoted to the *classroom organization* and *classroom management* for literacy. You may recall that in the section on *classroom management* we noted that Cambourne (1988) recommended a practice that he had seen working effectively. That practice required that the first two hours of the school day were to be devoted to language and that the time was divided among a number of literacy activities. This suggestion gives a good indication of the importance of language and literacy. However, some teachers of young children might argue that it does not go far enough. Many teachers argue that throughout the school day the arrangements for all the curriculum areas should be based on the need to encourage language and literacy. In this way, early years classrooms become literacy learning environments. Without a firm foundation in reading and writing, most subsequent learning could be restricted. Therefore, the classroom organization will include a substantial block devoted to language, or the whole day will be premised on the development of literacy, albeit that other subjects are studied in some depth within *thematic work/topic work*.

Within such a structure, teachers will hope to spend a substantial part of the day facilitating, guiding and supporting the children's literacy. In some literacy sessions, the role of the teacher is obvious. So in *story reading*, teachers will spend all of their time facilitating literacy. But when the children are engaged in other literacy activities (e.g. writing, thematic/topic work, play activities, etc.), the role of the teacher has to extend beyond the management and monitoring of the activities. Time has to be given to one-to-one literacy interactions with children, conferences with the children about their writing, and discussions with groups on some aspect of their literacy. Teachers need to be asking themselves how can the children be supported in their literacy development. And when that question is asked, the likely outcome will be that teachers will spend substantial parts of the day on literacy.

But the real need is to ensure that the children devote substantial parts of their day to literacy. And it is necessary for the teacher to monitor children's involvement with literacy. There is evidence to suggest that a high level of teacher involvement with literacy is not always matched by a high level of involvement on the part of the children (Southgate *et al.* 1981). Teachers should attempt to keep the children involved with literacy by ensuring that the classroom is organized for interesting literacy events which attract the children, managing the events of the classroom in a way which encourages and guides the children in their literacy, and interacting with the children individually, in groups and as a class in order to support the literacy learning. Monitoring the involvement with literacy of an individual child for a short period can be helpful in evaluating the literacy work within the classroom.

Because time for literacy is so obviously a need, there is the danger that we take it for granted. That would be a mistake. It would be useful if teachers checked, on a regular basis, the organization of the classroom for literacy, the time they spend themselves on literacy and, most important of all, the extent of the children's involvement with reading and writing.

Further reading

Cambourne, B. (1988) *The Whole Story: Natural Learning and the Acquisition of Literacy in the Classroom*. Auckland: Ashton Scholastic.

It should now be apparent, from the various references that have been made to this book by Brian Cambourne, that there are many practical points in the text. His recommendation that the first two hours of the school day should be devoted to language activities is a practical suggestion that also serves to emphasize the need to ensure that sufficient time is spent on language and literacy. And he also gives details of the ways in which the two hours might be arranged to provide a variety of language and literacy experiences for the children.

whole language

Whole language is not a method of teaching reading. It is a set of principles and beliefs about language, learning, teaching, curriculum and community which provide the framework for teachers to organize and manage the classroom in order to help children develop as literacy users. Kenneth Goodman (1986) has played a major part in furthering these ideas in recent years. However, he did not 'found whole language' (Goodman 1992), it was as he has argued a 'grassroots creation of professional educators, mostly classroom teachers' (p. 188). So teachers were developing their classroom practices and others were writing about those practices and the principles which lay behind them. Historically, that writing can be traced back to major figures such as Dewey (1916, 1938), although at that time the set of principles and beliefs would not have been described as whole language.

A basic feature of whole language is the view that language is indeed whole and it is best learnt as a whole with meaningful and relevant texts. For reading, therefore, *real books* written by someone with a story to tell or something to say are used rather than books which might have been written for other purposes, such as teaching phonics or systematically controlling the language in some way – often in reading schemes the controlled introduction of new words. The texts that are used should, therefore, be written typically in natural language. *Environmental print*, which provides an authentic and functional use of language, should be used alongside the stories and other books which are meaningful to the children.

The learning experiences that are provided for the children should recognize the active and constructive role of children in the learning process. Therefore, contexts which the children might perceive to be important and which require the need to communicate should be provided rather than the children being confronted by substantial periods of direct teaching. The learning should not be premised on the teaching of a sequence of skills, but should be based on learning to read by reading predictable texts, where the children are able to generate hypotheses as they transact with the text. (Reading as a transactional process, based on the ideas of Rosenblatt (1938/1976), which expresses the complex relationship between readers and their unique interpretation of the text, is a feature of whole language.) And the children can learn to write by writing, especially where the writing is for a clear purpose.

The teaching that is provided in whole language classrooms does not follow *laissez-faire* principles. The teachers will analyse needs, plan the teaching, develop the curriculum and monitor and evaluate progress. So that although whole language teachers use the notions of facilitating, guiding, supporting, encouraging and monitoring, rather than wishing to teach directly (although such teaching does occur at appropriate moments), they also ensure that learning takes place and in that sense they are teaching. Importantly within their planning, they ensure that they have created the necessary social settings for interactions – often teacher–child interactions – to occur. (Vygotsky's (1978) notion of the zone of proximal development gives support to the importance of the teacher–child interaction, in that the teacher can support the child in his or her learning so that once internalized the child can work independently at similar activities.) Inevitably, this means that a whole language teacher does not work merely as a technician following through the demands of a curriculum set by a textbook or an externally imposed curriculum, but has to work as a professional who knows about children and reading (as well as other curriculum areas).

Teachers should develop the curriculum by starting, whenever possible, from where the children are in their learning and then building out from there. And there needs to be an integration of language with the content of other subjects, so that finding out about some aspect of science leads to authentic speech and literacy activities. Thematic units or topics, with an emphasis on direct experiences in many instances, should be a common feature of whole language classrooms. Nevertheless, there are features in the classroom which most teachers recognize as being highly supportive of literacy development. The use of *environmental* and *classroom print*, a *library corner*, *listening area* and *writing centre*, *story reading*, *shared reading* and *sustained silent reading*, will all be evident because as many opportunities as possible for reading and writing are encouraged.

A whole language classroom attempts to create a community of learners in which the children support each other in their endeavours and the teacher is available to support and guide the learning and to learn alongside the children. On visiting whole language classrooms the teachers may not be immediately noticeable because instead of being at the front of the classroom teaching directly, they most frequently work alongside individual children or groups of children, although at certain times (e.g. story time, discussions, etc.) they may well work with the whole class. However, teachers still maintain order and there will be 'a set of rules, and a structure in their classroom' (Goodman 1986: 74). And the community will extend beyond the classroom and the school because the teachers like to ensure that there are productive *home–school links*.

Many British teachers who have worked within an integrated infant classroom will have a feel for the principles and beliefs of whole language. Indeed, as Kenneth Goodman (1992: 195) has stated, 'the basic concepts of whole language [largely without the term] have become institutionalized in British schools'. And those teachers who work to whole language principles and beliefs will understand that no two whole language classrooms are alike, because the teachers and children will respond to their own social and cultural contexts. In contrast, two classrooms which appear similar (at least superficially with story readings, writing, topic work, etc.), may in one case have a whole language teacher while the other works more didactically. It will be the way in which the language learning is maintained and the nature of the teacher–child interactions which will help the observer to detect the whole language teacher.

Further reading

Goodman, K. (1986) *What's Whole in Whole Language?* Portsmouth, NH: Heinemann Educational.

Although this short text provides a very readable and succinct statement about the nature and process of a whole language approach and therefore provides a good introduction to the subject, it does more than that. It indicates how that approach might be translated into classroom practice with a number of very practical suggestions. And despite being a short text, many teachers find that they can return constantly to it for support and ideas.

Goodman, K., Bird, L.B. and Goodman, Y. (1991) *The Whole Language Catalog*. Santa Rosa, CA: American School Publishers.

In complete contrast to Goodman's (1986) book, this compendium comprises some five hundred contributors from across the world, although most are from North America. Such diversity is held together by the numerous contributions that are provided by Ken or Yetta Goodman on learning, language, literature, teaching, curriculum and community. An interesting strand throughout the book is the drawing out of the historical foundations which provided a basis for the development of whole language.

Edelsky, C., Altwerger, B. and Flores, B. (1991) *Whole Language: What's the Difference?* Portsmouth, NH: Heinemann Educational.

Although Kenneth and Yetta Goodman's names are immediately associated with whole language, there are many other university staff and primary classroom teachers who have been and are developing whole language principles. And this inevitably means there are now many books on the subject. This book was developed from a 1987 article in *The Reading Teacher* by the same three authors. The sections in this text deal with: what whole language is; some misconceptions, including a warning about commercial programmes that have begun to appear in the USA under titles such as 'whole language basals' and 'whole language phonics programs'; historical perspectives; and some scenes of classroom life. The book does more than just provide practical examples, however, as it debates thoroughly the principles of whole language from a theoretical perspective. The authors argue that whole language teachers must have a theoretical base, 'a transactional, sociolinguistic model of language use and a social interactionist view of language acquisition' (p. 108), in order to develop the practical classroom.

writing

Although this book's title is *Reading in the Early Years Handbook* it is inevitable that writing will form part of the text, because the development of reading and writing are so closely linked. Therefore, although most of the sections in this handbook have a title which suggest some aspect of reading, there are some, like this one, which are more specifically focused on writing. But the link extends beyond these few sections on writing or aspects of writing because a number of the reading sections also make connections to writing. Perhaps we should remind ourselves of these connections.

We have noted that teachers who use a *language experience approach* emphasize the link between oral and written language and that children do, with teacher support, provide their own reading material by writing about that which has been experienced. For some teachers, these early attempts at writing can be facilitated, it is argued, by encouraging the children to use an *organic vocabulary*. But we can move away from the specific and recognize that teachers of young children will create a *classroom organization* in order to ensure that many opportunities for writing are made available. The *writing centre* is merely an obvious and named part of that provision; *play activities* are also organized in order to encourage writing by the children. However, the provision for writing can be encouraged before school is started and we have seen how one *home–school links* project emphasized writing, together with *environmental print* and *shared reading*, as a means of facilitating *emerging literacy*. Some emphasis upon writing in a book which is about reading should not surprise us, as a *real books approach* and *whole language* both argue for many opportunities for authentic writing in order to support children in their quest for meaning and an ability to communicate. Finally, writing is used within a *reading recovery* programme for those children perceived to need extra individual support, and it becomes a central part of *thematic work/topic work* where children are using writing as well as reading in order to assist their learning in other areas.

So writing is very much part of many of the literacy activities in the classroom. But the teacher will need to provide real purposes for writing and a variety of *audiences*. A starting point could be when children write about their experiences and that writing then forms part of a diary or journal. Additionally, writing letters can be employed usefully because there will be an obvious audience for the children. In the book *Writing with Reason* edited by Nigel Hall (1989), there are many interesting examples of children's letter-writing in chapters very much based on classroom practices. Furthermore, because so much of the children's initial involvement with reading is centred on stories that genre can also be used for some of their writing. Children can rewrite stories they have already heard as well as produce stories of their own; stories which can be shared with others in a number of ways. They can be included in the *library corner* as sheets on display, as book reviews, or new stories can be produced in a book format. Chris Burman (1990) includes sections on class and individual book-making in her writing about organizing for reading in the early years classroom.

Not all the writing will be in the expressive or poetic modes. The Bullock Report (DES 1975) made use of James Britton's model of writing, which suggested three main categories of writing: poetic, expressive and transactional. Children write in the transactional mode when they produce writing about observations that they have made, for example a record of the birds which visit the bird table (SCDC 1989) or as a report of a scientific experiment. And they can prepare plans for building with bricks or making a model. In such writing, the children soon understand that a story structure does not apply and they respond to this form of writing with different conventions. The children may have already written shopping lists with their parents at home and they can work alongside their teacher to do the same as they prepare for cooking. And they can conclude such sessions by writing up the recipe so that others can follow the instructions.

So the teacher will organize the classroom to provide for many opportunities for authentic writing for real audiences. And a variety of writing will be encouraged by the teacher. But what about the actual process of writing? The work of Donald Graves (1983) has been especially influential. In particular, he has popularized what has become known as 'process writing'. This suggests that writing involves a rehearsal (i.e. where ideas are sorted out), composing (i.e. where a first draft is prepared), redrafting (i.e. where the writing is developed and refined) and editing (i.e. where spelling, punctuation and presentation, which might include handwriting, are perfected).

This complete process, however, may not always apply. A shopping list is an example where although we might need to rehearse and compose the list, redrafting may or may not be required depending on whether items need to be added to or subtracted from the list, and an editing stage is most unlikely.

The number of stages to writing a letter may well depend upon the audience and our relationship with that audience. But how do young children learn about such a process? First, the teacher can demonstrate the process in the same way that *big books* are used to demonstrate reading. So with the whole class or a group of children, the teacher can construct a piece of writing on a large sheet of paper. During such writing, the teacher is able to demonstrate that the first attempts at writing often have to be refined in order to achieve what the writer wants to achieve. Second, *conferencing* on writing, between the teacher and an individual child, provides an opportunity for the teacher to bring to the child's attention the possibilities for redrafting and editing. Such teaching will enable the child to develop these writing strategies for use when writing independently.

Writing is a major part of the early years classroom because the ability to communicate to others is a crucial part of every child's learning. However, while writing, children have to attend very carefully to the letters, words, sentences, etc., that they write. This attention to the written language will support them subsequently when they read. Reading and writing are very closely linked and the teacher of young children will want to ensure that there are many opportunities to engage with both.

In the classroom

Teachers who provide many opportunities for young children to write find that those children develop a confidence when putting their thoughts on to paper. Of course, this means that the very youngest children may produce a page of vertical lines (|||||) as their writing emerges from earlier scribbles. Later, the children may produce writing such as that produced by four-year-old Kevin: 'u w g me'. He told his teacher that it said 'you won't get me'. Kevin's use of the sounds to produce his writing is typical of many young writers. Many teachers become extremely competent at deciphering such writing. For instance, three of Kevin's 'words' were represented by the first letter of those words, which is a common feature of children's writing initially. In addition, one word was written in a conventional form, 'me', and the first word was represented by the sound of the complete word. Being aware of the way in which young children construct their writing enables teachers to read much of what is written in the classroom. Furthermore, the children develop gradually towards more conventional representations of writing, which helps the teacher to read the writing and to support its further development.

Further reading

Graves, D.H. (1983) *Writing: Teachers and Children at Work*. Portsmouth NH: Heinemann Educational.

Many books on the teaching of writing have been published since this early work from Donald Graves. Yet it remains worth reading as it sets out the details of process writing. The purpose of the book was 'to assist classroom teachers with children's writing', and many teachers would attest that it did achieve that purpose. The five sections of the book – start to teach writing, make the writing conference work, help children learn the skills they need, understand how children develop as writers, and document children's writing development – are indicative of the broad sweep of the book.

SCDC (1989) *Becoming a Writer: The National Writing Project*. Walton-on-Thames: Nelson.

The School Curriculum Development Committee (SCDC) set up the National Writing Project as a basis to develop and extend children's competence as writers. The project involved numerous schools and hundreds of teachers and it was the work carried out in those classrooms which is reported in a number of publications. *Becoming a Writer* deals extensively with three- to seven-year-olds in the context of the classroom. There are three sections to the book and these deal with the writer's community outside the school (the role of the parent and home–school links are part of that section), the writer's environment inside the school (which considers among other things the role of the teacher) and the development of individual children as writers (with many delightful examples of the children's work provided). The final three pages are devoted to an overview of the book and the headings for that overview provide key areas for the teacher of young children to consider. The headings are: observe carefully, provide good writing models, write for a variety of audiences, teach planning, develop group work, build the children's confidence, encourage personal writing, provide real purposes for writing, encourage working with a partner, vary the formats used, give public value to the children's writing, and help them see writing as a process. The content under each of these headings provides a wealth of ideas for the encouragement of writing.

writing centre

As part of the classroom organization it is useful to have a writing centre. This is especially the case when the teacher is organizing some form of integrated day in the classroom, by which the children move from activity to activity throughout much of the day. In such circumstances, the teacher will want to ensure that many of the activities that the children spend time on encourage an involvement with literacy. The writing centre will be one of those areas that encourages literacy and, at least initially, will require little in the way of space and resources for it to be established.

To begin with, the writing centre will require a table and some chairs. However, as Morrow (1989) suggests, the addition of a message board is useful as it can be used to exchange messages between the teacher and the children, and the teacher can provide information for the class by posting notices. Importantly, the message/notice board can demonstrate the role of writing as a means of communication. The children can be attracted to the writing centre by the variety of writing materials that the teacher makes available. Therefore, adequate quantities of writing instruments (e.g. pencils, coloured pencils, crayons, felt-tipped pens and biros, as well as chalks and chalk boards) should be made available. Similarly, a range of materials to write on (e.g. lined and unlined paper in various sizes, shapes and colours) should be provided. It is also useful to introduce different materials from time to time in order to refresh the children's interest. The introduction of a typewriter and/or word processor is likely to increase the children's interest in writing. Often, such equipment encourages discussion and collaborative writing. In addition to the materials used directly for writing, it is helpful to have scissors, glue and other materials available, close by the centre, so that the children can produce greetings cards, posters and books where the purpose of the writing suggests that to be appropriate. Finally, as SCDC (1989) argued, the teacher should spend some time at the writing centre in order to encourage the purposeful use of the area. So brief visits to demonstrate writing, to observe, question and suggest might all be part of the teacher's role.

A wide variety of writing might be produced at the writing centre – stories, poems, letters, greetings cards and messages. Other writing might include lists, recipes, directions and notices as well as personal writing by the children in their own diaries or journals.

The writing is encouraged by the teacher's presence and by the authenticity of the writing, which has a purpose and an audience. Sheila Taylor, a reception class teacher, in her description of a writing table (or centre), notes the importance of an audience for the children's writing and she indicates the range of audiences that she developed (SCDC 1989). The importance of the other children in the class as an audience for the writing, as well as other classes, the head teacher and parents was demonstrated. The inclusion of her daughter at university, as a recipient for letters, indicated the ingenuity to which teachers will stretch in order to obtain an authentic audience – the children apparently knew her daughter.

Like most other literacy provision, the writing centre requires an initial careful organization. That organization then needs to be sustained by a sensitive management of the literacy events that take place. The writing centre, like other areas and activities in the early years classroom, requires support from the teacher. The teacher will act as a demonstrator of writing, but also as a guide and support for the children's own writing, which will facilitate the children's literacy development.

Further reading

SCDC (1989) *Becoming a Writer: The National Writing Project*. Walton-on-Thames: Nelson.

Although there is reference to writing centres in many books on the teaching and learning of writing with young children, it is seldom backed up with substantial information about the centre at work. The description by Sheila Taylor of the writing table (centre) in her reception classroom is one example where we do have more details of what might be involved in the setting up and subsequent management of a centre to encourage children's writing.

your classroom

At the end of this book it is appropriate to bring together some of the ideas from the various sections. However, before doing so we need to recognize that the sections contained: approaches or philosophies for the teaching and learning of literacy (e.g. *whole language*); aspects of *classroom organization* (e.g. *library corner*);

specific activities to encourage literacy development (e.g. *story reading*); as well as more detailed aspects of literacy learning (e.g. *invented spelling*). And although from time to time in the educational and national press a specific literacy activity might be offered by interested parties as the answer to all literacy learning, the reality is likely to be rather different. A range of activities needs to be provided in the classroom in order to support children's literacy learning. Of course, these activities are selected because they meet the requirements of the approach that has been adopted by the teacher. But it is a selection of activities rather than a reliance upon a single activity which is provided in the classroom.

However, as teachers we need to recognize that it is each one of us, rather than a method or activity, that is likely to be crucial in supporting children's learning. We need to be knowledgeable about children and about literacy, so that our decision making in the classroom is informed decision making. Undoubtedly, too, we need to be skilful organizers of the classroom and managers of events within the room. And our enthusiasm for literacy should be such that it motivates the children and makes them enthusiastic for literacy.

Clearly, the classroom should be a hive of activity related to literacy. Reading and writing should feature prominently throughout the day as the children engage with interesting print materials and write with a purpose for an authentic audience. I shall refrain from listing again all the activities, features and aspects of literacy which should be commonplace in the classroom, as that is what this book has been about. But each classroom has to be an area for literacy learning. This book has attempted to highlight the importance of that learning and to provide suggestions that will enhance children's literacy.

References

Adams, M.J. (1990) *Beginning to Read: Thinking and Learning about Print*. Cambridge, MA: MIT Press.

Alexander, R. (1992) *Policy and Practice in Primary Education*. London: Routledge.

Altwerger, B., Edelsky, C. and Flores, B. (1987) Whole language: What's new? *The Reading Teacher*, 41: 144–55.

Anderson, H. (1993) Creative full stop. *Times Educational Supplement*, 18 June, pp. vi–vii.

Anthony, R.J., Johnson, T.D., Mickelson, N.I. and Preece, A. (1991) *Evaluating Literacy: A Perspective for Change*. Portsmouth, NH: Heinemann.

Applebee, A.N. (1978) *The Child's Concept of Story*. Chicago, IL: Chicago University Press.

Arnold, H. (1982) *Listening to Children Reading*. Sevenoaks: Hodder and Stoughton.

Ashton-Warner, S. (1963) *Teacher*. London: Secker and Warburg.

Baghban, M. (1984) *Our Daughter Learns to Read and Write*. Newark, DE: International Reading Association.

Bain, R., Fitzgerald, B. and Taylor, M. (eds) (1992) *Looking into Language: Classroom Approaches to Knowledge about Language*. London: Hodder and Stoughton.

Barnes, D., Britton, J. and Rosen, H. (1969) *Language, the Learner and the School*. Harmondsworth: Penguin.

Barrs, M. and Johnson, G. (1993) *Record-keeping in the Primary School*. London: Hodder and Stoughton.

Bennett, J. (1991) *Learning to Read with Picture Books*, 4th edn. Stroud: Thimble Press.

Bettleheim, B. and Zelan, K. (1981) *On Learning to Read*. Harmondsworth: Penguin.

Beverton, S., Hunter-Carsch, M., Obrist, C. and Stuart, A. (1993) *Running Family Reading Groups*. Widnes: UK Reading Association.
Bloom, W. (1987) *Partnership with Parents in Reading*. Sevenoaks: Hodder and Stoughton.
Bryant, P. and Bradley, L. (1985) *Children's Reading Problems: Psychology and Education*. Oxford: Oxford University Press.
Burman, C. (1990) Organizing for reading 3–7. In B. Wade (ed.), *Reading for Real*. Buckingham: Open University Press.
Burt, M. (1893) Communications: Experiments in the teaching of reading. *The Dial*, 16 March, pp. 172–3.
Cambourne, B. (1988) *The Whole Story: Natural Learning and the Acquisition of Literacy in the Classroom*. Auckland: Ashton Scholastic.
Campbell, R. (1988) *Hearing Children Read*. London: Routledge.
Campbell, R. (1990a) *Reading Together*. Buckingham: Open University Press.
Campbell, R. (1990b) *Phonics, Standards and Real Books*. Exmouth: Rolle Faculty of Education, University of Plymouth.
Campbell, R. (1991) Reading assessment: The 1991 SATs. *Reading*, 26(1): 37–9.
Campbell, R. (1992) *Reading Real Books*. Buckingham: Open University Press.
Campbell, R. (1993a) *Miscue Analysis in the Classroom*. Widnes: UK Reading Association.
Campbell, R. (1993b) The importance of the teacher. *Reading Today*, 11: 34.
Campbell, R. (1994) The teacher response to children's miscues of substitution. *Journal of Research in Reading*, 17: 147–54.
Campbell, R. and Scrivens, G. (1995) The teacher role during sustained silent reading. *Reading*, 29(2).
Campbell, R. and Stott, G. (1994) Children's experience of learning to read. *Reading*, 28(3): 8–13.
Carter, R. (ed.) (1990) *Knowledge about Language and the Curriculum: The LINC Reader*. London: Hodder and Stoughton.
Chall, J. (1967) *Learning to Read: The Great Debate*. New York: McGraw-Hill.
Chalmers, G.S. (1976) *Reading Easy 1800–50*. London: The Broadsheet King.
Chapman, L.J. (1987) *Reading: From 5–11 Years*. Milton Keynes: Open University Press.
Cherrington, V. (1990) Developing contexts for writing non-narrative. In B. Wade (ed.), *Reading for Real*. Buckingham: Open University Press.
Clay, M. (1972) *Reading: The Patterning of Complex Behaviour*. London: Heinemann Educational.
Clay, M. (1985) *The Early Detection of Reading Difficulties*. Auckland: Heinemann Educational.
Clay, M. (1991) Introducing a new storybook to young readers. *The Reading Teacher*, 45: 264–73.

Clay, M. (1993) *Reading Recovery: A Guidebook for Teachers in Training*. London: Heinemann Educational.
CLPE (1988) *The Primary Language Record*. London: Centre for Language in Primary Education.
Clymer, T. (1963) The utility of phonic generalizations in the primary grades. *The Reading Teacher*, 16: 252–8.
Coleman, C. (1991) We're all going on a summer holiday. In N. Hall and L. Abbott (eds), *Play in the Primary Curriculum*. London: Hodder and Stoughton.
Coles, M. (1990) The 'real books' approach: Is apprenticeship a weak analogy? *Reading*, 24(2): 50–6.
Combs, M. (1987) Modeling the reading process with enlarged texts. *The Reading Teacher*, 40: 422–6.
Cullinan, B. (1989) Literature for young children. In D. Strickland and L.M. Morrow (eds), *Emerging Literacy: Young Children Learn to Read and Write*. Newark, DE: International Reading Association.
Davis, C. and Stubbs, R. (1988) *Shared Reading in Practice*. Milton Keynes: Open University Press.
Dearing, R. (1993) *The National Curriculum and its Assessment: An Interim Report*. London: National Curriculum Council.
DES (1967) *Children and their Primary Schools* (The Plowden Report). London: HMSO.
DES (1975) *A Language for Life* (The Bullock Report). London: HMSO.
DES (1988a) *Report of the Committee of Inquiry into the Teaching of English Language* (The Kingman Report). London: HMSO.
DES (1988b) *English for Ages 5 to 11* (The Cox Report). London: HMSO.
DES (1989) *English in the National Curriculum*. London: HMSO.
DES (1990) *English in the National Curriculum (No. 2)*. London: HMSO.
Dewey, J. (1916) *Democracy and Education*. New York: Macmillan.
Dewey, J. (1938) *Experience and Education*. New York: Macmillan.
Diack, H. (1965) *In Spite of the ALPHABET: A Study in the Teaching of Reading*. London: Chatto and Windus.
Dombey, H. (1988) Partners in the telling. In M. Meek and C. Mills (eds), *Language and Literacy in the Primary School*. Lewes: Falmer Press.
Donaldson, M. (1989) *Sense and Sensibility*. Reading: Reading and Language Information Centre, University of Reading School of Education.
Dutton, H. (1991) Play and writing. In N. Hall and L. Abbott (eds), *Play in the Primary Curriculum*. London: Hodder and Stoughton.
Edelsky, C., Altwerger, B. and Flores, B. (1991) *Whole Language: What's the Difference?* Portsmouth, NH: Heinemann Educational.
Ferreiro, E. and Teberosky, A. (1982) *Literacy before Schooling*. Portsmouth, NH: Heinemann Educational.
Fisher, R. (1992) *Early Literacy and the Teacher*. Sevenoaks: Hodder and Stoughton.
Fox, C. (1993) *At the Very Edge of the Forest: The Influence of Literature on Storytelling by Children*. London: Cassell.

Glynn, T. (1980) Parent–child interaction in remedial reading at home. In M.M. Clark and T. Glynn (eds), *Reading and Writing for the Child with Difficulties*. Birmingham: University of Birmingham, Educational Review.

Glynn, T., Crooks, T., Bethune, N., Ballard, K. and Smith, J. (1989) *Reading Recovery in Context*. Auckland: New Zealand Department of Education.

Goddard, N. (1974) *Literacy: Language Experience Approach*. London: Macmillan Educational.

Gollasch, F.V. (ed.) (1982a) *Language and Literacy: The Selected Writings of Kenneth S. Goodman. Vol. I: Process, Theory, Research*. London: Routledge.

Gollasch, F.V. (ed.) (1982b) *Language and Literacy: The Selected Writings of Kenneth S. Goodman. Vol. II: Reading, Language and the Classroom Teacher*. London: Routledge.

Goodacre, E.J. (1975) *METHODS: Including an Annotated Reading List and Glossary of Terms*. Reading: Centre for the Teaching of Reading, University of Reading.

Goodacre, E.J. (undated) *Hearing Children Read*. Reading: Centre for the Teaching of Reading, University of Reading.

Goodman, K. (1969) Analysis of reading miscues: Applied psycholinguistics. *Reading Research Quarterly*, 5: 652–8.

Goodman, K. (1986) *What's Whole in Whole Language?* Portsmouth, NH: Heinemann Educational.

Goodman, K. (1992) I didn't found whole language. *The Reading Teacher*, 46: 188–99.

Goodman, K. (1993) *Phonic Phacts*. Richmond Hill, Ontario: Scholastic Canada.

Goodman, K. (1994) Reading, writing and written texts: A transactional sociopsycholinguistic view. In R. Ruddell, M. Ruddell and H. Singer (eds), *Theoretical Models and Processes of Reading*. Newark, DE: International Reading Association.

Goodman, K., Bird, L.B. and Goodman, Y. (eds) (1991) *The Whole Language Catalog*. Santa Rosa, CA: American School Publishers.

Goodman, K., Shannon, P., Freeman, Y. and Murphy, S. (1988) *Report Card on Basal Readers*. New York: Richard C. Owen.

Goodman, Y. (1989) Evaluation of students. In K. Goodman, Y. Goodman and W. Hood (eds), *The Whole Language Evaluation Handbook*. Portsmouth, NH: Heinemann.

Goodman, Y. (1991) The history of whole language. In K. Goodman, L.B. Bird and Y. Goodman (eds), *The Whole Language Catalog*. Santa Rosa, CA: American School Publishers.

Goodman, Y. and Altwerger, B. (1981) *Print Awareness in Pre-School Children: A Working Paper*. Tucson, AZ: Arizona Centre for Research and Development, University of Arizona.

Goodman, Y., Watson, D. and Burke, C. (1987) *Reading Miscue Inventory: Alternative Procedures*. New York: Richard C. Owen.

Goswami, U.C. (1994) Phonological skills, analogies, and reading development. *Reading*, 28(2): 32–7.

Goswami, U.C. and Bryant, P. (1990) *Phonological Skills and Learning to Read*. Hove: Lawrence Erlbaum Associates Ltd.

Graham, J. (1991) *Pictures on the Page*. Sheffield: NATE.

Graves, D. H. (1983) *Writing: Teachers and Children at Work*. Portsmouth, NH: Heinemann Educational.

Hall, N. (1987) *The Emergence of Literacy*. Sevenoaks: Hodder and Stoughton.

Hall, N. (ed.) (1989) *Writing with Reason: The Emergence of Authorship in Young Children*. Sevenoaks: Hodder and Stoughton.

Hall, N. and Abbott, L. (eds) (1991) *Play in the Primary Curriculum*. London: Hodder and Stoughton.

Harris, A. J. (1979) The effective teacher of reading, revisited. *The Reading Teacher*, 33: 135–40.

Harrison, C. (1992) The reading process and learning to read. In C. Harrison and M. Coles (eds) *The Reading for Real Handbook*. London: Routledge.

Harste, J.C., Woodward, V.A. and Burke, C.L. (1984) *Language Stories & Literacy Lessons*. Portsmouth, NH: Heinemann Educational.

Heath, S.B. (1983) *Ways with Words: Language, Life and Work in Communities and Classrooms*. Cambridge: Cambridge University Press.

Hewison, J. and Tizard, S. (1980) Parental involvement and reading attainment. *British Journal of Educational Psychology*, 50: 209–15.

HMI (1991) *The Teaching and Learning of Reading in Primary Schools*. London: DES.

HMI (1992) *The Teaching and Learning of Reading in Primary Schools 1991*. London: DES.

Holdaway, D. (1979) *The Foundations of Literacy*. London: Ashton Scholastic.

Huey, E. (1908) (1972 reprint) *The Psychology and Pedagogy of Reading*. Cambridge, MA: MIT Press.

Hunt, L.C. (1970) The effect of self-selection, interest and motivation upon independent, instructional and frustrational levels. *The Reading Teacher*, 24: 146–51, 158.

Hutchinson, P. (1983) *Story Chest: Teacher's Book*. Leeds: Arnold-Wheaton.

Jones, J.K. (1967) *Colour Story Reading*. London: Pitman.

Kalman, J. (1991) Who invented invented spelling? In K. Goodman, L.B. Bird and Y. Goodman (eds), *The Whole Language Catalog*. Santa Rosa, CA: American School Publishers.

Lally, M. (1991) *The Nursery Teacher in Action*. London: Paul Chapman.

Laminack, L. (1991) *Learning with Zachary*. Richmond Hill, Ontario: Scholastic Canada.

Lefevre, C. (1964) *Linguistics and the Teaching of Reading*. London: McGraw-Hill.

Littlefair, A.B. (1991) *Reading All Types of Writing: The Importance of Genre and Register for Reading Development*. Buckingham: Open University Press.

Littlefair, A.B. (1992) *Genres in the Classroom*. Widnes: UK Reading Association.

Lunzer, E. and Gardner, K. (1979) *The Effective Use of Reading*. London: Heinemann Educational.

Mackay, D., Thompson, B. and Schaub, P. (1970) *Breakthrough to Literacy: Teacher's Manual*. London: Schools Council/Longman.

MacLeod, F. (1991) Down at the chippy. In N. Hall and L. Abbott (eds), *Play in the Primary Curriculum*. London: Hodder and Stoughton.

Manning, K. and Sharp, A. (1977) *Structuring Play in the Early Years at School*. London: Ward Lock Educational.

Mason, J.M., Peterman, C.L. and Kerr, B.M. (1989) Reading to kindergarten children. In D.S. Strickland and L.M. Morrow (eds), *Emerging Literacy: Young Children Learn to Read and Write*. Newark, DE: International Reading Association.

Matterson, E. (1969) *This Little Puffin . . . Finger Plays and Nursery Games*. London: Puffin.

McCracken, R.A. (1971) Initiating sustained silent reading. *Journal of Reading*, 14: 521–4, 582–3.

Meek, M. (1982) *Learning to Read*. London: Bodley Head.

Meek, M. (1988) *How Texts Teach What Readers Learn*. Stroud: Thimble Press.

Meek, M. (1990) What do we know about reading that helps us to teach? In R. Carter (ed.), *Knowledge about Language and the Curriculum*. London: Hodder and Stoughton.

Mills, H., O'Keefe, T. and Stephens, D. (1992) *Looking Closely: Exploring the Role of Phonics in One Whole Language Classroom*. Urbana, IL: National Council of Teachers of English.

Moore, P. and Tweddle, S. (1992) *The Integrated Classroom: Language, Learning and I.T.* London: Hodder and Stoughton.

Morgan, R.T.T. (1976) 'Paired reading' tuition: A preliminary report on a technique for cases of reading deficit. *Child Care Health and Development*, 2: 13–28.

Morrow, L.M. (1989) Designing the classroom to promote literacy development. In D.S. Strickland and L.M. Morrow (eds), *Emerging Literacy: Young Children Learn to Read and Write*. Newark, DE: International Reading Association.

Morrow, L.M. and Rand, M.K. (1991) Promoting literacy during play by designing early childhood classroom environments. *The Reading Teacher*, 44: 396–402.

Neate, B. (1992) *Finding Out About Finding Out: A Practical Guide to Children's Information Books*. Sevenoaks: Hodder and Stoughton.

Nicholson, T. (1992) Reading wars: A brief history and an update. *International Journal of Disability, Development and Education*, 39: 173–84.

NUT (1991) *Miss, the Rabbit Ate the 'Floating Apple'! The Case Against SATs*. London: National Union of Teachers.
Opie, I. and Opie, P. (1959) *The Lore and Language of School Children*. Oxford: Oxford University Press.
Phillips, M. (1990) Educashun still isn't working. *The Guardian*, 28 September.
Pitman, J. (1959) *The Enhardt Augmented (40-sound 42-character) Lower-Case Roman Alphabet*. London: Pitman.
Pluckrose, H. (1988) *School: A Place for Children?* London: Franklin Watts.
Price, J. (1989) The Ladybird Letters. In N. Hall (ed.), *Writing with Reason: The Emergence of Authorship in Young Children*. Sevenoaks: Hodder and Stoughton.
Read, C. (1971) Pre-school children's knowledge of English phonology. *Harvard Educational Review*, 41(4): 1–34.
Reid, J.F. (1974) *Breakthrough in Action: An Independent Evaluation of 'Breakthrough to Literacy'*. London: Schools Council/Longman.
Rhodes, L. (1981) I can read! Predictable books as resources for reading and writing instruction. *The Reading Teacher*, 34: 511–18.
Rosen, C. and Rosen, H. (1973) *The Language of Primary School Children*. Harmondsworth: Penguin.
Rosenblatt, L. (1938) *Literature through Explanation*. New York: Appleton-Century-Crofts (3rd edn, 1976, New York: Noble and Noble).
SCAA (1994) *English in the National Curriculum: Draft Proposals*. London: School Curriculum and Assessment Authority.
SCDC (1989) *Becoming a Writer: The National Writing Project*. Walton-on-Thames: Nelson.
SCDC (1990) *Writing and Micros*. Walton-on-Thames: Nelson.
Schickedanz, J.A. (1990) *Adam's Righting Revolutions*. Portsmouth, NH: Heinemann Educational.
Schonell, F. (1951) *The Psychology and Teaching of Reading*, 3rd edn. London: Oliver and Boyd.
SEAC (1991) *Standard Assessment Task: Teacher's Pack Key Stage 1. 1991*. London: HMSO.
Slaughter, J.P. (1992) *Beyond Storybooks: Young Children and Shared Book Experience*. Newark, DE: International Reading Association.
Smith, F. (1978) *Reading*. Cambridge: Cambridge University Press.
Smith, F. (1982) *Writing and the Writer*. London: Heinemann Educational.
Smith, F. (1992) Quotable. *Reading Today*, 10(2): 34.
Southgate, V. (1968) Formulae for beginning reading tuition. *Educational Research*, 11: 23–30.
Southgate, V., Arnold, H. and Johnson, S. (1981) *Extending Beginning Reading*. London: Heinemann Educational.
Start, K.B. and Wells, B.K. (1972) *The Trends of Reading Standards: 1970–71*. Slough: NFER.
Stauffer, R.G. (1970) *The Language-Experience Approach to the Teaching of Reading*. New York: Harper and Row.

Strickland, D.S. and Morrow, L.M. (eds) (1989a) *Emerging Literacy: Young Children Learn to Read and Write*. Newark, DE: International Reading Association.

Strickland, D.S. and Morrow, L.M. (1989b) Interactive experiences with storybook reading. *The Reading Teacher*, 42: 322–3.

Taylor, D. (1983) *Family Literacy: Young Children Learning to Read and Write*. Portsmouth, NH: Heinemann Educational.

Teale, W. (1984) Reading to young children: Its significance for literacy development. In H. Goelman, A. Oberg and F. Smith (eds), *Awakening to Literacy*. London: Heinemann Educational.

Teale, W. and Sulzby, E. (1989) Emergent literacy: New perspectives. In D.S. Strickland and L.M. Morrow (eds), *Emerging Literacy: Young Children Learn to Read and Write*. Newark, DE: International Reading Association.

Temple, C., Nathan, R., Temple, F. and Burris, N.A. (1988) *The Beginnings of Writing*. London: Allyn and Bacon.

Tizard, B. and Hughes, M. (1984) *Young Children Learning: Talking and Thinking at Home and at School*. London: Fontana.

Topping, K.J. and Lindsay, G.A. (1992) The structure and development of the paired reading technique. *Journal of Research in Reading*, 15: 120–36.

Topping, K.J. and Wolfendale, S. (eds) (1985) *Parental Involvement in Children's Reading*. London: Croom Helm.

Tough, Y.J. (1973) *Focus on Meaning: Talking to Some Purpose with Young Children*. London: Allen and Unwin.

Trelease, J. (1989) *The New Read-Aloud Handbook*, 2nd revised edn. London: Penguin.

Turner, M. (1990) *Sponsored Reading Failure*. Warlingham: IPSET Education Unit.

Upward, C. (1992a) *Cut Spelling: A Handbook to the Simplification of Written English by Omission of Redundant Letters*. Birmingham: Simplified Spelling Society.

Upward, C. (1992b) Is traditionl english spelng mor dificlt than jermn? *Journal of Research in Reading*, 15: 82–94.

Veatch, J. (1991) Whole language as I see it. In K. Goodman, L.B. Bird and Y. Goodman (eds), *The Whole Language Catalog*. Santa Rosa, CA: American School Publishers.

Vygotsky, L.S. (1962) *Thought and Language*. Cambridge, MA: MIT Press.

Vygotsky, L.S. (1978) *Mind in Society*. Cambridge, MA: Harvard University Press.

Wade, B. (ed.) (1990) *Reading for Real*. Buckingham: Open University Press.

Waterland. L. (1988) *Read with Me: An Apprenticeship Approach to Reading*. Stroud: Thimble Press.

Waterland, L. (ed.) (1989) *Apprenticeship in Action: Teachers Write about Read with Me*. Stroud: Thimble Press.

Weinberger, J., Hannon, P. and Nutbrown, C. (1990) *Ways of Working with*

Parents to Promote Literacy Development. Sheffield: University of Sheffield Division of Education.
Wells, G. (1986) *The Meaning Makers: Children Learning Language and Using Language to Learn*. London: Hodder and Stoughton.
Wheldall, K. and Entwistle, J. (1988) Back in the USSR: The effects of teacher modelling of silent reading on pupils' reading behaviour in the primary school classroom. *Educational Psychology*, 8: 51–66.
White, D. (1954/1984) *Books Before Five*. Portsmouth, NH: Heinemann.
Wray, D. and Medwell, J. (1991) *Literacy and Language in the Primary Years*. London: Routledge.

Children's books

Bourma, P. (1987) *Bertie at the Dentist's*. London: Bodley Head.
Carle, E. (1969) *The Very Hungry Caterpillar*. New York: Philomel Books.
Carle, E. (1982) *The Bad Tempered Ladybird*. London: Penguin.
Carle, E. (1988) *Do You Want to be My Friend?* Boston, MA: Houghton Mifflin.
Hill, E. (1983) *Where's Spot?* London: Penguin.
Hutchins, P. (1968) *Rosie's Walk*. London: Bodley Head.
Hutchins, P. (1972) *Good-Night Owl*. London: Bodley Head.
Keats, E. (1964) *Whistle for Willie*. London: Penguin.
Quest Books (1979) *Famous Cities: London*. London: Chambers.
Seuss, Dr (1957) *The Cat in the Hat*. New York: Beginner Books/Random House.
Sunshine Books (1980) *Dizzy Dog*. London: Frederick Warne.

READING TOGETHER

Robin Campbell

This book is about how adults can facilitate children's learning to read. It emphasizes that the crucial role of the teacher is to sustain, encourage and facilitate the child's self-activated learning. It is important that the adult and child are reading together from an interesting book, meaningful to both rather than being concerned with isolation and teaching of skills. The adult–child interaction has to be one of genuine sharing and this sharing provides the basis from which the child's literacy can emerge. Robin Campbell traces a sequence of reading together from story reading (adult reads to child) to shared reading (adult and child read together) on to hearing children read (child reads to adult) and finally to sustained silent reading (child reads to itself). To support this sequence he suggests practical activities for teachers and children, and provides a number of classroom case studies as exemplars.

Contents

96pp 0 335 09449 X (Paperback) 0 335 09450 3 (Hardback)

READING REAL BOOKS

Robin Campbell

'Real books' have been the focus of controversy as critics argue that the use of real books (rather than reading schemes) in primary schools has caused a downturn in reading standards. The evidence for this is, at best, questionable and the controversy has revealed widespread ignorance of what a real books approach means in practice.

Robin Campbell argues that, in fact, a real books approach is a very demanding one which requires subtle and sophisticated teaching strategies and prior careful planning of the classroom environment to facilitate the management of learning. It is based squarely on beliefs in the power of stories and in children as active constructors of learning as well as in the key role of the teacher. It also assumes that real books are but a significant starting point for a whole range of literacy activities in the classroom.

This is an important introduction to, and argument for, the use of real books as part of a whole language approach to teaching literacy.

Contents

96pp 0 335 15793 9 (Paperback) 0 335 15794 7 (Hardback)

READING THE CHANGES

Eleanor Anderson

In the context of changing perspectives on and experience of language, learning and schooling, Eleanor Anderson suggests a new model of the reading process and how it may be applied to classroom practice. She provides an overview of research and development in the field of language and literacy over the past forty years, a new framework for the reading process, and practical suggestions for use by teachers. She discusses, for instance, strategies for reading whole texts and complete texts, reading 'real books', reading and information handling, reading across the curriculum, and reading within national curricula. She also tackles how to develop a school reading policy, how to communicate such a policy within the community and to other professionals, and the challenge of reading for teacher education. She constructs a theoretically sound model which teachers may adapt to their own needs in trying to make sense of the myriad changes with which they are being asked to cope, and in the daily decision making in which they are involved.

Contents

Changing views of children's language and learning – Reading in this changing context – Applying a new model to classroom practice – Teaching and developing reading in this changing context – Teaching reading within national curricula – The challenge for teacher education – Communicating with colleagues, community, parents and other professionals – Epilogue – Appendices – References – Index.

128pp   0 335 15642 8 (Paperback)   0 335 15643 6 (Hardback)